Biodefence

NATO Science for Peace and Security Series

This Series presents the results of scientific meetings supported under the NATO Programme: Science for Peace and Security (SPS).

The NATO SPS Programme supports meetings in the following Key Priority areas: (1) Defence Against Terrorism; (2) Countering other Threats to Security and (3) NATO, Partner and Mediterranean Dialogue Country Priorities. The types of meeting supported are generally "Advanced Study Institutes" and "Advanced Research Workshops". The NATO SPS Series collects together the results of these meetings. The meetings are co-organized by scientists from NATO countries and scientists from NATO's "Partner" or "Mediterranean Dialogue" countries. The observations and recommendations made at the meetings, as well as the contents of the volumes in the Series, reflect those of participants and contributors only; they should not necessarily be regarded as reflecting NATO views or policy.

Advanced Study Institutes (ASI) are high-level tutorial courses intended to convey the latest developments in a subject to an advanced-level audience

Advanced Research Workshops (ARW) are expert meetings where an intense but informal exchange of views at the frontiers of a subject aims at identifying directions for future action

Following a transformation of the programme in 2006 the Series has been re-named and re-organised. Recent volumes on topics not related to security, which result from meetings supported under the programme earlier, may be found in the NATO Science Series.

The Series is published by IOS Press, Amsterdam, and Springer, Dordrecht, in conjunction with the NATO Emerging Security Challenges Division.

Sub-Series

A.	Chemistry and Biology	Springer
B.	Physics and Biophysics	Springer
C.	Environmental Security	Springer
D.	Information and Communication Security	IOS Press
E.	Human and Societal Dynamics	IOS Press

http://www.nato.int/science
http://www.springer.com
http://www.iospress.nl

Series A: Chemistry and Biology

Biodefence

Advanced Materials and Methods for Health Protection

edited by

Sergey Mikhalovsky
School of Pharmacy & Biomolecular Sciences, University of Brighton
United Kingdom

and

Abdukhakim Khajibaev
Republican Specialised Scientific Center for Emergency Medicine,
Ministry of Public Health, Tashkent, Uzbekistan

Springer

Published in Cooperation with NATO Emerging Security Challenges Division

Proceedings of the NATO Advanced Study Institute on Biodefence:
Advanced Materials and Methods for Health Protection
Bukhara, Uzbekistan
1-10 June 2009

ISBN 978-94-007-0219-6 (PB)
ISBN 978-94-007-0216-5 (HB)
ISBN 978-94-007-0217-2 (e-book)

Published by Springer,
P.O. Box 17, 3300 AA Dordrecht, The Netherlands.

www.springer.com

Printed on acid-free paper

Contents

Preface

At the beginning of the twenty-first century new threats to human well being have emerged, which stem from terrorist activities. Potential use of chemical, biological, radiological and nuclear warfare (CBRN) in terrorist events is considered to be very likely, and on a small scale it has already been used in the past. CBRN threat however is not limited to malicious intentions and can be caused by a careless attitude towards the use of technology and equipment, breach of safety rules, or triggered by natural disasters or environmental pollution.

The Chernobyl catastrophe of 1986, was caused entirely by human error although not intentional, can be considered, using modern vocabulary, a 'dirty bomb' on a large scale. Shrinking of the Aral Sea due to loss of water input diverted to irrigation caused serious, perhaps irreversible changes in the environment, which led to a deterioration in the health of the local population, particularly in the North-West of Uzbekistan. More recent outbreaks of 'bird flu' and 'swine flu', which fortunately have not led to epidemics, prove the vulnerability of the human race beyond terrorist activities. It is therefore of utmost importance to develop methods of detection, prevention and protection against warfare agents.

The NATO Advanced Study Institute, took place on 1st–10th June, 2009 in Tashkent and Samarkand, the Republic of Uzbekistan. It focused on defence against biological warfare with an emphasis on applications of modern technologies and advanced materials in detection, health protection and medical treatment of the population. These include high throughput sensitive detection methods, advanced nanostructured materials and techniques for external and internal protection of human health, as well as extracorporeal methods, adsorptive materials and bacteriophages decontaminating the human organism, and neutralising incorporated CBRN agents. The ASI served to disseminate information on recent developments in the field of biodefence not only to fight terrorism and terror related events, but also to seek broader solutions to many critical problems such as clean water supplies, health impact of environmental pollution and improved healthcare.

The choice of Uzbekistan was due to the particular concern of all strata of the Uzbek society – government, military, medical care providers, scientists and civil population about the threat of terrorist activities in this part of the world. This threat is very real, not only due to the geographical location and political situation in the region, but is also aggravated by the current state of environmental pollution and lack of proper sanitation in the area. Uzbekistan has a famous scientific and cultural heritage, which includes such great names as Abu Ali Ibn Sino (Avicenna), Ulugbek, Al-Bukhari and Al-Khorezmi to name but a few. The ASI was hosted by the Republican Specialised Scientific Centre for Emergency Medicine, which has direct scientific and practical interests in biodefence.

Scientists and medics from NATO, Partner Countries, Mediterranean dialogue countries and third countries attended the ASI. In total over 80 participants from 21 countries participated in our ASI making it a truly international event. It brought together specialists from different countries with the aim of fostering new developments and effective solutions to the current problems facing biodefence. 22 tutorial lectures, 16 short talks and over 30 posters were presented. These proceedings reflect their views on this highly inter- and multidisciplinary topic of biodefence.

This volume has been arranged in five chapters aimed at discussing nanostructured materials and methods of their characterization (Chapter I), advanced express-methods for detection and analysis of biological species (Chapter II), methods of protection (Chapter III) and medical treatment (Chapter IV) of patients with incorporated contaminants, and specifically extracorporeal methods of decontamination of the human body (Chapter V). All papers in this book have been peer reviewed prior to publication. We believe that this volume will be of major interest to researchers and students working in the area of materials science and engineering, chemistry, biosensors, biomaterials, extracorporeal methods, and therapeutics.

Acknowledgments

The Editors of this volume would like to express their sincere gratitude to the NATO Scientific Affairs Committee who provided financial support for this ASI and inspired us to organise it.

We would also like to recognise additional financial contributions from the University of Brighton, UK; the Republican Scientific Centre of Emergency Medicine, Tashkent; Samarkand Branch of the Centre of Emergency Medicine, Uzbekistan, and Arterium Ltd (Ukraine-Uzbekistan).

The contribution of Scientific Co-Chairmen of the ASI, Vladimir G. Nikolaev, Ukraine, and Thomas MS Chang, Canada, for their selection of the scientific presentations, which was instrumental to the ASI success.

We thank all authors and participants of the ASI for their enthusiasm and interest in its programme and for their presentations and discussions which maintained its high scientific level.

We would like to recognise the special role of Shukhrat Kasymov, V. Vakhidov Republican Specialised Centre of Surgery, Tashkent, for his contribution to the development and submission of a successful proposal to NATO.

A great number of staff in hospitable Uzbekistan are gratefully acknowledged for their efforts and ability to organise the event smoothly and efficiently: Abdunumon Sidikov and Bakhodir Rahimov, Ministry of Public Health; Munira Kamilova, Ministry of Foreign Affairs; Bokhodir Magrupov, Turakul Arzikulov and Agzam Ishankulov (Republican Specialised Scientific Centre for Emergency Medicine), Shukhrat Kasymov (V. Vakhidov Republican Specialised Centre of Surgery), Jamshed Ahtamov (Samarkand Branch for the Republican Centre for Emergency Medicine, Co-Chairman of the Local Organising Committee).

Help of other members of the Local Organising Committee in Tashkent and Samarkand is also acknowledged: Kamol Rizaev, Ravshan Yangiev, Shukur Isamukhamedov, Alisher Eshmuratov, Davron Tulyaganov, Shukhrat Atadjanov, Pulatoya Isakhanova, Marina Sizova, Dilorom Mirkhalilova, Davron Sabirov, Dmitriy Chebotarev, Evgeniy Mun, Murad Igamnazarov and Akmal Ahmedov.

Our special thanks are extended to Kamola Salmetova and Khikmat Anvarov of the Republican Scientific Centre of Emergency Medicine, who looked after the participants so well and remained calm even under stressful situations which they always resolved in the best interests of the participants.

Finally, we express our thanks to the University of Brighton team; Carol Howell, Ross Shevchenko and Irina Savina for their major contribution to the preparation of the Book of Abstracts, editing and proof reading of abstracts and manuscripts for this book, Steve Jones for IT support and maintaining the ASI website, and lastly senior management and Finance Department for their logistical support.

Contributors

Khadjibaev Abdukhakim M.
Scientific Centre of Emergency Medicine, Ministry of Public Health, Tashkent 1000115, Uzbekistan

Paiziev Adkham A.
Institute of Electronics, Uzbek Academy of Science, Durmon Yuli 33, Tashkent 100125, Uzbekistan

Kosenkov Aleksandr
I.M. Sechenov Moscow Academy of Medicine, 8-2, Trubetskaya Street, Moscow 119991, Russia

Kharlamov Aleksei
Frantsevich Institute for Problems of Materials Science, National Academy of Sciences of Ukraine, 3, Krjijanovskogo str., Kiev 03680, Ukraine

Gutnikova Alla R.
V.Vakhidov Republican Specialised Centre of Surgery, 10, Farkhadskaya Street, 100115 Tashkent, Uzbekistan

Saidkhanov Bois
V.Vakhidov Republican Specialised Centre of Surgery, 10, Farkhadskaya Street, Tashkent 100115, Uzbekistan

Vallières Cécile
Reactions and Process Engineering Laboratory, CNRS-Nancy University, 1, rue Grandville, 54001 Nancy, France

Geissler Eric
Laboratoire de Spectrométrie Physique CNRS UMR 5588, Université J. Fourier de Grenoble, BP 87, 38402, St Martin d'Hères cedex, Grenoble, France

Akbas Etem
Faculty of Medicine, Department of Medical Biology and Genetics, Mersin University, Çiftlikköy Merkez Campus 33343, Mezitli, Mersin, Turkey

Kushch Ievgeniia G.
Department of Pediatrics, Institute for Children and Adolescents Health Care, Academy of Medical Sciences of Ukraine, 52-A, 50 Let VLKSM Street, Kharkiv 61153, Ukraine

Baybekov Iskander M.
V.Vakhidov Republican Specialised Centre of Surgery, 10, Farkhadskaya Street, Tashkent 100115, Uzbekistan

Smart John D.
School of Pharmacy and Biomolecular Sciences, University of Brighton, Brighton BN2 4GJ, United Kingdom

László Krisztina
Department of Physical Chemistry and Materials Science, Budapest University of Technology and Economics, H-1521 Budapest, Hungary

Bajenov Leonid G.
V.Vakhidov Republican Specialised Centre of Surgery, 10, Farkhadskaya Street, Tashkent 100115, Uzbekistan

Kartel Mykola T.
Chuiko Institute of Surface Chemistry, National Academy of Sciences of Ukraine, 17 General Naumov Prospect, Kiev 03164, Ukraine

Starodub Nickolaj F.
National University of Life and Environmental Sciences, 15 Herojev Oboroni Str., Kiev 03041, Ukraine

Chanishvili Nino
Eliava Institute of Bacteriophage, Microbiology and Virology (IBMV), 3 Gotua street, Tbilisi 0160, Georgia

Gogotsi Yury
Department of Materials Science and Engineering, Drexel University, Philadelphia, PA 19104, USA

Ibadov Ravshan
V.Vakhidov Republican Specialised Centre of Surgery, 10, Farkhadskaya Street, Tashkent 100115, Uzbekistan

Khaydarov Renat R.
Institute of Nuclear Physics, Ulugbek township, Tashkent 100214, Uzbekistan

Kernchen Roman J.
Fraunhofer Institute for Technological Trend Analysis (INT), Appelsgarten 2, 53879 Euskirchen, Germany

Shevchenko Rostislav V.
School of Pharmacy and Biomolecular Sciences, University of Brighton, Brighton, BN2 4GJ, United Kingdom

Kudaibergenov Sarkyt E.
Laboratory of Engineering, K.I. Satpaev Kazakh National Technical University, Satpaev Street, 22, Almaty 050013, Kazakhstan

Mikhalovsky Sergey
School of Pharmacy and Biomolecular Sciences, University of Brighton, Lewes Road, Brighton, BN2 4GJ, UK

Kasimov Shukhrat
V.Vakhidov Republican Specialised Centre of Surgery, 10, Farkhadskaya Street, Tashkent 100115, Uzbekistan

Korraa Soheir
Egyptian Atomic Energy Authority National Center for Radiation Research and Technology, 3 Ahmed El Zomour Street, 8th Sector, Nasr City, P.O. Box 29, Cairo, Egypt

Kirkovsky Valeriy
Laboratory of Hemosorption, Byelorussian State Medical University, 28, Dzerzhinskogo Avenue, Minsk 220116, Belarus

Nikolaev Vladimir G.
R.E. Kavetsky Institute of Experimental Pathology, Oncology and Radiobiology, National Academy of Sciences of Ukraine, 45, Vasilkivska Street, Kiev 03022, Ukraine

Kryazhev Yury G.
Omsk Scientific Center, Institute of Hydrocarbons Processing, Siberian Branch of Russian Academy of Sciences, 54, Neftezavodskaya Street, Omsk 644040, Russia

Part I
Nanomaterials and Nanostructured Adsorbents

Chapter 1
Solvothermal Synthesis of Photocatalytic TiO_2 Nanoparticles Capable of Killing *Escherichia coli*

B.-Y. Lee, M. Kurtoglu, Y. Gogotsi, M. Wynosky-Dolfi, and R.F. Rest

Abstract A colloidal solution of titanium dioxide (TiO_2) nanoparticles was prepared by the solvothermal method and dip-coated onto a polypropylene fabric with TMOS binder. The prepared TiO_2 particles, colloidal solution and the coated fabrics were characterized by X-ray diffraction, SEM and TEM. The results showed that the TiO_2 particles prepared by the solvothermal method were composed of anatase which uniformly coated the substrate. Photocatalysis induced bactericidal properties of coated fabrics were tested by measuring the viability of *Escherichia coli*. It was found that solvothermally prepared TiO_2 coatings have the ability to kill *E. coli*. This unique property of TiO_2 makes it an ideal candidate in producing self-sterilizing protective masks and in providing bactericidal and self-cleaning properties to a variety of surfaces.

Keywords Solvothermal • Titania • Coated fabric • Photocatalyst • *E. coli*

1.1 Introduction

Photocatalysis based on TiO_2 has attracted much attention for environmental cleaning and antibacterial applications [1–3]. In order to synthesize TiO_2 nanoparticles, various modification of the sol–gel method have been widely used. However, sol–gel prepared TiO_2 requires a post-calcination process for crystallization [4], which limits the applicability of TiO_2 coatings to temperature resistant substrates. On the other hand, the solvothermal method, which does not need to be followed

B.-Y. Lee, M. Kurtoglu, and Y. Gogotsi (✉)
Department of Materials Science and Engineering, Drexel University,
Philadelphia, PA 19104, USA
e-mail: gogotsi@drexel.edu

M. Wynosky-Dolfi and R.F. Rest
Department of Microbiology and Immunology, Drexel University College of Medicine,
Philadelphia, PA 19129, USA

S. Mikhalovsky and A. Khajibaev (eds.), *Biodefence*, NATO Science for Peace and Security Series A: Chemistry and Biology, DOI 10.1007/978-94-007-0217-2_1,

by a high temperature calcination process, could be adopted to control particle size, shape, morphology, crystalline phase and surface chemistry by controlling composition, reaction temperature, pressure, solvents, additives, and aging time [5].

Escherichia coli (E. coli) is a common type of Gram-negative bacteria that is generally found in the lower gastrointestinal tract of mammals. These bacteria are also an environmental pathogen through contamination of water and soil. They are found in foods, on food handlers, and on most surfaces, including in hospitals [6]. *E. coli* contamination is a large problem with, according to the 2007 Center for Disease Control (CDC) statistics, approximately 73,000 cases of infections per year in the United States, resulting in an estimated 2,100 hospitalizations and about 60 deaths each year. This bacterium is the leading cause of food-borne illness in the United States each year. *E. coli* contamination remains a large problem that needs to be addressed. It is possible that TiO_2 could be used to decrease environmental contamination and thus transmission of these bacteria and potentially other environmental bacteria such as *Clostridium and Salmonella.*

In this paper, solvothermally prepared TiO_2 nanoparticle suspensions were successfully dip-coated onto fabric filters and their bactericidal properties against *E.coli* were analyzed and compared with that of Degussa P25 TiO_2 coated fabrics.

1.2 Experimental

1.2.1 Photocatalyst Preparation and Coating on Fabrics

TiO_2 colloidal solution was synthesized by a solvothermal process. Titanium tetraisopropoxide (99.9%, TTIP, Sigma Aldrich, USA) was used as a precursor for the synthesis of TiO_2 particles. Acetylacetone (99%, Sigma Aldrich, USA) was used as chelating agent to control the hydrolysis reaction and particle growth. The mixture was prepared by adding a mixture of acetylacetone and 0.15 mol of TTIP to 1 L of isopropyl alcohol. While stirring, 1.2 mol of deionized water and a specific amount of nitric acid (HNO_3, 70%) were added dropwise to the mixture, comprising about 1% by weight of the solution, and the mixture was stirred for 2 h to induce hydrolysis. Then the solution was placed into an autoclave and heated to 180 °C and the reactor temperature was kept constant for 3 h. The solution was subsequently peptized by a 0.3 M nitric acid solution. TiO_2 obtained by this method was designated as TiO_2 (ST). The preparation procedure is summarized and the schematic of autoclave apparatus is shown in Fig. 1.1. Colloidal silica was used as a binder in colloidal TiO_2 solutions in order to ensure a firm attachment of the nanoparticles on to the polypropylene substrate. Colloidal silica solution was prepared as follows: a given amount of tetramethylorthosilicate (99.9%, TMOS Sigma-Aldrich, USA) was mixed with ethanol and the mixture was stirred on a magnetic stirrer for an hour. Then a specific amount of water, ethanol and hydrochloric acid (37.5%) was added to the main solution while stirring. Solution pH was adjusted to pH = 2 followed by stirring for a further 6 h. The obtained colloidal

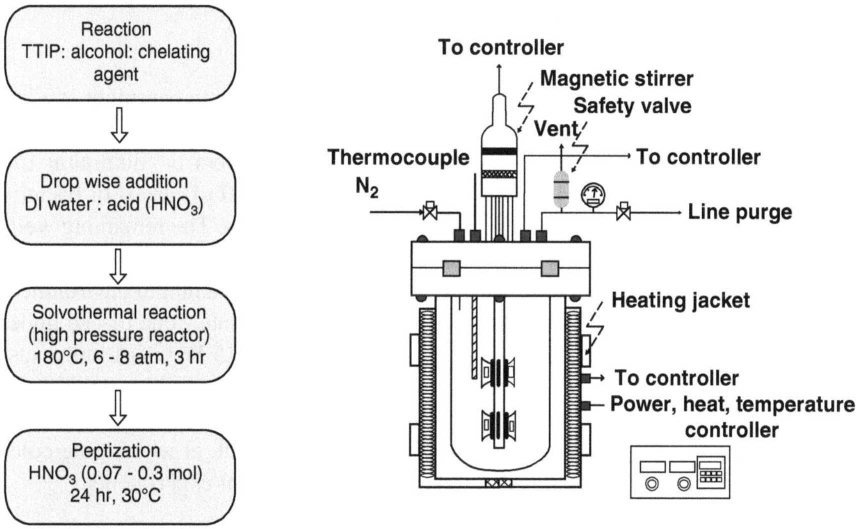

Fig. 1.1 Preparation of TiO_2 nanoparticles by the solvothermal method, and schematic of the apparatus

solutions of TiO_2 and SiO_2 were mixed, with a TiO_2:SiO_2 1.5:1 weight ratio, following a procedure modified from that reported in the literature [7].

A coating solution with Degussa P25 was prepared by dispersing 1 g powder in 500 ml of deionized water. Nitric acid was added to adjust the pH to 3. Then the dispersion was sonicated for 30 min in order to ensure a homogeneous particle distribution. Before coating, polypropylene fabrics (Global Protection/Amerinova, NJ) were thoroughly cleaned in an ultrasonic bath with ethanol and water and dried in an oven at 70°C. Then, the fabric was dipped into the selected TiO_2-SiO_2 colloidal solution for 30 min. Coated samples were dried at ambient temperature for an hour followed by a 20 min heating at 80°C. The coated fabric samples were washed in deionized water under sonication to remove loosely attached TiO_2 particles and then dried again at 70°C.

1.2.2 Characterization

Prepared samples were analyzed by powder X-ray diffraction (XRD) analysis using a Siemens D500 with nickel filtered Cu $K\alpha$ radiation (40 kV, 30 mA) in the 2θ range from 20° to 80°. The diffraction peak of the anatase (101) phase was selected to monitor the crystallinity of samples. The morphology of the TiO_2 particles and coated fabrics was studied using a field-emission SEM (Zeiss Supra 50VP). A high resolution transmission electron microscope (HR-TEM, JEOL-2010F) with a field emission gun at 200 kV was used to study particle morphology and crystallite size.

1.2.3 Antibacterial Test

Escherichia coli (*E. coli*) was grown in Luria Burtoni (LB) broth overnight at 37°C with shaking at 250 rpm. Bacteria were pelleted and re-suspended at the desired concentrations. One centimeter squares of TiO_2-coated filters or aluminum foil were placed in wells of a 24-well tissue culture plate and 50 μL drops of bacteria were carefully placed in the center of the filter or foil squares. The remaining wells of a 24-well plate were filled with water and a 2 mm thick, 10×15 cm Pyrex glass plate was placed on top of the tissue culture plate to maintain a humid environment and to avoid evaporation. This set-up was repeated in duplicate - one placed under UV light and the other not. Samples were irradiated with 215 W UV-A bulbs suspended 8 cm above the 24-well plate at room temperature. At 0, 30 and 120 min, bacteria were recovered from the filter or foil squares, diluted and plated on LB agar plates. LB agar plates were incubated at 37°C overnight, at which time colonies were counted. Data are represented as three independent experiments.

1.3 Results and Discussion

XRD patterns of the solvothermally prepared TiO_2 (ST), Degussa P25, and TiO_2 prepared by conventional sol-gel method (calcined at 600°C) are shown in Fig. 1.2. The solvothermal titania powder was obtained by drying at 60°C. In the case of P25

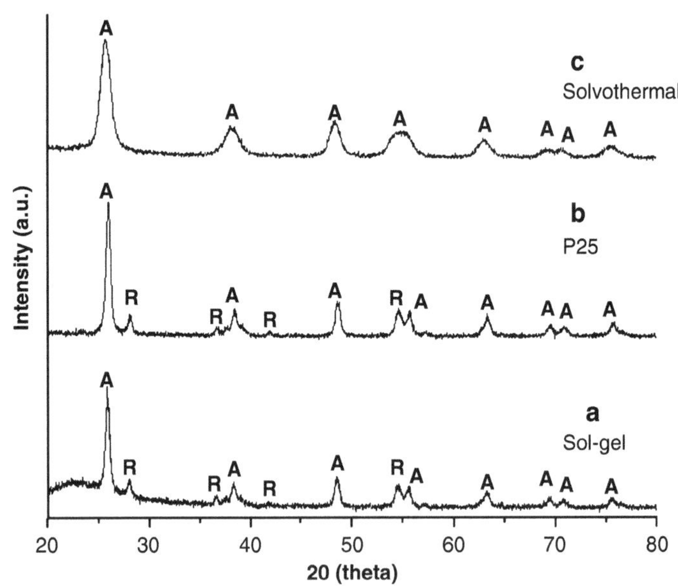

Fig. 1.2 X-ray diffraction patterns of TiO_2 powders: (**a**) sol–gel preparation, (**b**) commercial TiO_2 (Degussa P25), and (**c**) solvothermal preparation. (A: anatase, R: rutile)

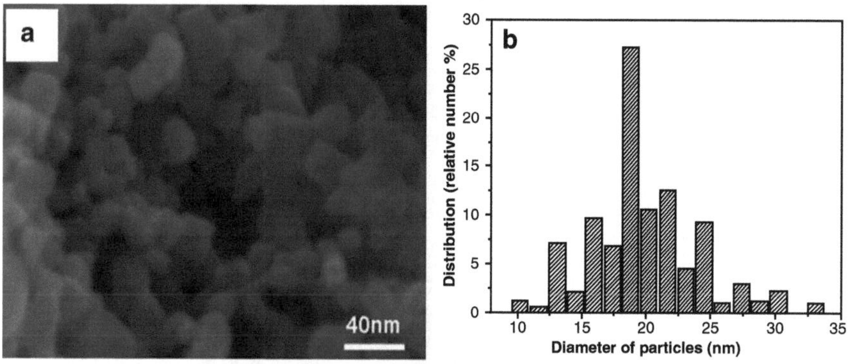

Fig. 1.3 SEM image of TiO_2 (ST) nanoparticles (**a**), and calculated particle size distribution (**b**)

TiO_2, both anatase and rutile structures were found. On the contrary, the TiO_2 (ST) sample showed only anatase structure. The average crystallite size was 9.3 nm for TiO_2 (ST) samples by using Scherrer's equation [8], which was significantly smaller compared to the P25 powder, with an average crystallite size between 15 and 25 nm [9].

Crystallization in the anatase structure was reported to occur in the sol–gel processed TiO_2 after calcination between 350°C and 500°C [5]. However, crystallized TiO_2 particles can be produced by using the solvothermal method without any post-treatment.

Crystallization of TiO_2 occurs during solvothermal treatment at high pressure, and the crystals grow to primary particle size through homo-coagulation. At this point, excess solvent partially suppresses further crystal growth; as a result, the particle size becomes smaller than that in the sol–gel method. However, hydrolysis and condensation reactions occur very rapidly in sol–gel synthesis of transition metal oxides, therefore uniform and ultrafine products are difficult to obtain.

The morphology and the calculated particle size distribution (PSD) of TiO_2 (ST) particles are shown in Fig. 1.3 (a) and (b). It was observed that the PSD is between 10 and 33 nm with a mean diameter of 17 – 19 nm, which is somewhat larger than the one determined from XRD. However, SEM does not allow us to see the smallest particles and particles that look like single crystals in SEM may indeed be twinned or polycrystalline. Thus, we expect SEM analysis to give overestimated values of the particle size.

TEM images of TiO_2 (ST) nanoparticles are shown in Fig. 1.4a and give a clear view of the smallest particles that could not be seen in SEM. The average particle size of the as-synthesized (ST) nanoparticles was 5–8 nm with a spherical morphology. TiO_2 particles are observed to be homogeneously dispersed in the amorphous silica matrix (Fig. 1.4b). The lattice fringes of 0.35 nm were observed, corresponding to the lattice spacing of (101) plane in the anatase phase (Fig. 1.4(c)).

Surface morphologies of the as-received fabric filters before coating, and after coating with Degussa P25 and TiO_2 (ST) dispersions were observed with SEM as shown in Fig. 1.5 (a) to (c), respectively. The SEM images show that the

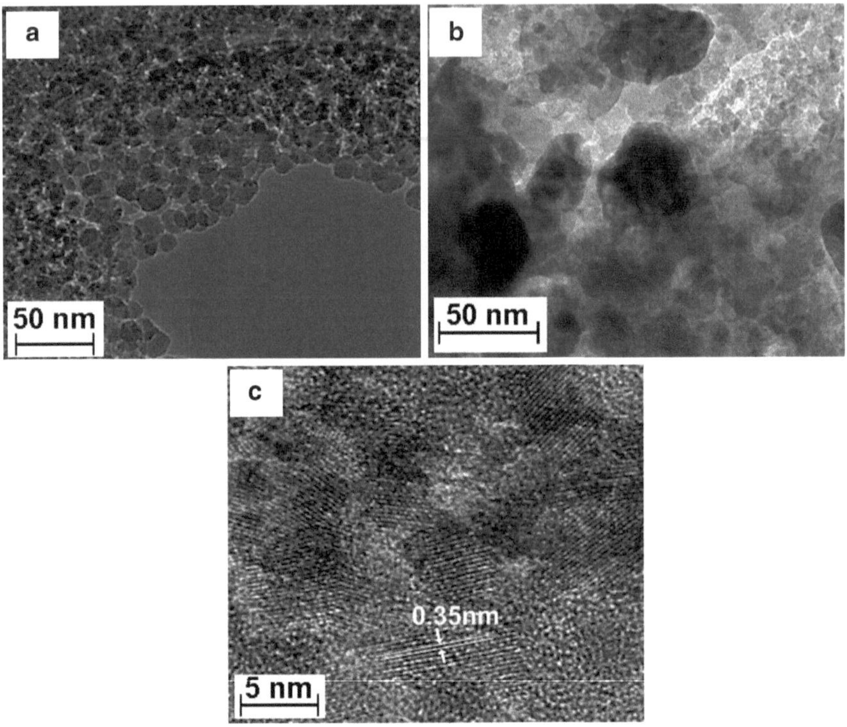

Fig. 1.4 TEM images of (**a**) as prepared TiO_2, and (**b**) TiO_2-SiO_2 particles prepared by the solvothermal method. (**c**) HRTEM image of TiO_2 prepared by the solvothermal method

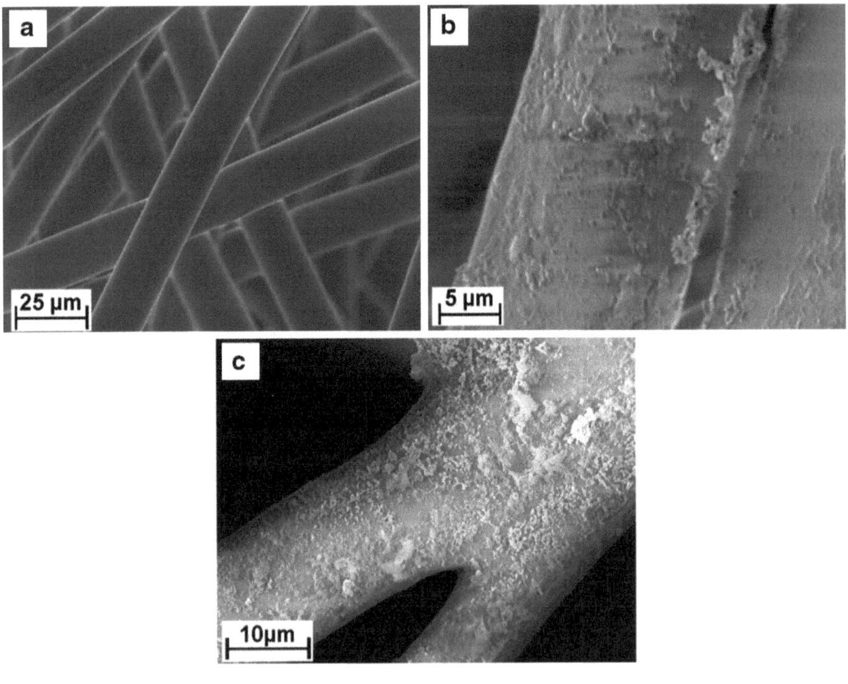

Fig. 1.5 SEM images of the polypropylene fabric: (**a**) as-received, and after coating with (**b**) TiO_2 (ST) and (**c**) P25 particles

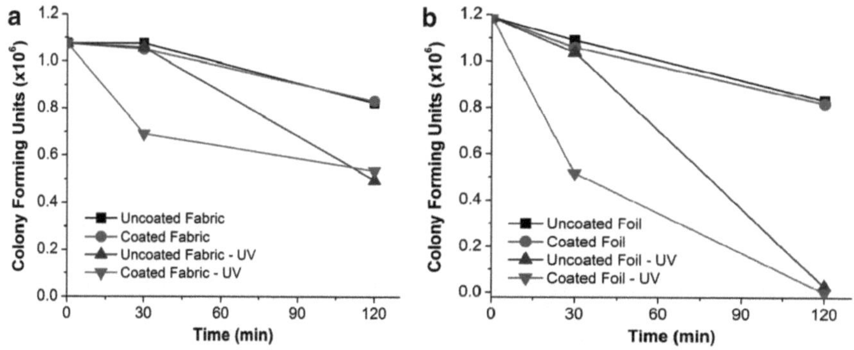

Fig. 1.6 Photocatalytic killing of *E. coli* on TiO_2 electrosprayed samples (**a** - fabric and **b** - aluminum foil) in comparison with uncoated (control) samples irradiated with UV-A light

TiO_2 particles are largely aggregated on the surface, which indicates that the primary TiO_2 particles coagulated into larger particles during the coating and drying. The morphology of P25 coated fabric shows somewhat larger particles, agglomeration and areas of uncovered surface. The layer of TiO_2 (ST) on the fibers was, in average, much more uniform and continuous than that of Degussa P25.

Photocatalytic bactericidal activity experiments were performed using *E. coli* with untreated and TiO_2-coated fabric and aluminum foil (Fig. 1.6) and with or without UV-A irradiation. Photocatalytic bactericidal properties of TiO_2-coated fabric and foil were observed after 30 min. The most distinctive difference between coated and UV-irradiated materials was observed initially. This is a clear demonstration of the photocatalytic ability of TiO_2 and accelerated surface decontamination. We observed complete bacteria killing only on aluminum foil coated with TiO_2, and partial killing on the coated fabric. These results suggest that TiO_2 coated materials have bactericidal properties.

1.4 Conclusions

TiO_2 coated fabric filters were prepared in a one-step process by the solvothermal method, and their properties were compared with those electrosprayed with Degussa P25. Filters coated with TiO_2 nanoparticles prepared by the solvothermal method were superior to the commercial TiO_2 powder in terms of particle size and homogeneity. A significant amount of bactericidal activity towards *E. coli* was successfully implanted into fabric filters by dip coating a solvothermally prepared TiO_2 dispersion.

Acknowledgments This work was supported by Global Protection LLC and Amerinova. TEM analysis was done by Patricia Reddington at the Centralized Research Facility of Drexel

University. The authors are grateful to L. Schiliro and S. Guarino (Amerinova) for providing the polypropylene fabrics and helpful discussion.

References

1. Fujishima A, Rao TN, Tryk DA (2000) Titanium dioxide photocatalysis. J Photochem Photobiol, C 1:1–21
2. Choi W (2006) Pure and modified TiO_2 photocatalysts and their environmental applications. Catal Surv Asia 10:16–28
3. Kaneko M, Okura I (2002) Photocatalysis: science and technology. Springer, Tokyo
4. Kang M, Lee S-Y, Chung C-H, Cho SM, Han GY, Kim B-W, Yoon KJ (2001) Characterization of a TiO_2 photocatalyst synthesized by the solvothermal method and its catalytic performance for $CHCl_3$ decomposition. J Photochem Photobiol, A 144:185–191
5. Tomita K, Petrykin V, Kobayashi M, Shiro M, Yoshimura M, Kakihana MA (2006) Water-soluble titanium complex for the selective synthesis of nanocrystalline brookite, rutile, and anatase by a hydrothermal method. Angew Chem Int Edit 118:2438–2441
6. Feng P, Weagant SD, Grant MA (1998) Enumeration of Escherichia coli and the Coliform Bacteria, in Bacteriological Analytical Manual, Edn. 8 - Revision A, Chapter 4, US Food and Drug Administration
7. Kwon CH, Kim JH, Jung IS, Shin H, Yoon KH (2003) Preparation and characterization of TiO_2-SiO_2 nano-composite thin films. Ceram Int 29:851–856
8. Zhang Q, Gao L, Guo J (2000) Effects of calcination on the photocatalytic properties of nano-sized TiO_2 powders prepared by $TiCl_4$ hydrolysis. Appl Catal, B 26:207–215
9. Porter JF, Li Y-G, Chan CK (1999) The effect of calcination on the microstructural characteristics and photoreactivity of Degussa P-25 TiO_2. J Mater Sci 34:1523–1531

Chapter 2
Carbon Nanotubes: Biorisks and Biodefence

M.T. Kartel, L.V. Ivanov, S.N. Kovalenko, and V.P. Tereschenko

Abstract From the time of the discovery of carbon nanotubes (CNT) the question of their toxicity remains of key importance. The practical use of these unique nanomaterials in biotechnology, molecular biology and medicine can be complicated because of possible adverse effect of CNT on subcellular and cellular structures, tissues and whole organs. Similarly to any other nanoparticles, CNT toxicity is defined by their form, size, purity, charge, dose, entry route into the body, concentration in the target organ, duration of contact and other factors. The research on toxicity and biocompatibility of CNT of different origin, structure and purity began in 2001. It has been conducted with various biological components, performing experiments both *in vitro* and *in vivo*.

Here some aspects of cytotoxicity and potential for medical use of CNT are discussed.

Keywords Carbon nanotubes • Cytotoxicity • Cytocompatibility • Medical applications of CNT

2.1 Introduction

From the time of Iijima's publication on carbon nanotubes, CNT [1] (which were probably discovered earlier [2]), the question of their toxicity remains of key importance. The practical use of these unique nanomaterials in biotechnology, molecular biology and medicine can naturally be complicated because of possible

M.T. Kartel (✉)
Chuiko Institute of Surface Chemistry, NASU, Kiev, Ukraine
e-mail: nikar@kartel.kiev.ua

L.V. Ivanov and S.N. Kovalenko
National Pharmaceutical University, Kharkov, Ukraine

V.P. Tereschenko
Institute for Ecological Pathology of Humans, Kiev, Ukraine

S. Mikhalovsky and A. Khajibaev (eds.), *Biodefence*, NATO Science for Peace and Security Series A: Chemistry and Biology, DOI 10.1007/978-94-007-0217-2_2,

adverse effect of CNT on subcellular and cellular structures, tissues and whole organs. Similarly to any other nanoparticles, CNT toxicity is dependent on their shape, size, purity, charge, dose, entry route into the body, concentration in the field of body-target, duration of influence and other factors. The research on toxicity and biocompatibility of CNT of different origin, structure and chemical purity has been performed since 2001. It has been conducted with various biological components, performing experiments both *in vitro* and *in vivo*. A number of original papers and reviews on this subject are available [3–8].

Carbon nanotubes are among the most interesting objects of nanotechnology. They have cylindrical structure with a diameter in the range of one to several dozen nanometres and length of several nanometres to several microns. CNT are built of one or several graphene layers with hexagonal arrangement of carbon atoms. Tubes have a tip in the shape of a hemispherical head with a chemical structure of a half fullerene. Unlike fullerenes, which represent the molecular form of carbon, CNT combine properties of nanoclusters and a massive solid body. This leads to an occurrence of specific, sometimes unexpected mechanical, optical, electric, magnetic and physico-chemical properties, which attract the attention of researchers and end-users:

Mechanical properties: hardening of metals and alloys, creation of novel polymeric composites, special additives to lubricants and oils, etc.

Electronic properties: semiconductor and metal conductivity, magneto-resistance, emission of electrons, electronic devices of the molecular size, information recording, diodes, field transistors, cold cathodes, materials for displays, quantum wires and dots, cathodes for X-ray radiation, electric probes, etc.

Optical properties: light-emitting diodes, resonance absorption of near IR-radiation;

Physical and chemical properties: large specific surface and possibility of surface chemical modification, adsorbents, catalysts, chemical sensors, materials for electrodes, chemical batteries, fuel elements and super condensers.

Biological properties: ability to migrate into biological cells, biosensors, prosthetics, drug delivery, medical nanodevices, application in gene engineering.

The industrial production of CNT has now achieved several tons per year and it is continually increasing. During their production, conditioning and applications, CNT can penetrate into the human body by inhalation, contact with skin, with food and drinking water, or deliberate introduction into the blood and under the skin if used for medical applications. They can also influence microorganisms, plants, animals, when they are released into the environment in significant amounts. However despite the vast knowledge generated about CNT, their impact on biological objects is still not clear.

2.2 Biorisks Associated with CNT

A variety of new materials had been produced using nanoparticles before scientists became concerned about their possible negative impact and consequences for the human body and the environment. The toxicology of carbon nanomaterials, in particular nanotubes, has emerged only recently and it is at a stage of accumulating primary data. There are three main factors which define the ability of carbon nanoparticles to cause possible damage:

- A high surface area-to-mass ratio and as a result a large area of contact between the nanoparticle and the cellular membrane, and significant influence on adsorption and transport of toxic substances.
- Contact time: the longer CNT contact with the cell membrane, the higher probability of cell damage. However, this factor also includes the mobility of nanoparticles, which can migrate to the surrounding tissue and be removed from the organism.
- The reactivity or inherent toxicity of chemical substances introduced together with CNT. They can be located inside nanotubes or attached to their external surface. This factor is related to the surface area-to-mass ratio of nanoparticles. The higher the ratio, the more likely is the negative impact.

Studying toxicity and biocompatibility of CNT is very important. Smart et al. [9] outlined directions of future research in this field. It includes pulmonary toxicity, skin irritability, macrophage response, interrelation of CNT with their toxicity, absorption, distribution and excretion, and influence of chemical functionalization of CNT on their biocompatibility.

It is not clear yet to what extent the mechanical damage of cell membranes caused by nanotubes and the effect of CNT on biochemical processes in subcellular organelles (mitochondria and nuclei) contribute to nanotubes toxicity. While the influence of CNT on DNA and cell nuclei was experimentally proved [10, 11], there is no data on the effect of nanotubes on the activity of mitochondria, which play a key role in viability of cells. The data currently available on pulmonary toxicity, skin irritability, cytotoxicity, biocompatibility, influence on environment, and therapeutic action of CNT are inconsistent and do not give a clear picture about level of safety of such nanomaterials for living organisms. It has become clear only that purified single-walled nanotubes of small length and chemically modified nanotubes with functionalized surfaces have lower toxicity and better biocompatibility. It is known that CNT are capable of entering the membrane of biological cells, to reach the cytoplasm, and in some cases into the nucleus. It has been established empirically that concentration limit of cytotoxicity of CNT suspension is about 0.01 mg/mL.

Some data on CNT cytotoxicity and cytocompatibility are summarized in Tables 2.1 and 2.2 [12–28].

To study the mechanism of cytotoxic action of CNT we used a modified method of spin labels [20], which allows the quantitative determination of CNT influence on membrane integrity of human blood erythrocytes, and mitochondrial activity of hepatocytes in rat liver homogenate, without extraction of mitochondria from cells.

Water-soluble iminoxyl free radical – 2,2,6,6,-tetramethyl-4-oxo-piperidin-1-oxyl (commercial trade name TEMPON) was used as a paramagnetic probe.

Table 2.1 Cytotoxicity of CNT

Authors	Material	Type of cell	Result
Shvedova et al. [12]	SW CNT, Fe-catalyst	Human keratinocytes (HaCaT) in solution with 0.06–0.24 mg/mL CNT, contact time 8 h	Accelerated oxidative stress (production of free radicals and peroxides, exhaustion of general antioxidant reserves); decrease of cell viability, morphological changes
Monteiro-Riviere et al. [13]	MW CNT, (CVD-method), purified	Human keratinocytes of (HEK) in solution with 0.1–0.4 mg/mL CNT, contact time 48 h	Production of inflammatory cytokines (IL); reduction of cells viability depending on time and dose of exposure
Tamura et al. [14]	CNT, purified	Human blood neutrophils in contact with CNT for 1 h	Increase of superoxide anion-radicals and inflammatory cytokine (TNF- α) production; decrease of cells viability
Cherukuri et al. [15]	SW CNT, purified	Phagocytic cells of mice (J774.1)	Catching ~50% of nanotubes, no cytotoxic effect
Shvedova et al. [16]	SW CNT, Fe-catalyst	Macrophagic murine cells (RAW264.7)	Increase of pro-fibrotic mediator TGF-β1; no oxidative burst, nitric oxide production or apoptosis was observed
Muller et al. [17]	MW CNT, purified	Peritoneal macrophages of rats – incubation in solution with 20, 50 and 100 mg/mL CNT, contact time 24 h	Release of lactate dehydrogenase and inflammatory cytokines (мRNA squirrel TNF-α)
Jia et al. [18]	SW and MW CNT (arc, CVD), purified	Alveolar macrophages – solution of SW CNT (conc. 1.41–226 mg/cm^2) and MW CNT (conc. 1.41–22.6 mg/cm^2), contact 6 h	Reduction of cells viability and macrophages functional ability decrease
Cui et al. [19]	SW CNT	Human embryonic kidney cells (HEK 293) in solution with 0.78–200 mg/mL of SW CNT	Induction of apoptosis and reduction of adhesion ability (and corresponding genes), reduction of cellular proliferation

SW- single wall, MW- multiwall

Table 2.2 Cytocompatibility of CNT

Author	Material	Type of cell	Results
Elias et al. [21]	CNT-containing orthopedic materials	Osteoblasts – inoculation on material	Increase of osteoblast proliferation, increase of alkaline phosphatase activity, absence of cytotoxicity
Supronowicz et al. [22]	PLA/CNT – nano-composites	Osteoblasts – contact with nanocomposites, effect of electric current	Increase of osteoblast proliferation
Price et al. [23]	PU/CNT – nano-composites	Osteoblasts, chondrocytes, fibroblasts, plain muscular cells – contact with PU/CNT	Adhesion increased only for osteoblasts; absence of cytotoxicity
Correa-Duarte et al. [24]	MW CNT, oxidized	Fibroblasts of mice (L929) – inoculation to CNT, observation – 7 days	Formation of the isolated cells, fusion after 7 days, absence of cytotoxicity
McKenzie et al. [25]	MW CNT, purified, different diameter	Astrocytes (cells which are responsible for reduction of nervous tissue damages) – contact with CNT surface	Normal proliferation, adhesion and functional activity on tubes, especially with a diameter less than 100 nm
Hu et al. [26]	PU/CNT – nano-composites	Astrocytes, axons of rats – contact with PU/CNT nanocomposites	Reduction of astrocyte adhesion, increased inhibition of axons. Cytotoxicity is absent
Gabay et al. [27]	MW CNT, purified and chemically modified	Neurons – inoculation on CNT, observation – 4 days	Localization on CNT, proliferation of aksons. Cytotoxicity is absent
McKnight et al. [28]	Vertically oriented nanofibers+DNA	Chinese hamster ovary (CHO) cells – centrifugation and compression	Part of cells was lost, small production of GFP; cytotoxic response was not observed

PLA - polylactic acid, PU - polyurethane

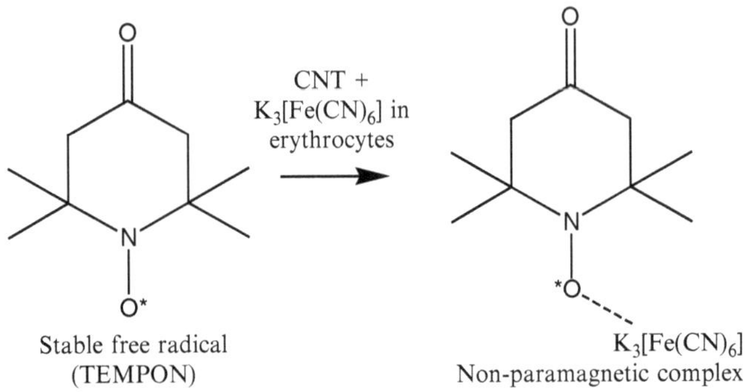

(2.1)

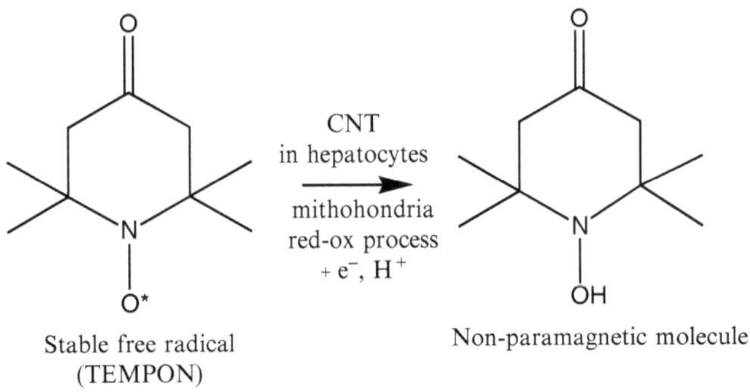

(2.2)

ESR-spectra of TEMPON degradation in erythrocytes and hepatocytes were studied. The degradation was caused by the chemical processes presented in Schemes 2.1 and 2.2.

The erythrocyte membrane damage caused by CNT increased with time (Fig. 2.1a). Introduction of CNT suspension at concentrations from 0.01 to 0.2 mg/mL during the first step did not lead to erythrocyte membrane infringement. However after 2 days of exposure to CNT at concentrations ranging from 0.01, 0.05, 0.1 and 0.2 mg/mL and at temperature 6°C the quantity of damaged erythrocytes was 4, 10, 16 and 25%, respectively.

The incubation of liver homogenate with CNT for 4 h at 0°C leads to considerable decrease of mitochondrial activity (perhaps due to inhibition of chain transfer of electrons in mitochondria). The data obtained showed (Fig. 2.1b) that the cytotoxicity caused by CNT is associated with not only structural changes in the cell membrane, but also with CNT influence on their functional properties.

We have studied CNT influence on growth rate and proliferation of some cellular colonies [29]. Interesting results were obtained in case of bread-making yeast-like fungi *Saccharomyces cerevisiae* (strain 608) and hamster kidney cells. Introduction of small amounts of CNT (~3 μg/mL) in fungal suspensions led to 2-fold increase in *Saccharomyces cerevisiae* colonies number compared to the control, after 48 h of incubation at 30°C (Fig. 2.2). Similar results were obtained for colonies of hamster kidney cells. Presence of CNT activated cell proliferation and increased cell growth rate by 1.5 times.

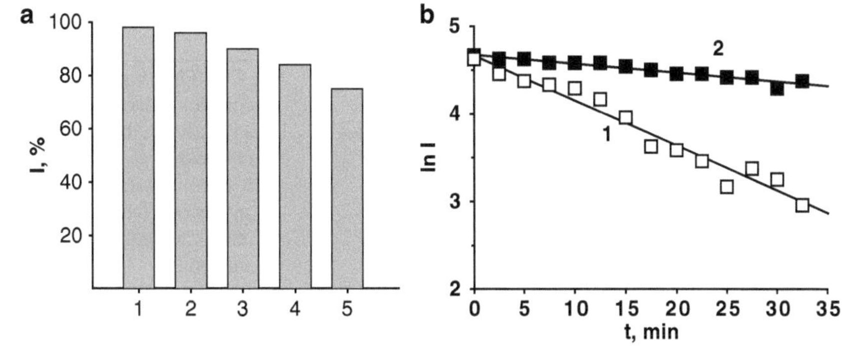

Fig. 2.1 (**a**) Influence of CNT concentration in presence of $K_3[Fe(CN)_6]$ on intensity of the ESR spectra of the paramagnetic label TEMPON: control (without CNT) (*1*) and adding CNT to blood erythrocytes at 0.01 (*2*), 0.05 (*3*), 0.1 (*4*) and 0.2 (*5*) mg/mL; (**b**) kinetics of the ESR signal intensity decay of the paramagnetic label in liver homogenate after 4 h inoculation: *1* – control (without CNT), *2* – in presence of CNT with concentration 0.2 mg/mL

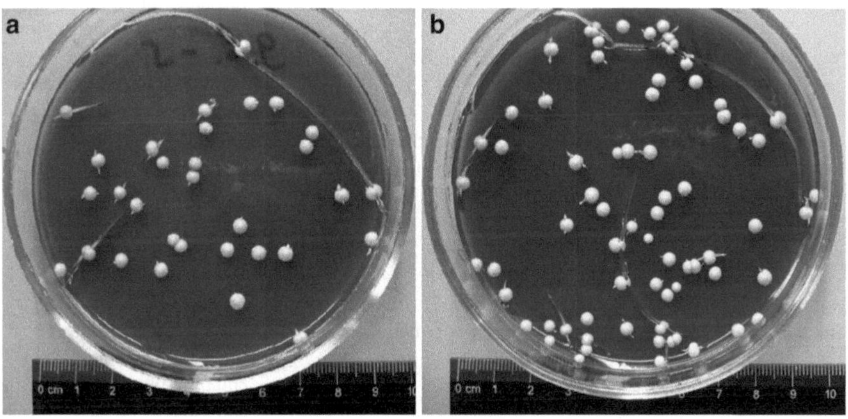

Fig. 2.2 Influence of adding CNT into a nutrient medium on growth of Saccharomyces cerevisiae colonies after 48 h of incubation: (**a**) control (without CNT), (**b**) in the presence of CNT (~3 μg/mL)

2.3 Biomedical Applications of CNT

Nanotubes are functionalised to improve their solubility in water or to attach to their surface biologically active substances such as peptides and drugs. The ability to attach biological substances has raised an interest in using nanotubes as carriers for delivery of drugs and vaccines. A number of researchers performed functionalization of CNT with physiologically active molecules and macro-objects. These results are summarized in Table 2.3 [30–40].

Compared to classical drug delivery systems such as liposomes or peptides, nanotubes have a higher efficiency [41] and this can be used for the further development of delivery systems. Stability and diversity of nanotube forms provide long time circulation and biocompatibility that result in more efficient transport of substances.

Table 2.3 Use of CNT as carriers of bioactive substances

Author	CNT conjugate	Results
Pantarotto et al. [30]	Functionalized SW CNT+small peptide sequence from the foot-and-mouth disease virus (FMDV)	SW CNT-FMDV peptide complex induced a specific antibody response *in vivo*. It was maintained and recognized by mono- and polyclonal antibodies
Pantarotto et al. [31]	Functionalized SW CNT+peptide fragment from the α-subunit of the Gs protein (αs)	SWCN-αs complex was able to cross the cellular and nuclear membranes (human 3 T6 and murine 3 T3 cells)
Kam et al. [32]	Purified and shortened SW CNT+streptavidin	SW CNT-streptavidin conjugate caused extensive cell death, which was attributed to the delivery of streptavidin to the cells (proleukemia cells of human and T-lymphocytes)
Wu et al. [33]	CNT+amphotericin B	Amphotericin B entered various cells and increased its activity
Bianco et al. [34]	CNT+proteins (fibrinogen, protein A, erythropoietin, and apolipoprotein)	CNT-TEG-short protein complex quickly entered fibroblasts and other cells, sometimes migrated to their nuclei. Proteins executed their normal biological functions
Lu et al. [35]	SW CNT+RNA polymer	Successful transportation of SW CNT-RNA polymer complex into cytoplasm and nucleus of cell
Pantarotto et al. [26]	SW CNT and MW CNT+plasmid DNA	All conjugates influenced regulative expression of marker genes in human cells
Cai et al. [37]	SW CNT+plasmid DNA, with nickel under the influence of a magnetic field	High efficiency of transduction of SW CNT-DNA conjugates in lymphoma cells (Ball 7 B-lymphoma)
Kam et al. [38–40]	SW CNT+cytochrome C,RNA, DNA	CNT transferred cytochrome C to the cancer cells; accumulation of SW CNT-RNA conjugates in cytoplasm and nucleus of HeLa cells

By using nanotubes for drug delivery the problem of poor solubility of a considerable number of substances such as many medicines could be overcome. Furthermore, nanotubes can be modified to improve their contact and penetration into target cells. In conclusion, using nanotubes for drug delivery should increase efficiency of the latter and can reduce their side-effects.

SW CNT functionalized with DNA showed a 10 times more effective penetration and expression of genes *in vitro*, in comparison with molecular DNA. Other charged macromolecules such as polypeptides and liposomes, can provide more effective transport, but they can cause destabilization of the cellular membrane exhibiting a cytotoxic effect. Whereas, using nanotubes for gene delivery has not caused any cytotoxic effects.

Successful gene therapy demands an effective system for therapeutic gene delivery into organs and tissues. Therefore gene delivery is based on the development of a non-viral delivery system. Such vector systems have the ability to introduce the alien genetic information into a cell. Carbon nanotubes can be used for creation of new vectors for gene transportation.

2.4 CNT: Pros and Cons

Carbon nanotubes are unique materials with specific properties [42]. There is a considerable application potential for using nanotubes in the biomedical field. However, when such materials are considered for application in biomedical implants, transport of medicines and vaccines or as biosensors, their biocompatibility needs to be established. Other carbon materials show remarkable long-term biocompatibility and biological action for use as medical devices. Preliminary data on biocompatibility of nanotubes and other novel nanostructured materials demonstrate that we have to pay attention to their possible adverse effects when their biomedical applications are considered.

Despite the need to know how nanotubes may affect or cause toxicity for live organisms, only a small number of studies have been dedicated to this problem. Furthermore, results of these studies have been inconsistent and not fully understood. The data obtained show that crude nanotubes possess a certain level of toxicity (in both *in vivo* and *in vitro* studies) associated mainly with the presence of metals, which are used as catalysts in nanotube synthesis. For purified nanotubes minimal toxic effects were seen even at high concentrations, and chemically functionalized nanotubes used for drug delivery did not show any toxic effects. However, the ability of nanotubes to form aggregates requires further research in this area.

From the data obtained so far one could conclude that work with nanotubes should be done with precaution, and certain safety actions need to be considered working with nanotubes in laboratories and during their manufacture. The success of nanotechnologies will depend on continuing research in the area of toxicology of carbon nanotubes and the materials based on them.

In the study conducted by Hurt et al. [43], toxicology of nanoparticles (nanotoxicology) with a special emphasis on CNT was considered. The necessity of carrying out toxicology research as well as the lack of such work in this area was highlighted. It was considered that the future development of nanotoxicology is associated with the following:

- Materials should be characterized and described in as many details as possible, because the nanotube toxicity can depend on by-products of their synthesis as well as on their design. It would be desirable to provide at least information on their composition (including metals and heteroatoms, which are present in a quantity higher than 0.1%), detailed description of morphology, data on surface chemistry, crystallinity, and spatial organization of graphene planes;
- Better understanding of mechanism of nanotube interaction with biological objects is required; the possible toxicity will depend on dose and exposure time;
- Methods for tracking nanotubes in biological materials are needed to measure the rate of nanotube transport, distance of penetration from places of introduction at inhalation, with food and water, and implantation of nanotubes;
- Methods for dose measurement;
- Determination of the main indicators of toxicity, as carbon nanotubes can cause different toxic effects.

It was concluded that the overarching objective of nanotube toxicology is to find materials that will have no harmful effect on nature and humans.

The progressive growth of technologies of production and applications of nanomaterials, in particular on the basis of nanocarbons (fullerenes, nanotubes, nanodiamonds, aerogels, etc.) is observed all over the world. Physical, chemical and mechanical properties of such substances are capable of exerting an unpredictable impact on biological objects. In this review, we have offered approaches to formation of identification methodology, toxicological research and assessment of risks for human organisms and the environment posed by manufacture and use of nanosized substances [44]. In course of our study, the experience gained from the Chernobyl catastrophy, and the effect of small doses and low intensity of technogenic pollution on a human body has been used.

It is obvious that we are at the stage of accumulating the knowledge of how to handle safely nanosized objects. Carbon nanotubes are currently and will be in the future at the forefront among other known nanomaterials, in terms of volumes of research, manufacturing and applications in various fields of practical activities, including medicine and biology.

References

1. Iijima S (1991) Helical microtubules of graphitic carbon. Nature 354:56–58
2. Radushkevich LV, Lukyanovich VM (1952) About structure of carbon created at thermal decomposition of carbon monoxide on iron contact. J Phys Chem 26:88–95

3. Sinha N, Yeow JT-W (2005) Carbon nanotubes for biomedical applications. IEEE Trans Nanobiosci 4:180–195
4. Kohli P, Martin CR (2005) Smart nanotubes for biotechnology. Curr Pharm Biotech 6:35–47
5. Toxicology of Carbon Nanomaterials. Special Issue (2006) Carbon 44:1027–1120
6. Rey DA, Batt CA, Miller JC (2006) Carbon nanotubes in biomedical applications. Nanotech Law Business 3:263–292
7. Yang W, Thordarson P, Gooding JJ et al (2007) Carbon nanotubes for biological and biomedical application. Nanotechnology 18:1–12
8. Porter AE, Gass M, Muller K et al (2007) Direct imaging of single-walled carbon nanotubes in cells. Nature Nanotech 2:713–717
9. Smart SK, Cassady AI, Lu GQ et al (2006) The biocompatibility of carbon nanotubes. Carbon 44:1034–1047
10. Schipper ML, Nakayama-Ratchford N, Davis CR et al (2008) A pilot toxicology study of single-walled carbon nanotubes in a small sample of mice. Nature Nanotech 3:216–221
11. Zhu L, Chang DW, Dai L et al (2007) DNA Damage induced by multiwalled carbon nanotubes in mouse embryonic stem cells. Nano Lett 7:3592–3597
12. Shvedova AA, Castranova V (2003) Exposure to carbon nanotube material: Assessment of nanotube cytotoxicity using human keratinocyte cells. J Toxicol Environ Health A 66: 1909–1926
13. Monteiro-Riviere NA, Nemanich RJ, Inman AO et al (2005) Multi-walled carbon nanotube interactionwith human epidermal keratinocytes. Toxicol Lett 155:377–384
14. Tamura K, Takashi N, Akasaka T et al (2004) Effect of micro/nano particle size on cell function and morphology. Key Eng Mater 254:919–922
15. Cherukuri P, Bachilo SM, Litovsky SH et al (2004) Near-infrared fluorescence microscopy of single-walled carbon nanotubes in phagocytic cells. J Am Chem Soc 126:15638–15639
16. Shvedova AA, Kisin ER, Mercer RR et al (2005) Unusual inflammatory and fibrogenic pulmonary responses to single walled carbon nanotubes in mice. Am J Physiol Lung Cell Mol Physiol 289:698–708
17. Muller J, Huaux F, Moreau N et al (2005) Respiratory toxicity of multi-walled carbon nanotubes. Toxicol Appl Pharmacol 207:221–231
18. Jia G, Wang H, Yan L et al (2005) Cytotoxicity of carbon nanomaterials: Single-wall nanotube, multi-wall nanotube and fullerene. Environ Sci Technol 39:1378–1383
19. Cui D, Tian F, Ozkan CS et al (2005) Effect of single wall carbon nanotubes on human HEK293 cells. Toxicol Lett 155:73–85
20. Kartel NT, Grischenko VI, Chernykh VP et al (2008) A study of cytotoxicity of carbon nanotubes by spin probe method. In: Kartel MT (ed) Chemistry, Physics and Technology of Surface 14. Naukova dumka, Kiev, pp 557–564
21. Elias KL, Price RL, Webster TJ (2002) Enhanced functions of osteoblasts on nanometer diameter carbon fibers. Biomaterials 23:3279–3287
22. Supronowicz PR, Adjayan PM, Ullman KR et al (2002) Novel current conducting composite substrates for exposing osteoblasts to alternating current stimulation. J Biomed Mater Res 59A:499–506
23. Price RL, Waid MC, Haberstroh KM et al (2003) Selective bone cell adhesion on formulations containing carbon nano-fibers. Biomaterials 24:1877–1887
24. Correa-Duarte MA, Wagner N, Rojas-Chapana J et al (2004) Fabrication and biocompatibility of carbon nanotube-based 3D networks as scaffolds for cell seeding and growth. Nano Lett 4:2233–2236
25. McKenzie JL, Waid MC, Shi R et al (2004) Decreased functions of astrocytes on carbon nanofibre materials. Biomaterials 25:1309–1317
26. Hu H, Ni Y, Montana V et al (2004) Chemically functionalized carbon nanotubes as substrates for neuronal growth. Nano Lett 4:507–511
27. Gabay T, Jakobs E, Ben-Jacob E et al (2005) Engineered self-organisation of neural networks using carbon nanotube clusters. Physica A 350:611–621

28. McKnight TE, Melechko AV, Griffin GD et al (2003) Intracellular integration of synthetic nanostructures with viable cells for controlled biochemical manipulation. Nanotechnology 14:551–556
29. Ivanov LV, Chernykh VP, Kartel NT et al (2008) Study of mechanisms of carbon nanotubes cytotoxicity. In: Chemistry, Physics and Technology of Surface Modification. Proceedings of. ISC, Kiev: 34–36
30. Pantarotto D, Partidos CD, Hoebeke J et al (2003) Immunisation with peptide-functionalized carbon nanotubes enhanced virus-specific neutralising antibody response. Chem Biol 10:961–966
31. Pantarotto D, Briand J-P, Prato M et al (2004) Translocation bioactive peptides across cell membranes by carbon nanotubes. Chem Commun 1:16–17
32. Kam NWS, Jessop TC, Wender PA et al (2004) Nanotube molecular transporters: Internalization of carbon nanotube-protein conjugates into mammalian cells. J Am Chem Soc 126:6850–6851
33. Wu W, Wieckowski S, Pastorin G et al (2005) Targeted delivery of amphotericin B to cells by using functionalized carbon nanotubes. Angew Chem Int Edit 44:6358–6362
34. Bianco A, Kostarelos K, Prato M (2005) Application of carbon nanotubes in drug delivery. Curr Opin Chem Biol 9:647–649
35. Lu G, Moore JM, Huang G et al (2004) RNA polymer translocation with single-walled carbon nanotubes. Nano Lett 4:2473–2477
36. Pantarotto D, Singh R, McCarthy D et al (2004) Functionalized carbon nanotubes for plasmid DNA gene delivery. Angew Chem Int Edit 43:5242–5246
37. Cai D, Mataraza JM, Huang Z et al (2005) Highly efficient molecular delivery into mammalian cells using carbon nanotubes spearing. Nat Methods 2:449–454
38. Kam NWS, Dai HJ (2005) Carbon nanotubes as intracellular protein transporters: generality and biological functionality. J Am Chem Soc 127:6021–6026
39. Kam NWS, Liu Z, Dai HJ (2005) Functionalization of carbon nanotubes via cleavable disulfide bonds for efficient intracellular delivery of siRNA and potent gene silencing. J Am Chem Soc 127:12492–12493
40. Kam NWS, Liu ZA, Dai HJ (2006) Carbon nanotubes as intracellular transporter for proteins and DNA: An investigation of the uptake mechanism and pathway. Angew Chem Int Edit 45:577–581
41. Drug delivery and biomolecular transport. Carbon nanotubes monthly 3 Nov 2005. http://www.nanosprint.com/information_products/cnt_monthly/index.php?id=131
42. Rakov EG (2001) Chemistry and application of carbon nanotubes. Usp Khim 70:934–973
43. Hurt RH, Montioux M, Kane A (2006) Toxicology of carbon nanomaterials: Status, trends and perspectives on the special issue. Carbon 44:1028–1033
44. Kartel MT, Tereschenko VP (2008) Conception for methodology of identification and toxicological tests of nanomaterials and estimation of risk for human organism and environment at their production and application. In: Kartel MT (ed) Chemistry, Physics and Technology of Surface 14. Naukova dumka, Kiev, pp 565–583

Chapter 3
Toxicology of Nano-Objects: Nanoparticles, Nanostructures and Nanophases

A. Kharlamov, A. Skripnichenko, N. Gubareny, M. Bondarenko, N. Kirillova, G. Kharlamova, and V. Fomenko

Abstract The present paper discusses classification of nano-objects, which is based on their size, morphology and chemical nature. The subject of nanochemistry includes those nano-objects whose chemical properties depend on size and morphology, such as spheroidal molecules, anisotropic (2D) and isotropic (1D) nanoparticles, nano-clusters and nanophases. Nanophase is a nano-dimensional part of the microphase whose properties depend on its size. The potential health hazards of nano-objects are associated with their capability of penetrating the body through inhalation, digestion or the skin.

Keywords Nanochemistry • Nanotechnology • Nanotoxicology • Nanoparticles • Nanostructures, "micrographene sheet"

3.1 Introduction

At the end of the twentieth century, in the area of physics, and later in the area of chemistry extraordinarily important experimental results were produced, which gave rise to a new concept of nano-world. Development of high resolution electron microscopes allows detection of not only nano-dimensional particles but also large molecules. New types of matter such as spheroidal molecules with a hollow core (fullerenes and nanotubes), nanosized phases formed by a few atoms of metals

---

A. Kharlamov (✉), A. Skripnichenko, N. Gubareny, and M. Bondarenko
Frantsevich Institute for Problems of Materials Science, National Academy of Science of Ukraine, 3 Krjijanovskogo str, Kiev 03680, Ukraine
e-mail: dep73@ipms.kiev.ua; akharlamov@ukr.net

N. Kirillova and G. Kharlamova
Kiev National Taras Shevchenko University, 64 Volodimirska str, Kiev 03001, Ukraine

V. Fomenko
National University of Food Technology, 68 Volodimirska str, Kiev 03001, Ukraine

S. Mikhalovsky and A. Khajibaev (eds.), *Biodefence*, NATO Science for Peace and Security Series A: Chemistry and Biology, DOI 10.1007/978-94-007-0217-2_3,

(nanophases) and clusters formed by a few molecules were discovered. The special features and properties of these materials depend on their size and morphology and differ from currently known substances. In the macro-world, properties of macro- and micro-dimensional substances depend on their nature and structure but not on their size. The possibility to manipulate nano-dimensional objects and to create nanorobots at the molecular level is expected to substantially influence technical progress. With appearing of new branches of science and technology, such as nanotechnology and nanomedicine, one can talk about a "nano" era, an era of formation of new science – nanology [1], a science about the nano-world. Nanology has changed the paradigm of all scientific and manufacturing activity. The traditional technology deals with large objects which can be reduced in size whereas nanotechnology constructs its products from individual atoms and molecules "upwards".

3.2 History of Discovery, Classification and Chemistry of Nano-Objects

Before discussing any adverse effects of nano-objects on humans and the environment, it is necessary to classify nano-objects, identify their main sources and understand their chemical properties. Nano-objects certainly existed in nature long before they attracted interest of researchers. Carbon nanoparticles have been continuously generated and released in the atmosphere by forest fires and volcanic eruption. Nature has also designed unique living nano-tools. For instance the gecko – a beautiful lizard, can move easily on a ceiling or a window pane due to adhesive pads on its digits, each of which contains hundreds of spade-like tips of a diameter less than 200 nm.

First scientific research of nano-objects, probably, goes back to the nineteenth century, when Faraday (in 1856) discovered that the colour of highly dispersed colloid gold solutions depends on the particle size of gold. This unique feature of gold solutions was actually known much earlier, in the alchemistry era, and even the word "alchemistry" probably originates from the Chinese term meaning "gold juice" because of the red colour of some colloid gold solutions.

Other examples of using nano-objects in technology are the unique Lycurgus, King of the Thracian's glass cup, and the legendary Damascus steel made in fourth and eighth century, respectively. Their secrets were unveiled only recently. It appears that a sabre made of Damascus steel is reinforced by anisotropic nanoparticles of carbon nanotubes. Etching of the saber blade by carbon nanotubes creates a superhard surface. The enigmatic change of the Lycurgus cup colour from green to crimson under sunlight is associated with presence of gold and silver nanoparticles in the glass.

Emission of nanoparticles in the atmosphere from anthropogenic sources (machines, aero engines, power stations, smelters, plasma, welding and heat treatment processes) has been continuously increasing ever since the beginning of the industrial revolution.

At present a great variety of nano-objects, which have no analogues in nature, are produced in large quantities. Their potential impact on the environment and

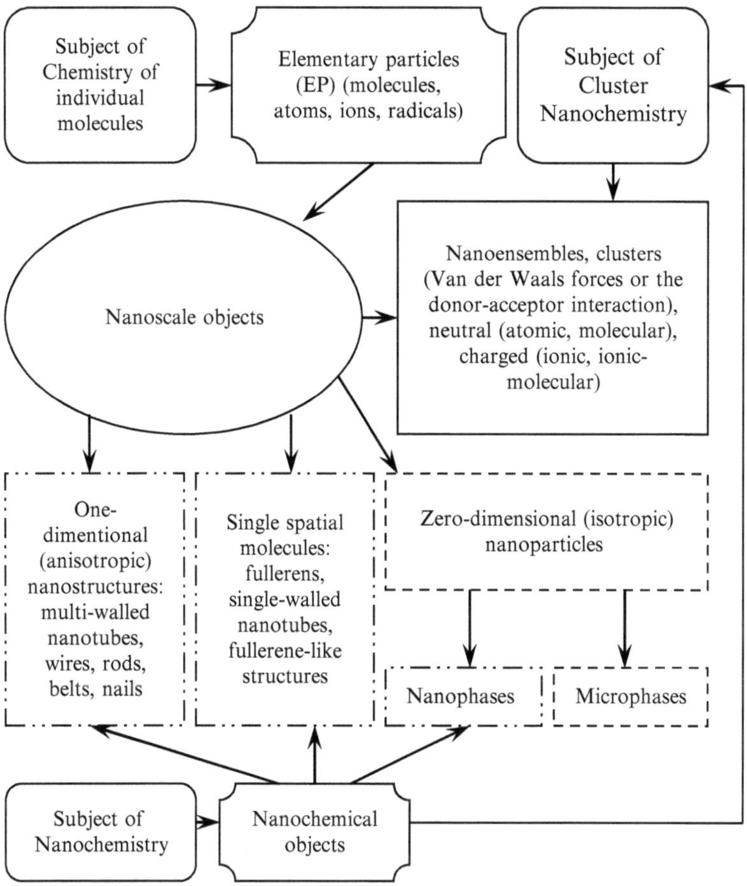

Fig. 3.1 Classification of nano-objects based on their dimension, morphology, structure and chemistry

humans is unknown. Thus studying possible adverse effects of these nano-objects is an extraordinarily important task. On the other hand, because nano-dimensional objects are extremely various in their chemical nature, composition, structure and morphology, it is necessary to classify them (Fig. 3.1). Such a classification would be a logical starting point for a systematic approach to assessing environmental and health effects of nano-objects.

It is especially important to create and develop terminology of nanochemistry as a part of a new area of science – nanology, or the "science of the nanoworld" (nanologists prefer this term to a more widely used word nanoscience). Figures 3.2–3.8, show the diversity of the morphology of nanostructures of carbon, silicon and boron carbides, which were synthesised via hydrocarbon pyrolysis [2–5] or from elemental substances [6–10]. Morphologies of carbon nanotubes thus obtained are very unusual (Fig. 3.2).

Carbon nanotubes with armchair shape present a special interest because it is possible to see that the metal catalyst is not always located at the top of nanotube. Therefore it is evident that the growth of graphene layers may occur not only from a surface of a metal nanoparticle, as it is usually understood. Among the products

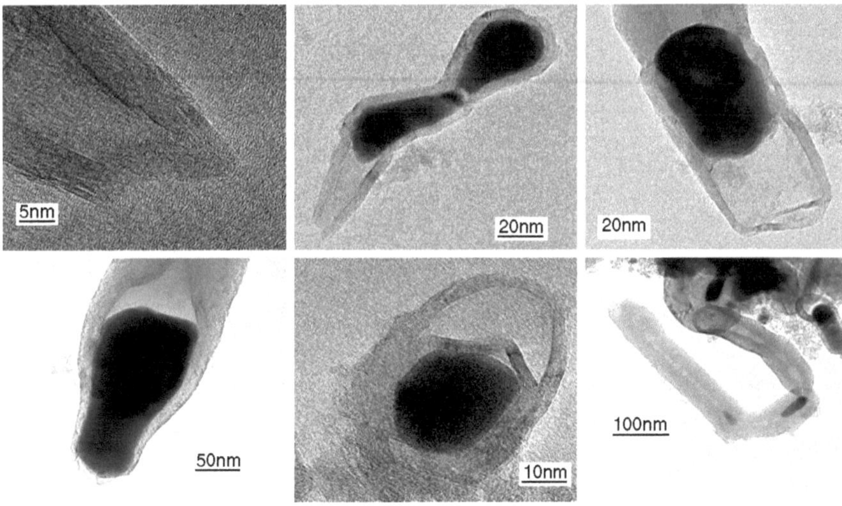

Fig. 3.2 Unusual morphologies of carbon nanotubes containing metallic nanoparticles inside

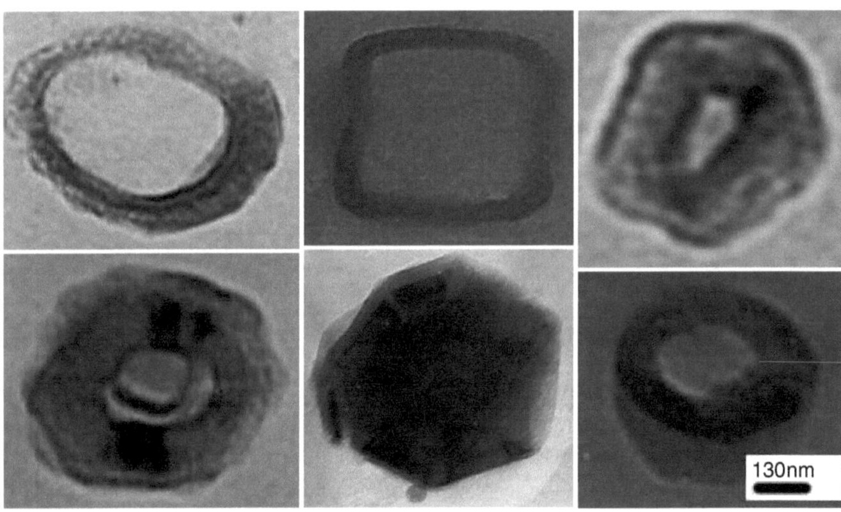

Fig. 3.3 Carbon toroids formed simultaneously with the growth of carbon nanotubes and carbon onions

of pyrolysis other unique carbon nanostructures such as various polygons, a ring with a hollow core and onion structures were found (Figs. 3.3 and 3.4).

The growth of such structures is possible only from a gas phase and probably occurs as a result of dehydropolymerisation (polycondensation) [4,11]. Under more harsh reaction conditions multi-walled nanotubes grow as a loop on ceramic reactor walls (Fig. 3.4). We suggest that the benzene molecule could be the main fragment in the graphene network formation. At temperatures>600°C benzene rapidly undergoes dehydrogenation followed by diphenyl formation that can be considered

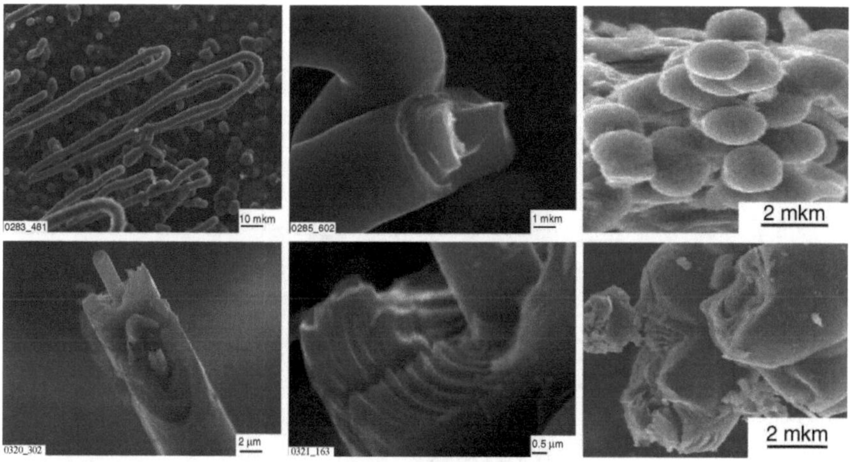

Fig. 3.4 SEM images of multi-walled carbon nanotubes and carbon onions

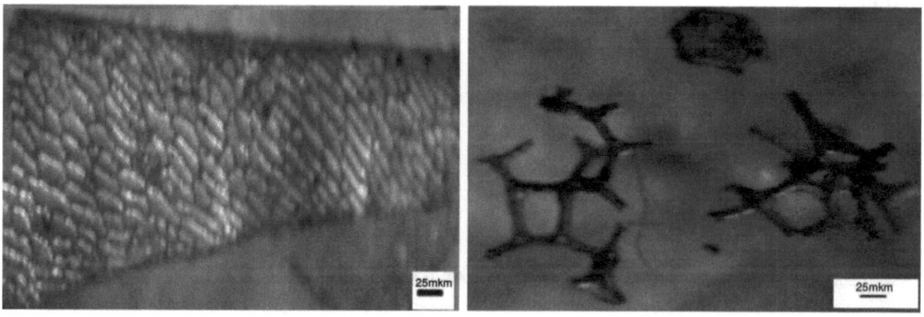

Fig. 3.5 Optical microscopy images of "micrographene sheet" and "carbon microclusters"

as the first stage of a graphene network formation. Further condensation of benzene and diphenyl expands the number of condensed carbon hexagons leading to formation of the graphene network. The network is formed from planar molecules but because of sp^3- hybridisation of peripheral carbon atoms, convolution of the formed carbon structure occurs. This mechanism has been confirmed by discovery of unique structures in the shape of "micrographene" sheet and "carbon microclusters" (Fig. 3.5), which we have found in hydrocarbon pyrolysis products.

For the first time we have discovered transparent (painted in various colours) thread-like crystals of carbon among the products of hydrocarbon pyrolysis and during synthesis of silicon and boron carbides (Fig. 3.6) [12]. The X-ray spectral analysis has shown that the transparent threads consist of carbon (Fig. 3.7).

Growth of anisotropic silicon and boron carbide nanoparticles from powdered reagents was performed using a process of exothermic nanosynthesis [6,7] (Fig. 3.8).

Such nanostructures are formed as a result of fast growth at temperatures, at which the equilibrium pressure of silicon, boron and especially carbon vapour is

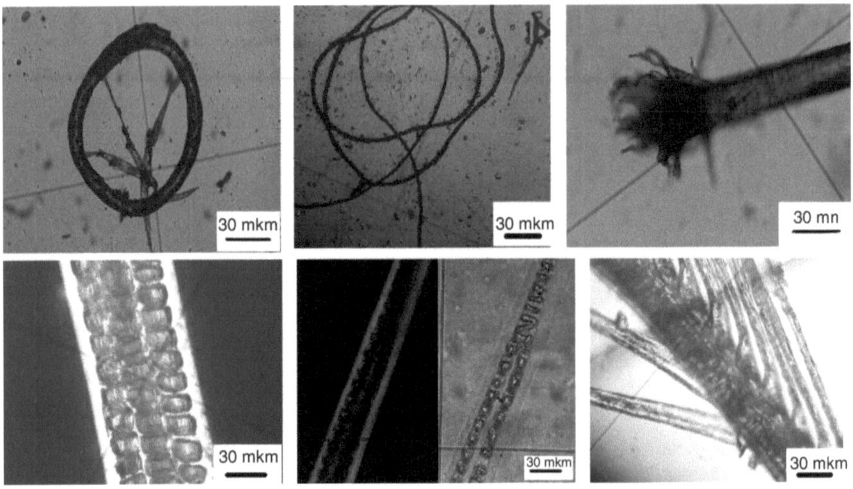

Fig. 3.6 Optical microscopy images of transparent carbon crystalline threads obtained in polarised light

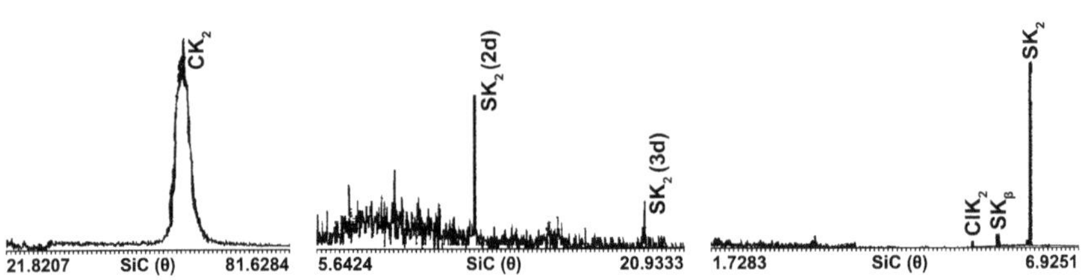

Fig. 3.7 The X-ray spectral analysis of carbon threads shown in Fig. 3.6

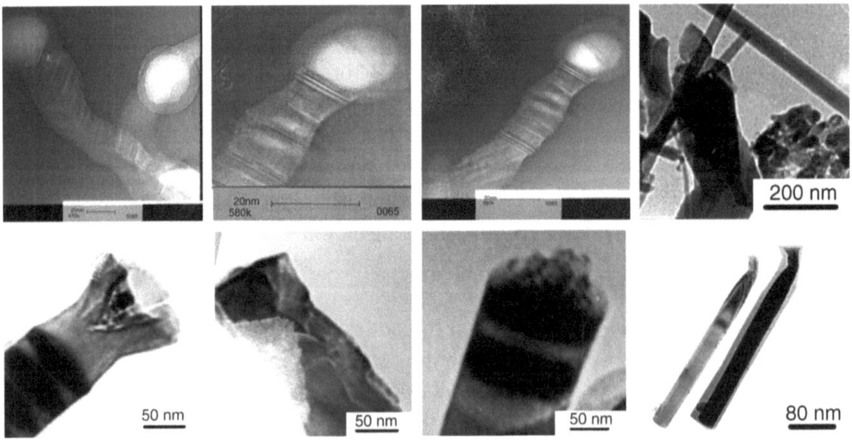

Fig. 3.8 TEM images of the tips of silicon carbide nanothreads

negligible. The reaction occurs because the local temperature and respective vapour pressure in the vicinity of the reactive zone is much higher than the temperature and vapour pressure across the reactor creating a nanocentre of growth of an isotropic particle. Melting of the nanocentre and sublimation of the reagents in its vicinity is facilitated by the heat of the exothermic reaction. The evaporating atoms are mainly transported in the direction of the molten nanocentre forming a carbide product.

Nanostructures of various morphologies and nanoparticles can be considered as objects of nanochemistry, as their properties are mainly determined by their "nano" dimensions. Thus nanoparticles, being a nano-dimensional part of a microphase, have essentially different physical, chemical and electronic properties, and sometimes even a different crystal structure. They should therefore be described as a nanophase, as opposed to a microphase. For example, the melting temperature (T_m) of nanoparticles (5–10 nm) of gold is hundreds of degrees lower than T_m of the gold microphase [13]. Moreover gold nanoparticles of such dimensions have a crystal structure completely different from that of the gold microphase. Contrary to microphases, nanophases are limited in their size to nano-dimensions. The geometrical dimensions of a nanophase are strictly individual and determined by other characteristics of the object. Each characteristic of a nanophase such as its electronic, optical and magnetic properties, or melting temperature could have a different limiting size which distinguishes it from a microphase.

Nano-clusters are also nano-dimensional objects. They can be neutral (atomic or molecular) or charged (ionic or ionic-molecular) complexes or ensembles of molecules, atoms and ions.

Chemical properties of nano-objects are related to their:

(a) nano-dimensions, which are comparable to the size of individual molecules;
(b) dependence of nanophase properties on particle size;
(c) unusual shape (tubes, tapes, rods, spheres);
(d) large surface area, etc.

3.3 Toxicity of Nano-Objects

At present nanotechnology is often perceived as a panacea for solving many global problems. However few systematic studies have been carried out to elucidate effects of nano-objects on health and the environment. Even specialists are practically unaware of the possible impact of nano-objects they are dealing with. However some of the results of studying toxicity of nanoparticles are alarming [14]. Penetration of nanoparticles into biosphere can cause many problems. The unique feature of nano-objects is that they are capable of easily overcoming biological barriers of the living organism, and can interfere with normal physiological and biochemical processes causing various pathologies (Fig. 3.9). It seems that the nature does not have natural protection mechanisms against damaging effects of novel nano-objects already produced in substantial quantities.

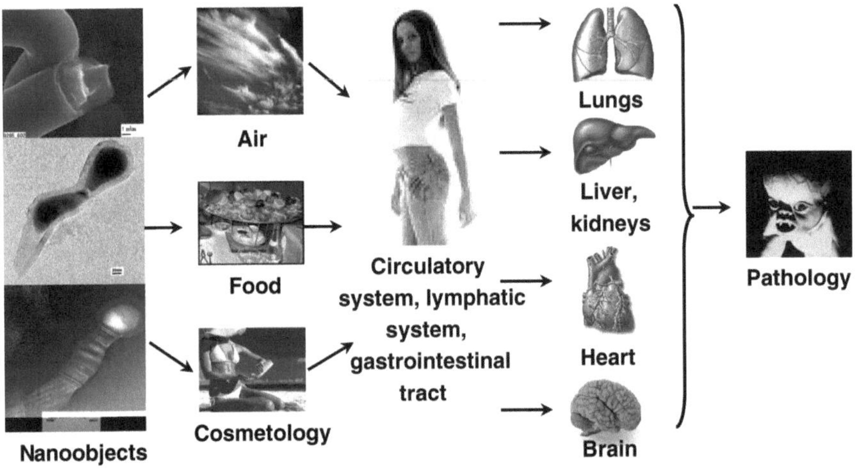

Fig. 3.9 The main routes of nano-object penetration into the human organism

The main routes of nano-objects penetration into the organism are (Fig. 3.9):

- Through inhalation (adsorbed by the huge surface of the lungs and thence transfer into the blood stream);
- By digestion (easily transferred into the blood via intestines, and passing into the liver as a protecting barrier);
- Through the skin (especially if it is damaged).

Experiments on animals and fish have demonstrated a big danger of uncontrolled distribution of nanoparticles in the environment: nanoparticles can get directly into brain tissue from the circulatory system. Inhalation of polystyrene nanoparticles causes an inflammation of the pulmonary tissue and initiates thrombosis of blood vessels. Impact of carbon nanotubes on the lungs is comparable with toxicity of asbestos and benzpyrene; it has been suggested that carbon nanotubes can suppress the immune response of the body. Through the respiratory pathway nanoparticles can influence the nervous system [15]. The experiments on dogs and aquarium fish have shown that fullerenes penetrate the brain. Having a large surface area, carbon nanoparticles, especially those partially destroyed or with imperfect morphology (Fig. 3.4), can become containers/carriers for the adsorbed carcinogenic substances - products of hydrocarbon pyrolysis. Thus both morphology and structure of nanoparticles and the chemical nature of the adsorbed chemicals can have an adverse effect on human health.

Environmental behaviour of carbon nanostructures is extremely difficult to predict because they contain on their surface a number of adsorbed substances such as polyaromatic hydrocarbons (PAH), which are known carcinogenic substances. Carbon nanoparticles generated by combustion processes, in particular from cigarette smoke contain thousands of different chemicals, which may be toxic to living species [16].

The number of studies on the health effects of fullerenes and carbon nanotubes is rapidly increasing. However, the data on their toxicity are often mutually contradictory. For example, the researchers from universities of Rice and Georgia (USA) found that in aqueous fullerene solutions colloidal "nano-C_{60}" particles were formed, which even at low concentration (approximately 2 molecules of fullerene per 108 molecules of water) negatively influence the liver and skin cells [17–19]. The toxicity of this "nano-C_{60}" aqueous dispersion was comparable to that of dioxins. In another study, however, it was shown that fullerene C_{60} had no adverse effects and, on the contrary, had anti-oxidant activity [20]. Solutions of C_{60} prepared by a variety of methods up to 200 mg/mL were not cytotoxic to a number of cell types [21]. The contradiction between the data of different authors could be explained by different "nano-C_{60}" particles composition and dispersion used in research.

In other publications single-walled carbon nanotubes were shown to promote neoplasm formation in kidneys [22, 23]. Contrary to [20], other authors found that carbon nanostructures were capable of inducing reactive oxygen species (oxygen radicals) that could damage cellular structures [24–26].

3.4 Conclusions

Our current state of knowledge is insufficient to fully assess potential health hazards associated with the use of nano-objects and relate health effects to their chemical, structural and morphological properties. The main danger of nano-objects is that they are capable of easily penetrating the blood stream and internal organs via inhalation, ingestion and through the skin. Further systematic research of "structure-properties" of nano-objects is required.

References

1. Kharlamov AI, Kirillova NV (2009) Fullerenes and fullerenes hydrides as products of transformation (polycondensation) of aromatic hydrocarbons. Proc Ukr Acad Sci 5:112–120
2. Kharlamov AI, Kirillova NV, Ushkalov LN (2006) Simultaneous growth of spheroidal and tubular carbon structures during the pyrolysis of benzene. Theor Exp Chem 42(2):90–95
3. Kharlamov AI, Ushkalov LN,K Kirillova NV, Fomenko VV, Gubareny NI, Skripnichenko AV (2006) Synthesis of onion nanostructures of carbon at pyrolysys of aromatic hydrocarbons. Proc Ukr Acad Sci 3:97–103
4. Kharlamov AI, Loythenko SV,K Kirillova NV, Kaverina SV, Fomenko VV (2004) Toroidal nanostructures of carbon. Single-walled 4 -, 5 – and 6 hedrons and nanorings. Proc Ukr Acad Sci 1:95–100
5. Kharlamov AI, Ushkalov LM, Kirillova NV (2007) Novel method of obtaining of new type of nanotubes of vanadium oxide. Proc Ukr Acad Sci 4:148–156
6. Kharlamov AI, Kirillova NV, Karachevtseva LA, Kharlamova AA (2003) Low-temperature reactions between vaporizing silicon and carbon. Theor Exp Chem 39(6):374–379

7. Kholmanov IN, Kharlamov AI, Barborini E, Lenardi C, Li Bassi A, Bottani CE, Ducati C, Maffi S, Kirillova NV, Milani P (2002) A simple method for the synthesis of silicon carbide nanorods. J Nanosci Nanotechnol 2(5):453–456
8. Kharlamov AI, Kirillova NV, Kaverina SV (2003) Hollow and thread-like nanostructures of boron carbide. Theor Exp Chem 39(3):141–146
9. Kharlamov AI, Kirillova NV (2002) Gas-phase reactions of formation of silicon carbide nanofilaments from silicon and carbon powders. Theor Exp Chem 38(1):59–63
10. Kharlamov AI, Kirillova NV, Loytchenko SV (2002) Synthesis of elongated nanostructures of silicon carbide from powdery silicon and carbon. Proc Ukr Acad Sci 10:98–105
11. Kharlamov AI, Kharlamova GA, Kirillova NV, Fomenko VV (2008) Persistent organic pollutants at nanotechnology and their impact on people health. In: Mehmetli E, Koumanova B (eds) The fate of persistent organic pollutants in the environment. Springer, pp 425–441
12. Kharlamov AI,K Kirillova NV, Zaytseva ZA (2007) Novel state of carbon: transparent thread-like anisotropic crystals. Proc Ukr Acad Sci 5:101–106
13. Pul Ch, Owens F (2005) Nanotechnology. Tekhnosfera, Moscow, Russia
14. Hoet P, Bruske-Holfeld I, Salata O (2004) Nanoparticles – known and unknown health risks. J Nanobiotech 2:12–18
15. Oberdörster G, Oberdörster E, Oberdörster J (2005) Nanotoxicology: an emerging discipline from studies of ultrafine particles. Environ Health Perspect 113:823–839
16. Siegmann K, Siegmann HC (1997) The formation of carbon in combustion and how to quantify the impact on human health. Europhys News 28:50–57
17. Oberdörster E (2004) Manufactured nanomaterials (fullerenes, C60) induce oxidative stress in the brain of juvenile largemouth bass. Environ Health Perspect 112:1058–1062
18. Sayes CM, Fortner JD, Guo W et al (2004) The differential cytotoxicity of water-soluble fullerenes. Nano Lett 4:1881–1887
19. Sayes CM, Gobin AM, Ausman KD et al (2005) Nano-C60 cytotoxicity is due to lipid peroxidation. Biomaterials 26:7587–7595
20. Andrievsky GV, Klochkov VK, Bordyuh AB, Dovbeshko GI (2002) Comparative analysis of two aqueous-colloidal solutions of C- 60 fullerene with help of FTIR reflectance and UV-Vis spectroscopy. Chem Phys Lett 364:8–17
21. Levi N, Hantgan RR, Lively MO et al (2006) C60-Fullerenes: detection of intracellular photoluminescence and lack of cytotoxic effects. J Nanobiotech 4:14–17
22. Donaldson K, Aitken R, Tran L et al (2006) Carbon nanotubes: review of their properties in relation to pulmonary toxicology and workplace safety. Toxicol Sci 92(1):5–22
23. Ostiguy C, Lapointe G, Trottier M et al (2006) Health effects of nanoparticles. Studies and research projects. IRSST 52
24. Zhua S, Oberdörster E, Haascha ML (2006) Toxicity of an engineered nanoparticle (fullerene, C60) in two aquatic species, Daphnia and fathead minnow. Mar Environ Res 62:5–9
25. Markovic Z, Todorovic-Markovic B, Kleut D et al (2007) The mechanism of cell-damaging reactive oxygen generation by colloidal fullerenes. Biomaterials 28(36):5437–5448
26. Schranda AM, Daia L, Schlager JJ et al (2007) Differential biocompatibility of carbon nanotubes and nanodiamonds. Diamond Relat Mater 16(12):2118–2123

Chapter 4
Carbon Adsorbents with Adjustable Porous Structure Formed in the Chemical Dehydro-Halogenation of Halogenated Polymers

Yu G. Kryazhev, V.S. Solodovnichenko, V.A. Drozdov, and V.A. Likholobov

Abstract Synthesis of carbon adsorbents with controlled pore size and surface chemistry adapted for application in medicine and health protection was explored. Conjugated polymers were used as carbon precursors. These polymers with conjugated double bonds C=C have high thermal stability. Formation of sp^2 carbon structures occurs via condensation and aromatization of macromolecules. The structure of carbon materials obtained is related to the structure of the original conjugated polymer, thus the porous structure of carbon adsorbents could be controlled by variation of the conjugated polymer precursor.

Dehydrochlorination of polyvinylidene chloride and chlorinated polyvinyl chloride was carried out. High chlorine content in the polymers (more than 60%) provides the formation of chlorinated conjugated polymers, polychlorovinylenes. The reactivity of chlorinated polyvinylenes contributes to the sp^2 carbon material formation during heat treatment. Synthesis of porous carbon has been carried out in three stages: low-temperature dehydrohalogenation of the polymer precursor by strong bases, carbonization in the inert atmosphere at 400–600°C and activation up to 950°C.

Keywords Activated carbon • Halogenated polymers • Mesopores • Ultra-Micropores

4.1 Introduction

Activated carbons are widely used for treatment of acute and chronic poisoning as oral adsorbents and for blood purification. However, medical carbons currently available are predominantly microporous and their use is therefore limited to

Y.G. Kryazhev (✉), V.S. Solodovnichenko, V.A. Drozdov, and V.A. Likholobov
Omsk Scientific Center, Institute of Hydrocarbons Processing, Siberian Branch of Russian Academy of Sciences, Omsk, Russia
e-mail: carbonfibre@yandex.ru

S. Mikhalovsky and A. Khajibaev (eds.), *Biodefence*, NATO Science for Peace and Security Series A: Chemistry and Biology, DOI 10.1007/978-94-007-0217-2_4,

adsorption of small molecules (chemical toxins) rather than large molecules such as biotoxins, which require larger meso- and macropores. Producing activated carbon with controlled meso- and narrow macropore size presents a challenge. In this paper we describe a new approach to synthesis of micro-/mesoporous activated carbon.

4.2 Experimental

The initial halogenated polymeric materials were obtained from the polyvinyl chloride-polyvinylidene chloride, PVC-PVDC (Rovil® fiber) and chlorinated polyvinyl chloride, PVC. Dehydrochlorination was performed in the presence of a base solution in a polar organic solvent (dimethylsulfoxide, acetone or tetrahydrofurane). The products were filtered and extracted with water in a Soxhlet apparatus until all chloride ions were removed. Thermal treatment was performed in a tubular furnace in CO_2 flow at 10 $cm^3 min^{-1}$.

The Raman spectra were obtained on a LabRAM (Jobin-Yvon) Raman spectrometer. The Raman spectra were excited by a He-Ne laser generating laser beam at 632.8 nm. The laser radiation power was 1 mW. The Raman spectrum regions containing *D, G,* and *T* lines characteristic of carbonaceous materials were analyzed.

Synchronous thermal analysis was carried out with STA 449C Jupiter thermal analyzer (Netzsch) in argon at flow rate 15 $cm^3{\cdot}min^{-1}$. Polymer samples were heated from 20 to 700°C at a rate of 10°C$\cdot$$min^{-1}$ and then allowed to cool down. Gaseous products were analyzed with a QMS 403C Aeolos quadrupole mass spectrometer (MS) connected to the main analyzer. MS data were collected for lines with given m/e values.

Nitrogen adsorption was measured at 77.4 K using an ASAP-2020 instrument, Micromeritics. Prior to analysis the samples were degassed under vacuum at 573 K overnight and additionally in the measuring port at 623 K for 6 h (the residual pressure was $\sim 3 \times 10^{-5}$ torr). Nitrogen was introduced in doses of 1 cm^3 STP/g in the region of initial fillings (up to the equilibrium pressure $P/P_0 = 0.01$). The actual time for establishing adsorption equilibrium at each adsorption point at very low P/P_0 values was as long as 40–50 min. During the adsorption experiments, the P_0 pressure was measured every 2 h, and P/P_0 calculations at 77.4 K were corrected accordingly. The dead volume of the burette was measured with the sample using helium at room temperature and 77.4 K to obtain more accurate results. The gases used (N_2 and He) were 99.999 vol.% pure.

The structural characteristics of samples were calculated from adsorption-desorption isotherms using various approaches: micro- and mesopores were estimated by using equations of the theory of volume filling of micropores (TVFM), the Horvath-Kavazoe method (HK), the comparative t-method, the non-local density functional theory (NL DFT) for estimating the structural characteristics; mesopore parameters were estimated using Barrett-Joyner-Halenda (BJH), Dollimor-Hill (DH) and Derjaguin-Brukhoff-de Boer (DBdB) methods based on the classic thermodynamic concepts; the effective (apparent) specific surface area was estimated using the Brunauer-Emmett-Teller method (BET-equation).

4.3 Results and Discussion

Dehydrohalogenation of polyvinylidene fluoride and polyvinylidene chloride was used previously for synthesis of a new form of a linear chain carbon - carbyne [1, 2]. We have found that dehydrochlorination proceeded with a decreasing rate and completed in 6 h at 80°C. According to potentiometric data for chloride ions, only 31% of chlorine contained in the initial polymer system reacted under these conditions (Fig. 4.1).

It should be expected that further thermal treatment of the partially dehydrochlorinated polymer will result in easy elimination of HCl and enrichment of the product with carbon. Indeed, TGA data (Fig. 4.2, curve 1) show that the dehydrochlorinated polymer loses some weight even at 150°C.

According to MS data, volatile products of thermal degradation contain HCl. The mass spectra exhibit two diffuse peaks in the ranges of the highest weight loss rate.

Taking this data into account, we subjected the chemically dehydrochlorinated polymer to thermal treatment firstly at 200°C for 2 h to enrich the product with carbon via thermal dehydrochlorination and then at 350°C for 30 min to allow the formation of carbon-like structures.

Raman microspectroscopy [3] allows the observation of the transformation of a polyene structure to a carbon one. The formation of conjugate polyene units under the conditions of chemical dehydrochlorination of the polymer was confirmed by the presence of characteristic narrow peaks at 1,107 and 1,490 cm^{-1} in the Raman spectra. The products obtained by thermal treatment at elevated temperatures are highly disordered sp^2-carbon materials, in which the porous structure has developed upon subsequent gasification (Fig. 4.3).

This is a result of polyene formation from PVC and PVDC, as shown in Scheme 4.1:

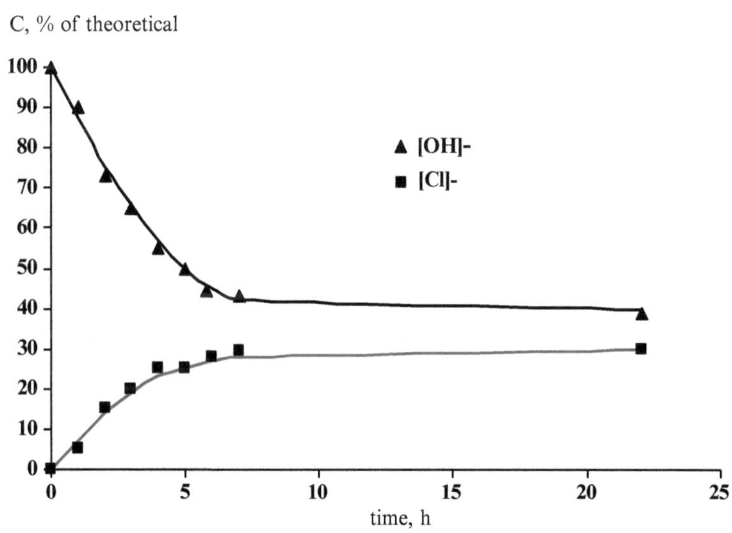

Fig. 4.1 Kinetics of Cl^- ions release and OH^- ions consumption during dehydroclorination of PVDC-PVC composition. Experimental conditions: (80°C, KOH in DMSO–propan-2-ol, 1:1 w/w)

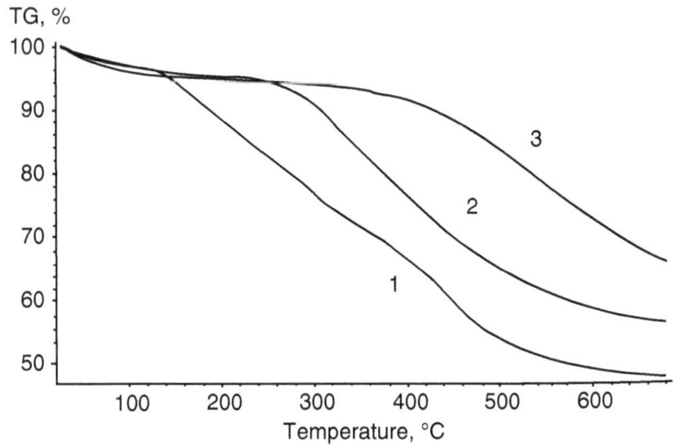

Fig. 4.2 Thermogravimetric analysis of the chemically dehydrochlorinated olyvinylidene chloride: *1* – not subjected to thermal treatment; *2* – heated at 200°C (for 2 h); *3* – heated at 200°C (2 h) and then at 350°C (0.5 h)

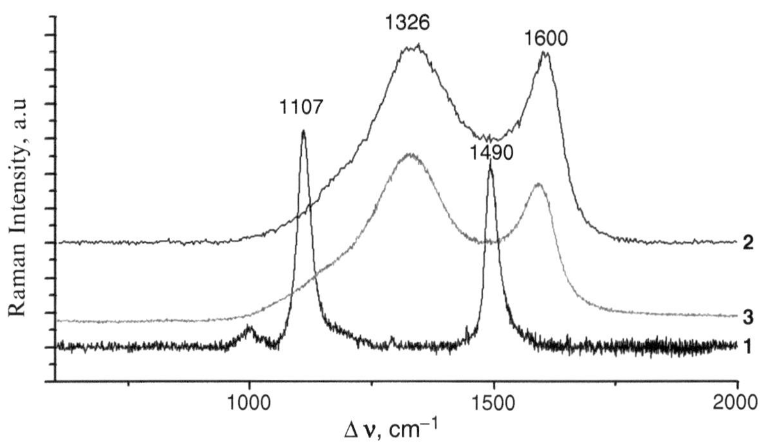

Fig. 4.3 Data of Raman spectroscopy (He-Ne laser, $\lambda = 632{,}8$ nm) for the following samples: *1* – polyvinyl chloride-polyvinylidene chloride composition after chemical dehydrochlorination (80°C, KOH in dimethyl sulfoxide –propan-2-ol 1 : 1, w/w); *2* – chemically dehydrochlorinated polymer carbonized in CO_2 at 350°C; *3* – carbonized product activated in CO_2 at 950°C

Interchain dehydrochlorination at increased temperatures leads to fused aromatic structures (Scheme 4.2):

TGA data confirm transformation of the polyene structure into the carbon one. Thus isothermal heating at 200°C resulted in almost complete dehydrochlorination of the polymer, and intense weight loss occurs only at 300°C (Fig. 4.2, curve 2).

According to MS data, HCl does not evolve at any temperature studied. The weight loss due to the thermal treatment at 200°C was 39%. According to our calculation, this percentage corresponds to the elimination of 94% of the theoretically pos-

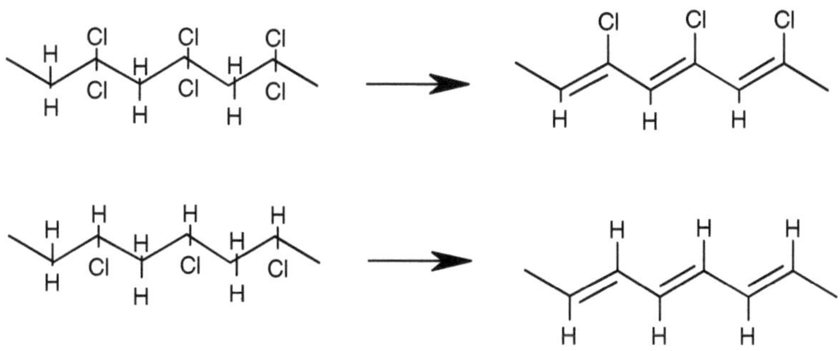

Scheme 4.1 Polyene formation from PVC and PVDC

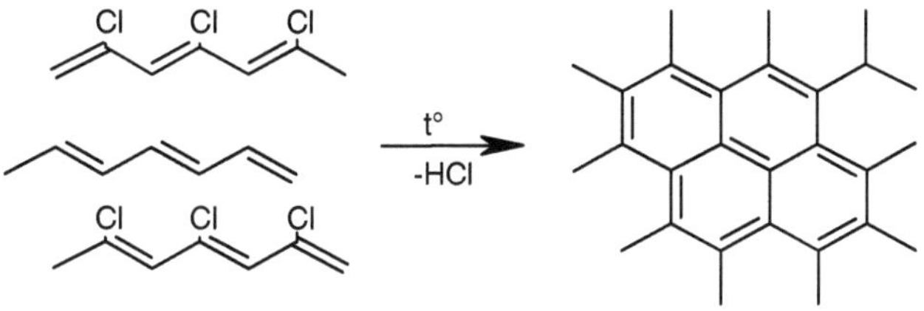

Scheme 4.2 Possible reaction of formation of fused aromatic structures from polyenes and chlorinated polyenes

sible amount of HCl (considering its amount in the reaction mixture at the chemical dehydrochlorination stage as determined from potentiometric data). The weight loss in the pyrolysis of a fully dehydrochlorinated sample can be a result of aromatization and condensation of unsaturated macrochains with elimination of hydrogen and low molecular weight hydrocarbons, or with de-polymerization of the macromolecules. For the sample treated at 200°C and then at 350°C, no significant weight loss was observed up to 400°C (Fig. 4.2).

The results obtained are consistent with the existing views on the tendency of polyconjugated systems towards spontaneous stabilization upon thermal treatment: heating makes the system more resistant to thermal degradation. TGA curves (Fig. 4.2) of the samples subjected to thermal treatment at 200 and 350°C are shifted to higher temperatures, with retention of the general pattern of weight loss. Thus, the carbon-rich structures were formed at relatively low temperatures.

On the basis of these results it is concluded that porous carbon materials could be obtained via various routes. By selecting reagents, catalysts, and temperature-time regimes, the density of three-dimensional carbon-carbon grid and the length of polyconjugated domains can be regulated. Further opportunities for regulating the porous structure and surface chemistry of activated carbon arise at the activation stage at high temperatures.

Highly porous sorbents were obtained by dehydrochlorination of Rovil® fiber in LiOH solution in dimethylsulfoxide at 160°C followed by activation with carbon dioxide at 950°C (Fig. 4.4).

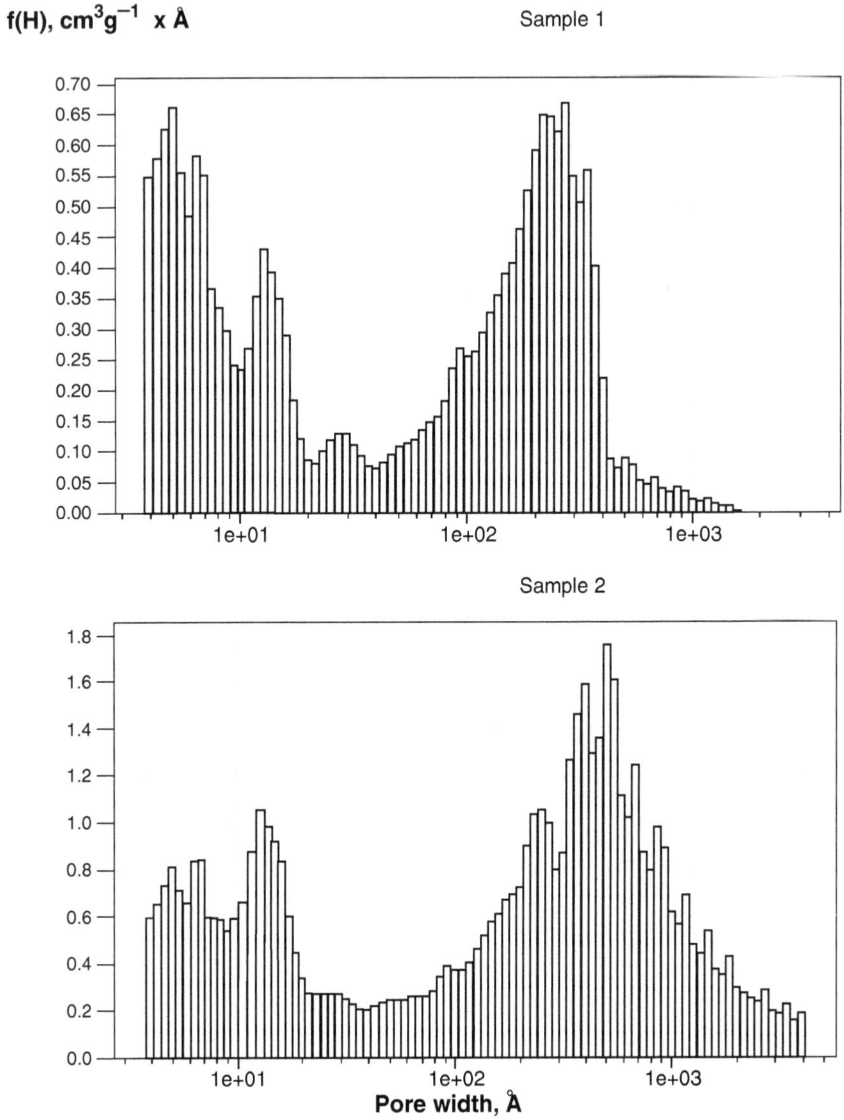

Fig. 4.4 NLDFT Pore size distribution (NLDFT-PSD) in porous carbons with high volume of ultra- and super-micropores (V_{mi}=0.4–0.7 cm^3g^{-1}), and mesopores (V_{meso}=1.2–1.4 cm^3g^{-1}).Li/Cl atomic ratio was 1:1 for sample 1 and 0.75:1 for sample 2

Their pore size distribution and S_{BET} were dependent on the nature of the organic solvent (Table 4.1).

Addition of nanodispersed SiO_2 decreased the formation of mesopores (Fig. 4.5). Addition of 5% of SiO_2 preserved the volume of micropores, while the volume of mesopores reduced four-fold. In this case the formation of mesopores was possibly

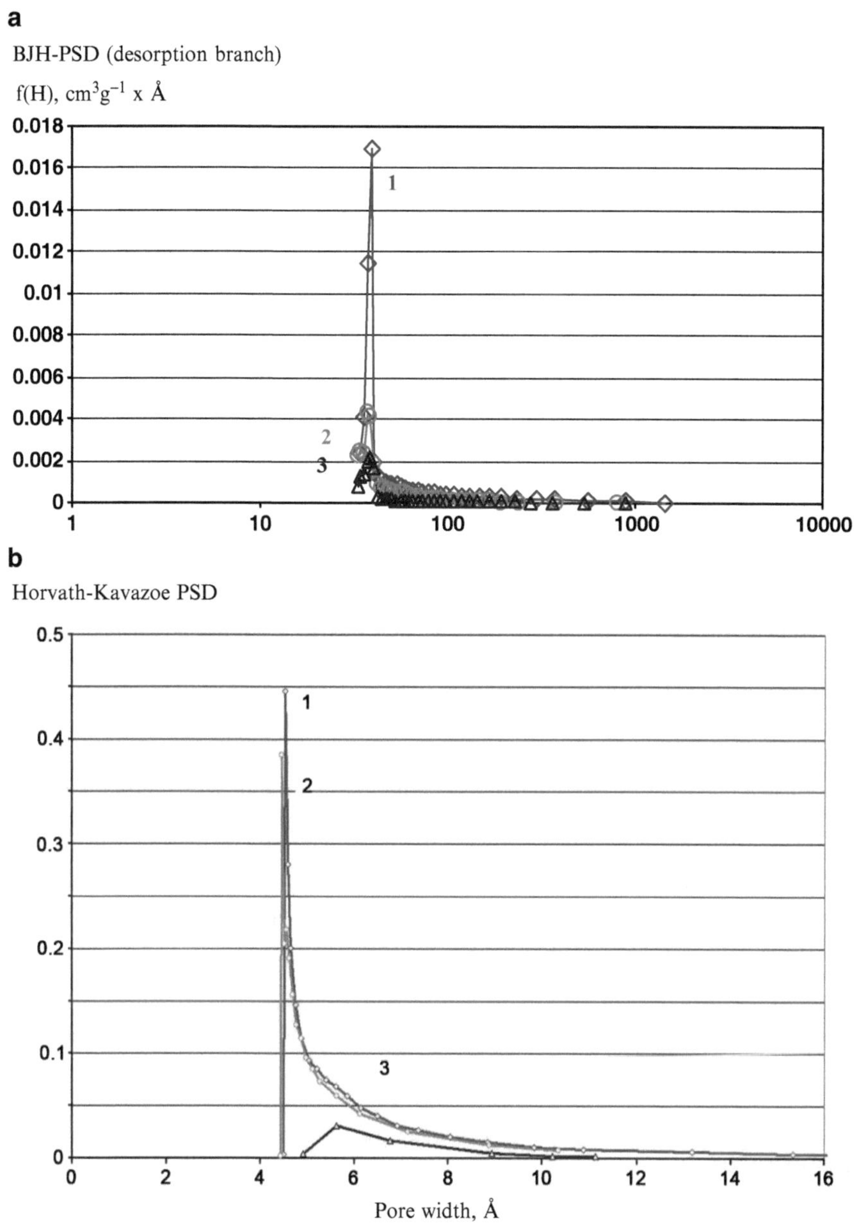

Fig. 4.5 Effect of adding SiO_2 nanodispersion on the pore size distribution in products of polymer dehydrochlorination. *1* – initial sample; *2* – with 5% of SiO_2; *3* – with 25% of SiO_2

Table 4.1 Effect of solvent used for dehydrochlorination of the polymer precursor on pore size distribution in activated carbon. Experimental conditions: chlorinated PVC was treated with KOH at 20°C for 5 h; thermal treatment conditions: carbonization at 400°C for 30 min followed by activation with CO_2 at 900°C for 5 min

		HK calculations		Adsorption branch		Desorption branch	
Solvent	S_{BET}, $m^2 g^{-1}$	V_{micro}, $cm^3 g^{-1}$	H, Å	V_{meso}, $cm^3 g^{-1}$	D_{meso}, Å	V_{meso}, $cm^3 g^{-1}$	D_{meso}, Å
Dimethyl sulfoxide	1009	0.40	5.8	0.79	184	0.84	150
Tetrahydro furane	733	0.29	5.6	0.25	173	0.27	99
Acetone	766	0.30	5.2	0.19	300	0.20	212

prevented by the presence of nanoparticles, which size was similar to the diameter of mesopores.

4.4 Conclusions

Carbon materials were obtained from polymeric precursors produced by chemical dehydrochlorination of polyvinyl chloride–polyvinylidene chloride and chlorinated polyvinyl chloride in the presence of a strong base, followed by subsequent thermal treatment under relatively mild conditions. The sorbents obtained have three types of pores: ultra-micropores, micropores, and mesopores. In this respect, they differ substantially from microporous activated carbons such as Saran, conventionally prepared from chlorinated polymers by thermal treatment without chemical dehydrochlorination.

The adsorbent structure was dependent on the structure of the conjugated polymer precursor and carbon formation conditions.

The activated carbons obtained have a potential for medical applications in treatment of chemical and biological poisoning as oral adsorbents and in extracorporeal blood detoxication.

Acknowledgements This work is a continuation of the research performed in 2000–2004 with support by NATO "Science for Peace" program, Project SfP 973472 – "Scientific and Technological Development of Advanced Carbon Fibers and Coatings".

References

1. Sladkov AM (2003) Carbyne: the third allotropic form of carbon. Nauka, Moscow [in Russian]
2. Korshak VV, Kudryavtsev YuP, Korshak YuV et al (1988) Formation of beta-carbyne by dehydrohalogenation. Makromol Chem Rapid Comm 9(3):135–143
3. Bukalov SS, Mikhalitsyn LA, Zubavichus YaV et al (2006) Investigation of the structure of graphite and other sp2 materials by means of micro-Raman spectroscopy and x-ray diffraction. Russian Khim Zh 1(1):83–87 [in Russian]

Chapter 5
Applications of Small Angle X-Ray Scattering Techniques for Characterizing High Surface Area Carbons

E. Geissler and K. László

Abstract Small angle X-ray or neutron scattering (SAXS or SANS) techniques offer a powerful means of investigating the adsorption of vapour by high surface area carbons. While traditional vapour phase adsorption methods yield overall adsorbed amounts, scattering observations give complementary direct information on the location of the adsorption sites as well as an independent measure of the internal surface area of the substrate. Data collected from the traditional small angle region (range of transfer momentum $q < 1$ Å^{-1}) may be used to calculate the density of the condensed phase in the micropores, while that collected from the higher resolution range ($q > 1$ Å^{-1}) contains information both on the adsorbed amount and on spatial correlations within the adsorbed phase, as well as between it and the substrate. The effects of adsorption of a single species of molecule can be monitored by SAXS alone. The presence of more than one species, however, requires the use of SANS combined with contrast variation, i.e., employing selective isotopic substitution, for instance by replacing hydrogen by deuterium. In this article we discuss the adsorption of water vapour on two nanoporous carbons.

Keywords Small angle x-ray scattering • High surface area carbons

List of Abbreviations

AC	Activated carbon
APET	Activated carbon from poly(ethylene terephthalate)
BET	Brunauer-Emmett-Teller model [5]

E. Geissler (✉)
Laboratoire de Spectrométrie Physique CNRS UMR 5588, Université J. Fourier de Grenoble, BP 87, 38402, St Martin d'Hères cedex, Grenoble, France
e-mail: erik.geissler@ujf-grenoble.fr

K. László
Department of Physical Chemistry and Materials Science, Budapest University of Technology and Economics, H-1521 Budapest, Hungary

S. Mikhalovsky and A. Khajibaev (eds.), *Biodefence*, NATO Science for Peace and Security Series A: Chemistry and Biology, DOI 10.1007/978-94-007-0217-2_5,

BM2	Bending magnet #2 at ESRF
CRG	Collaborative research group
ESRF	European Synchrotron Radiation Facility
NPC	Nanoporous carbon
RH	Relative humidity
SAXS	Small angle X-ray scattering
SANS	Small angle neutron scattering
WAXS	Wide angle X-ray scattering

5.1 Introduction

High surface area nanoporous carbon (NPC) is a sorbent used almost ubiquitously both in liquid and gas phase applications ranging from drinking/waste water treatment, industrial or chemical/biological warfare protection to clinical treatment of acute poisoning cases by haemoadsorption. Different types of molecule occupy adsorption sites that depend on the polarity and on the surface treatment of the substrate. Furthermore, extraneous molecules, notably water vapour, can compete with other target molecules, hence compromising the role of the carbon. While standard gas adsorption techniques give complementary information on these processes, scattering measurements, such as small angle X-ray scattering (SAXS), offer two important advantages, namely direct spatial information on the distribution of the adsorbate, and measurements on samples at equilibrium. In addition, small angle neutron scattering (SANS) offers the possibility of discriminating between two or more adsorbed species. This article describes the use of SAXS and wide angle X-ray scattering (WAXS) to detect the adsorption of water vapour on two different NPCs.

5.2 Theory

The scattering of light (including X-rays and neutrons) by a sample is determined by the angular dependence of the phase difference φ of the light re-emitted by all pairs of points in the sample that are illuminated by the incident beam.

$$\phi_{j,k} = \mathbf{q}.\mathbf{r}_{j,k}, \tag{5.1}$$

where $\mathbf{r}_{j,k}$ is the vector connecting the two points j and k and $\mathbf{q}$ is the transfer wave vector, with magnitude

$$|\mathbf{q}| = q = (4\pi / \lambda)\sin(\theta / 2) \tag{5.2}$$

In this expression, λ is the wavelength of the incident light (for X-rays $\lambda \approx 1$ Å) and θ is the angle through which the light is scattered. To calculate the scattering from the whole sample, the product $E_j E_k \exp(i\varphi_{j,k})$ of electric fields from all pairs of points in the sample must be summed, giving a total *structure factor* $S(q)$, the q dependence of which is characteristic of the particular sample. When molecules adsorb on an internal surface, the scattering properties of the whole sample are modified. Not only does the angular dependence of the scattering intensity vary, but also its absolute value changes. Thus, for a carbon of electron density $\rho_C = Zd_{He}N_A/M$ (in which Z is the atomic number and M the molar mass of carbon, N_A is Avogadro's number and d_{He} the mass density of the carbon skeleton, measured by helium pycnometry) the scattered intensity is

$$I(q) = r_0^2(\rho_C - \rho_a)^2 S(q). \tag{5.3}$$

In Eq. 5.3, r_0 is the classical radius of the electron (2.82×10^{-13} cm), and ρ_a is the electron density of the adsorbate in the pores. When the pores are only partially filled, then Eq. 5.3 becomes

$$I(q) = r_0^2(\rho_C - p(q)\rho_a)^2 S(q) \tag{5.4}$$

$p(q)$ is the relative density with respect to the bulk state of the molecules adsorbed in the pores, i.e., the occupation density. $p(q)$ is expected to vary between 0 and 1. It is assumed that the adsorbed species does not change the structure of the carbon matrix, i.e., $S(q)$. Eq. 5.4 works well in the micropore region of the SAXS response, but in the low q region the binary character of the system becomes uncertain, since bubbles may develop, generating liquid-air interfaces. These give rise to extra scattering that can be handled only by considering the system as fully ternary. Although SAXS alone cannot resolve ternary systems, complementary information can be found by applying contrast variation techniques involving isotopic substitution using SANS (see next contribution in this volume). For the present case, however, the ternary nature of the system is no obstacle, since in the higher q range air-liquid-carbon interfaces do not arise, and also because the pores are randomly arranged with no spatial correlation.

From Eq. 5.4 it follows that the ratio of the intensity scattered by the sample containing adsorbed molecules to that in the dry state is

$$u(q) = I_a(q) / I_{dry}(q) = [\rho_C - p(q)\rho_a]^2 / \rho_C^2 \tag{5.5}$$

Hence

$$p(q) = (\rho_C / \rho_a) \cdot \left[1 - u(q)^{1/2}\right] \tag{5.6}$$

5.3 Experimental

Two high surface area carbons were investigated. The first carbon, derived from activation of carbonized poly(ethylene terephthalate) (APET) was ash-free [1]. The second, a commercially available carbon in wide use (R1 Extra, Norit), had an ash content of 6.2%.

Gravimetry measurements were kindly performed by P. Lodewyckx (Royal Military Academy, Brussels, Belgium). Approximately 50 g of the carbons were placed in contact with air of known RH at 20.0 ± 1.5°C. Exposure times were approximately 1 week per RH point.

For the X-ray scattering observations the samples were powdered and placed in Lindemann glass capillary tubes. The capillaries were held for 8 weeks at 293 K in closed containers in contact either with hexane vapour or with aqueous salt solutions of different relative humidity. At the end of the preparation, the capillary tubes were flame-sealed. X-ray measurements were made at the BM2 bending magnet beam line at the ESRF, Grenoble, France. With incident energy 18 keV, the wave vector range explored was $6\times 10^{-3} \leq q \leq 6\,\text{Å}^{-1}$.

5.4 Results and Discussion

Figure 5.1 illustrates the scattering response of a typical NPC. The extended power-law behaviour at low q comes from the interfaces between large grains in the system. The slope of about –3.2, which differs substantially from the value – 4 characteristic of smooth surfaces [2], implies that these interfaces are extremely rough [3]. The shoulder at $q \approx 0.1\,\text{Å}^{-1}$ is the signature of micropores. The scattering intensity at low q is determined by the large-scale average density of the carbon material, d_{av} which is low, owing to the high porosity. As the resolution q increases the signal responds to the difference in density between the micropores and that of the carbon skeleton, d_{He}, which is higher. The steep slope following the shoulder is the scattering from the walls of the micropores. Its intensity is proportional to the surface area of the carbon, and from its intensity the X-ray surface area S_X can be evaluated [4]. In the WAXS region of the spectrum ($q > 1\,\text{Å}$) the residual order of the carbon atoms becomes visible. Bragg reflections from the carbon are not detected, demonstrating the amorphous nature of this sample.

When molecules adsorb onto the carbon as seen in Fig. 5.1, the intensity in the WAXS region increases, owing to the larger number of scattering centres. In the SAXS micropore region, however, since $p(q) > 0$ in Eq. 5.4, the intensity decreases with respect to the dry carbon. At values of q below the shoulder, on the other hand, the presence of solvent in the micropores *increases* the average large-scale density of the carbon and the signal intensity exceeds that of the dry sample. In Fig. 5.2 the effect on the occupation density $p(q)$ of two different species of adsorbed molecules is shown for the ash-free high surface area carbon APET. In the sample exposed to hexane vapour at partial pressure $P/P_0 = 0.4$, $p(q) = 1$ in the micropore region, while, at smaller q, decreases to zero : this shows that the smallest pores are full, while the larger pores are empty. When, however, the sample is immersed in liquid hexane the solvent occupies the larger pores as well. The small overshoot of $p(q)$ beyond 1 in this region may be due to a ternary character of the system.

The response of the system to water vapour is different to that of hexane. At relative humidity RH = 0.5, Fig. 5.2 shows that the micropores ($q \approx 0.4\,\text{Å}^{-1}$) are filled only to

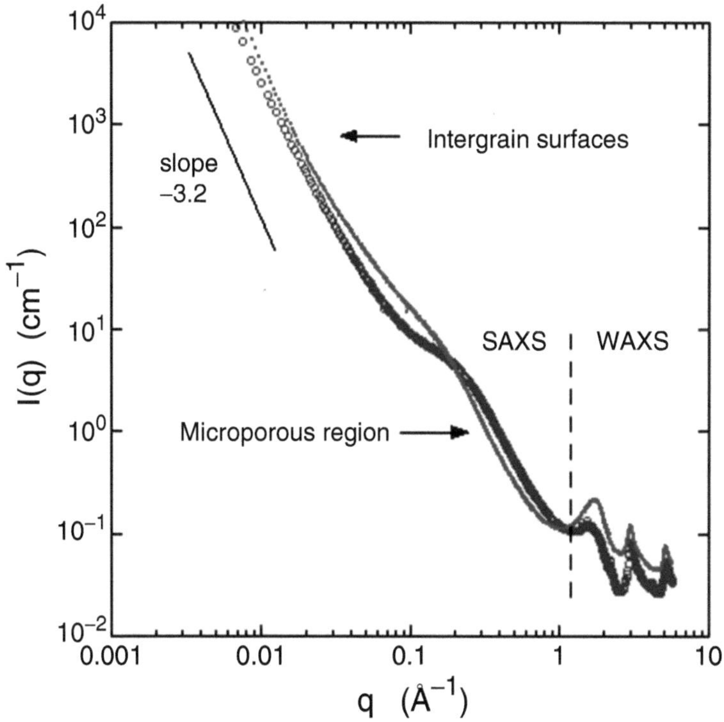

Fig. 5.1 Typical SAXS/WAXS spectrum of a high surface area carbon in the dry state (o) and after exposure to water vapour at RH = 0.54 (•)

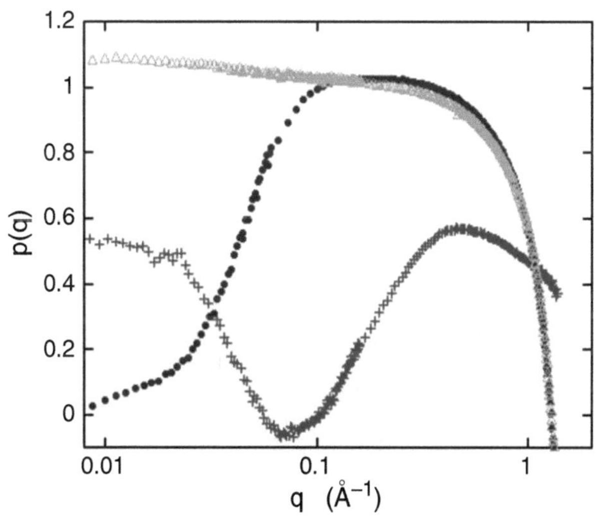

Fig. 5.2 Occupation density $p(q)$ of hexane vapour in APET at partial pressure $P/P_0 = 0.4$ (•), and immersed in liquid hexane (Δ). With water vapour at relative humidity RH = 0.5 (+), the occupation density does not exceed 0.6 in the micropores

60%. At lower q, in the larger size range $\pi/q \approx 30$ Å the pores are empty. At $q \approx 0.08$ Å^{-1}, $p(q)$ even becomes slightly negative. Such behaviour can be understood in terms of clusters of water molecules that exhibit water-air interfaces. Figure 5.2 illustrates the qualitative difference in the adsorption characteristics of hexane and water.

The surface area of the micropores S_X can be found from the Porod scattering region of Fig. 5.1 (0. 2 Å$^{-1} \leq q \leq 1$ Å^{-1}), where the scattering intensity varies as q^{-4} [2]:

$$I(q) = Kq^{-4} + b \tag{5.7}$$

In Eq. 7, the constant intensity b stems from the atomic disorder of the carbon atoms in the amorphous matrix. The expression for S_X then becomes

$$S_X = \frac{\pi K}{Q} \frac{V_{tot}}{1 + V_{tot} d_{He}} \tag{5.8}$$

where V_{tot} is the total pore volume of the sample and Q is the second moment of the scattering curve,

$$Q = \int_0^{\infty} I(q) q^2 dq \tag{5.9}$$

Table 5.1 lists the values of V_{tot}, d_{He}, and the BET surface area S_{BET} [5] derived from the low temperature nitrogen absorption curves [6,7], as well as the values of S_X calculated from the scattering curves for the two samples APETA and R1. It is noticeable that in both cases S_X is appreciably larger than S_{BET}, a result that is generally attributed to kinetic hindrance, whereby the nitrogen molecules at 77 K do not possess sufficient thermal energy to penetrate into the narrowest micropores.

Above $q = 1$ Å^{-1}, the scattering signal in the WAXS region displays excess intensity over that of the dry carbon. Figure 5.3 shows the excess intensity in this range for sample R1, i.e., the difference in intensity scattered by the sample exposed to water vapour and that of the dry carbon. The irregular form of the difference signal in this q range stems from Bragg reflections due to microcrystalline inorganic impurities in this commercial carbon. The carbon itself, however, is amorphous. It is noteworthy

Table 5.1 Characteristic data derived from low temperature N2 isotherms, from He pycnometry and from SAXS for the two samples studied

	R1	APET
V_{tot}, cm^3/g	0.72	0.48
d_{He}, g/cm^3	2.21	1.82
d_{av}, g/cm^3	0.854	0.965
S_{BET}, m^2/g	1,519	1,114
S_X, m^2/g	1,710	1,810

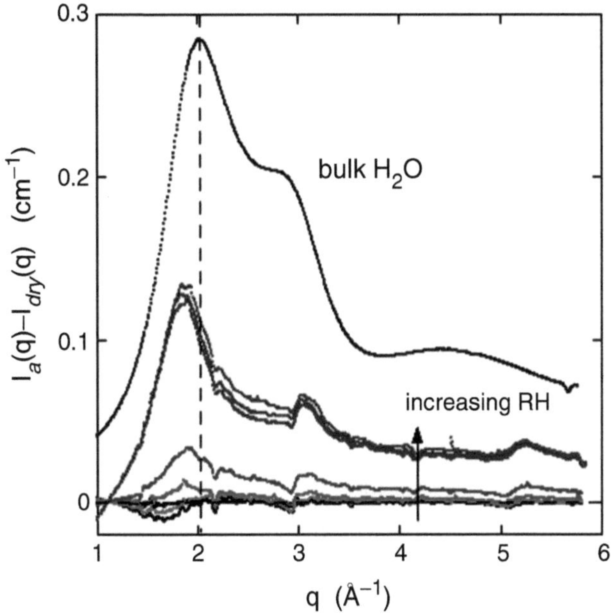

Fig. 5.3 Difference in intensity between dry carbon R1 and the same carbon with adsorbed water at different relative humidity, compared to the signal from bulk water. The "noise" in the difference signal is due to microcrystalline impurities in this commercial carbon

that treatment of this sample with nitric acid removes most of the micro crystallites and equivalent measurements of the adsorbed water appear much smoother. Figure 5.3 also displays the signal from bulk water. The positions of the peaks of the adsorbed water are clearly displaced with respect to the characteristic features in bulk water. The arrangement of the water molecules adsorbed in the carbon matrix therefore differs notably from that in the bulk. The broad peaks at 1.8, 3.0 and 5.2 $Å^{-1}$correspond more closely to those of the disordered carbon substrate than to bulk water, which suggests that the water molecules tend to occupy vacant sites in the carbon lattice.

The amount of adsorbed water is obtained by comparing the amplitudes of the signals of adsorbed and bulk water, with the assumption that the filling factor of the carbon powder in the capillary is 2/3. The result of this comparison is shown in Fig. 5.4. This Figure compares the results obtained from the WAXS intensity curves of Fig. 5.3 with direct measurements by gravimetry of the amount of adsorbed water at 20°C. Agreement between these two sets of results is satisfactory. It is shown elsewhere [7] that measurements of water uptake made by a traditional adsorption instrument on much shorter times scale, e.g., a few days, can grossly underestimate the longer term water adsorption capacity, exemplified by the times scale of the present experiments (3 months).

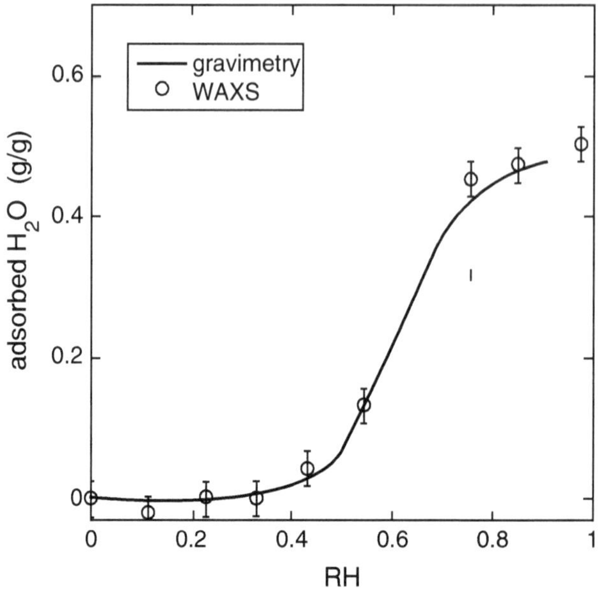

Fig. 5.4 Amount of adsorbed water on carbon R1 measured by WAXS, compared to gravimetric measurements conducted over a long time period (several months)

5.5 Conclusions

The combination of SAXS and WAXS employed here provides information not only on the total internal surface area in highly microporous systems but also on the nature and distribution of polar or non-polar molecules in the pores. The method is especially valuable in situations where the adsorption process may be slow, such as with water vapour.

Acknowledgments We are grateful to the European Synchrotron Radiation Facility, Grenoble, for access to the French CRG beamline BM2, and to Norit for providing the carbon samples. We express our gratitude to Cyrille Rochas, Jean-François Bérar, György Bosznai and Orsolya Czakkel for their assistance. This research was supported by the EU – Hungarian Government joint fund (GVOP – 3.2.2 – 2004 – 07 – 0006/3.0).

References

1. László K, Geissler E (2006) Surface chemistry and contrast-modified SAXS in polymer-based activated carbons. Carbon 44:2437–2444
2. Glatter O, Kratky O (eds) (1982) G. Porod in small angle X-ray scattering. Academic, London
3. Pfeifer P, Avnir D, Farin D (1983) Ideally irregular surfaces, of dimension greater than two, in theory and practice. Surf Sci 126:569–572

4. László K, Czakkel O, Josepovits K, Rochas C, Geissler E (2005) Influence of surface chemistry on the SAXS response of polymer-based activated carbons. Langmuir 21:8443–8451
5. Brunauer S, Emmett P, Teller E (1938) Adsorption of gases in multimolecular layers. J Amer Chem Soc 60:309–319
6. László K, Bóta A, Nagy LG (1997) Characterization of activated carbons from waste materials by adsorption from aqueous solutions. Carbon 35:593
7. László K, Czakkel O, Dobos G, Lodewyckx P, Rochas C, Geissler E (2010) Water vapour adsorption in highly porous carbons as seen by small and wide angle X-ray scattering. Carbon 48:1038–1048

Chapter 6
The Competitive Role of Water in Sorption Processes on Porous Carbon Surfaces

K. László and E. Geissler

Abstract Concurrent equilibrium adsorption on a highly porous activated carbon of both water vapour and toluene was studied to determine the extent and the location of toluene adsorption in the presence of water. We report small angle neutron scattering (SANS) measurements in which the H/D ratio of both the water and toluene components is varied. Measurements are made both in the lower transfer wave vector region ($5 \times 10^{-2} \leq q \leq 1$ Å^{-1}) and in the high q region >1 Å^{-1}. Just below the Porod scattering region (0.3–1 Å^{-1}), the liquid/vapour interface contributes significantly. To solve the intrinsic ternary character of the signal in this region, contrast variation measurements with H_2O/D_2O mixtures alone and with toluene-D and toluene-H mixtures alone at constant relative pressure were performed. The carbon samples, of commercial origin (Norit R1), were previously treated with nitric acid to reduce the ash content, which simplifies the data treatment in the diffraction region at high q.

Keywords Sorption • Activated carbon • Porous carbon surfaces

List of Abbreviations

AC	Activated carbon
RH	Relative humidity
RP	Relative pressure
SWNT	Single wall nanotube

K. László (✉)
Department of Physical Chemistry and Materials Science, Budapest University of Technology and Economics, H-1521 Budapest, Hungary
e-mail: klaszlo@mail.bme.hu

E. Geissler
Laboratoire de Spectrométrie Physique CNRS UMR 5588, Université J. Fourier de Grenoble, BP 87, 38402 St Martin d'Hères cedex, Grenoble, France

S. Mikhalovsky and A. Khajibaev (eds.), *Biodefence*, NATO Science for Peace and Security Series A: Chemistry and Biology, DOI 10.1007/978-94-007-0217-2_6,

GCMC	Grand canonical Monte Carlo calculation
SAXS	Small angle X-ray scattering
SANS	Small angle neutron scattering
WAXS	Wide angle X-ray scattering
TH	Hydrogenated toluene C_7H_8
TD	Deuterated toluene C_7D_8
THD	50:50 v/v mixture of toluene H and toluene D
ILL	Institut Laue Langevin
b_a	Scattering length of the adsorbate
b_C	Scattering length of carbon
b_D	Scattering length of deuterium
b_H	Scattering length of hydrogen
d_a	Mass density of the adsorbate
d_C	Mass density of carbon
I	Intensity of neutrons
I_{inc}	Intensity from incoherent scattering
M_a	Molecular weight of the adsorbate
M_C	Molecular weight of carbon
q	Transfer wave vector
$S(q)$	Structure factor
S_{BET}	Specific surface area
λ	Wavelength of the incident neutron beam
ρ_a	Scattering length density of the adsorbate
ρ_C	Scattering length density of the carbon
θ	Scattering angle

6.1 Introduction

By virtue of their versatility, activated carbons (ACs) are the most frequently employed adsorbents. Since ancient times the high affinity of carbon for a wide diversity of chemical species has established it as a multi-purpose adsorbent. They are used extensively not only in daily life in domestic or office air filters but also on an industrial scale for gas purification. As they are general adsorbents they are the first choice for dealing with industrial accidents or terrorist attacks.

The outstanding performance of ACs stems from a unique combination of geometrical and chemical characteristics. Nowadays carbon adsorbents with tailor-made surface area and pore hierarchy are commercially available [1–3]. Chemical treatment, in addition to impregnation or doping techniques, is often used to enhance the performance of porous carbons. Introduction of heteroatoms into the carbon skeleton renders the carbon surface more attractive to polar molecules [4].

The affinity between the carbon surface and the fluid phase plays a major role in adsorption processes, as the generally non-specific interaction substantially affects the distribution of the adsorbed molecules within the pores. Non-polar vapour molecules are attracted to the carbon matrix through a strong dispersion interaction, which favours adsorption even at low relative pressure (RP), while the adsorption of water on the carbon surface is hindered by the strong hydrogen bonding among the water molecules in the fluid [5, 6]. At very low surface coverage water adsorption is governed both by the surface chemistry and the porosity of the carbons. Water uptake at low relative humidity (RH) may be enhanced by introducing oxygen functionalities into the carbon, since through a cooperative bonding mechanism they have the same effect as pre-adsorbed water [7, 8]. Such surface functional groups act as nucleation centres that ripen into clusters already at low RH [9]. Pore filling for water does not begin until about RH = 0.50. The kinetics of water vapour adsorption in high surface area carbons is also slower and more complex than that of small non-polar molecules [10].

Under real operating conditions, water molecules from the ambient RH tend to infiltrate and preempt adsorption sites reserved for other target molecules, thereby compromising the role of the carbon. Competition can be concurrent (e.g., in gas masks) and/or consecutive (application after storage). The recognition of the role of water therefore has particular relevance in AC – mixed vapour phase interactions.

Sequential adsorption of binary mixtures of water and organic vapours on single-walled carbon nanotubes (SWNTs) has been studied both experimentally and by grand canonical Monte Carlo (GCMC) simulation to elucidate the distinct interactions between adsorbates and the nanoporous structure of SWNTs [11]. Adsorption of pure water left the outer surface of the SWNTs free, but filled the nanotubes. When the water-filled SWNTs were exposed to organic vapour, the adsorbed water remained intact and the organic vapour adsorbed only on the outer surface. If the organic vapour was adsorbed first, it occupied both the inside of the tubes and the external surface. On further exposure to water the organic adsorbate was substituted inside the tubes but left the organic outer layer unaffected. This conclusion does not necessarily apply, however, to ACs owing to their complex pore structure and their heterogeneous chemical composition. Consecutive equilibrium adsorption studies of similar binary mixtures on a commercial AC at 25 °C showed improved total pore filling (larger than 100%) near the water saturation pressure, possibly as a result of high molecular packing density within the pores. Organic pre-loadings were held constant. At low water loadings, molecular interaction of adsorbates was noteworthy, while at high water loadings, competition for adsorption sites and pore volume became significant. Slight cooperative adsorption was observed both with water-miscible and water-immiscible organic compounds. [12].

These techniques give information on the equilibrium uptake and the overall composition of the adsorbed layer, but not on the spatial distribution of the two adsorbates. Such observations are difficult to make by traditional adsorption techniques [13–15]. Small angle X-ray scattering (SAXS) observations can yield model-independent information on pore filling by any adsorbed molecule. It was recently reported that water vapour isotherms can be generated from combined SAXS and wide angle X-ray scattering (WAXS) experiments, based on the change in the contrast due to the adsorbate. Moreover, the spatial distribution of the adsorbed water also can be deduced from the same data set [10]. This method, however, is not applicable to binary vapour phases since it does not discriminate between different types of adsorbates. In this work we intend to show that small angle neutron scattering (SANS) offers a means of determining the extent to which two adsorbates are adsorbed in each other's presence, since the contrast of both molecules can be varied by changing their degree of deuteration [16, 17].

6.2 Experimental

A commercial high surface area carbon (Norit R1 Extra) was exposed to concentrated nitric acid for 3 h at room temperature, then thoroughly washed with distilled water and dried (S_{BET} = 1,450 m^2/g, surface carbon/oxygen ratio = 9.4 atomic%). The ash content of the resulting material was 2.2% w/w. This process affects only the surface chemistry of the carbon, not the porosity [10]. Powdered samples were exposed to the two sets of vapour simultaneously at two different values of RH, 0.11 (above supersaturated H_2O or D_2O solutions of LiCl) and 0.87 (supersaturated aqueous solutions of KCl), and also in contact with the vapour of the toluene in a separate vial at 20°C. At this temperature the RP of the toluene is 0.037 [18] (The isotope effect was neglected). Two degrees of deuteration were selected, both for the water and for the toluene (TH and TD), namely 0.5 and 1 (v/v). The carbon samples, contained in low boron glass NMR tubes of 5 mm external diameter, were flame-sealed after exposure for 3 months to the corresponding vapour mixture. SANS measurements were made on the D16 instrument at the Institut Laue Langevin (ILL), Grenoble, in the transfer wave vector region $0.05\,\text{Å}^{-1} < q \leq 2.5\,\text{Å}^{-1}$, where $q = (4\pi/\lambda)\sin(\theta/2)$, θ being the scattering angle and $\lambda = 4.75\,\text{Å}$ the wavelength of the incident neutron beam.

6.3 Results and Discussion

The intensity I of neutrons of wavelength λ scattered through angle θ by a carbon sample in dry air is governed both by the structure factor, $S(q)$, and the scattering length density ρ_C of the carbon. The scattering length density of the air can be neglected. Thus,

$$I(q) = \rho_C^{\,2} \cdot S(q) + I_{inc} \tag{6.1}$$

In Eq. 6.1, $\rho_C = (b_C d_C / M_C)$, where b_C is the scattering length of carbon, d_C its mass density, and M_C the molecular weight. q is the magnitude of the transfer wave vector, $q = (4\pi/\lambda)\sin(\theta/2)$. An important difference between SAXS and SANS is the contribution in the latter case from incoherent scattering, I_{inc}. This originates principally from the protons in the sample, but also, to a lesser extent, from deuterium as well as any impurities that the sample may contain.

The incoherent signal thus contains valuable information on the amount of protonated material in the sample. Furthermore, as the evaluation of the incoherent component is critical in the higher q region of the scattering response where the coherent signal becomes weak, it is advantageous to compare the SANS signal of a given sample with that of SAXS, where incoherent scattering is negligible. Figure 6.1 shows this comparison for the dry carbon, in which, to give agreement, a constant signal of 0.06 cm^{-1} has been subtracted from the SANS signal. This is the incoherent background of the dry sample. Figure 6.1 displays the main features of the scattering response of this carbon: the shoulder at $q \approx 0.2$ Å^{-1} is the signal from the nanopores; the Porod region (0.3 Å$^{-1} \leq q \leq 0.8$ Å^{-1}) is the scattering from the pore walls; finally the broad amorphous peak at $q \approx 1.7$ Å^{-1} is the disordered analogue of the interlayer spacing of crystalline graphite (002 Bragg peak). Apart from residual impurities, this sample exhibits no crystallinity [10].

When molecules are adsorbed in the nanopores, the neutron scattering contrast of the carbon decreases from its value in the dry state (i.e., in air) to

$$\rho_C - \rho_a = \left(\frac{b_C d_C}{M_C} - \frac{b_a d_a}{M_a} \right) \tag{6.2}$$

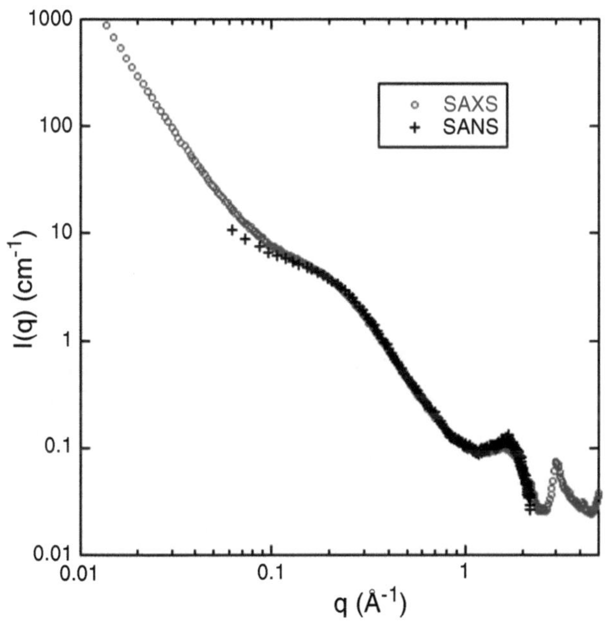

Fig. 6.1 SAXS response of dry carbon (o) compared with that of SANS (+). For agreement at high q, I_{inc} = 0.06 cm^{-1} was subtracted from the SANS signal

ρ_a, b_a, d_a and M_a are respectively the scattering length density, scattering length, mass density and molecular weight of the adsorbate molecules. $\rho_C \approx \rho_{D20} \approx 0.105 \times 10^{-12}$ mole cm^{-2}, while $\rho_{TD} \approx 0.094 \times 10^{-12}$ mole cm^{-2}. The value of b_a is defined by the degree of deuteration. According to Eq. 6.2, condensation of molecules in the pores reduces the scattering intensity in the region $q < 1$ Å^{-1}. If the bulk value is taken for d_a, then Eq. 6.2 would imply complete pore filling, which is not necessarily the case [17]. In the scattering vector range $q > 0.2$ Å^{-1}, effects due to the ternary (or quaternary) nature of the system are not expected to be significant because of the random distribution of the pores and also because of the reduced probability, at this length scale, of significant interfaces between the two solvents as well as with air. In contrast to the scattering behaviour at small q, where Eqs. 6.1 and 6.2 apply, in the region above $q \approx 1$ Å^{-1}, individual molecules become resolved and instead of reducing the contrast, they add to the signal.

Figures 6.2 and 6.3 compare the SANS scattering responses, for RH = 0.11 and RH = 0.87, of the dry carbon, the carbon + TD, carbon + D_2O, and carbon + D_2O + TD. The loss of intensity due to the reduced contrast factor is evident in the region 0.2 Å$^{-1} \le q \le 1$ Å^{-1}, except for D_2O at RH = 0.11. In the latter case (Fig. 6.2) the adsorbed amount is very small, which is consistent with the mainly hydrophobic character of this carbon and with recent SAXS measurements on the same system [10]. At RH = 0.87, Figs. 6.2 and 6.3 also show that in the region 0.2 Å$^{-1} \le q \le 1$ Å^{-1}

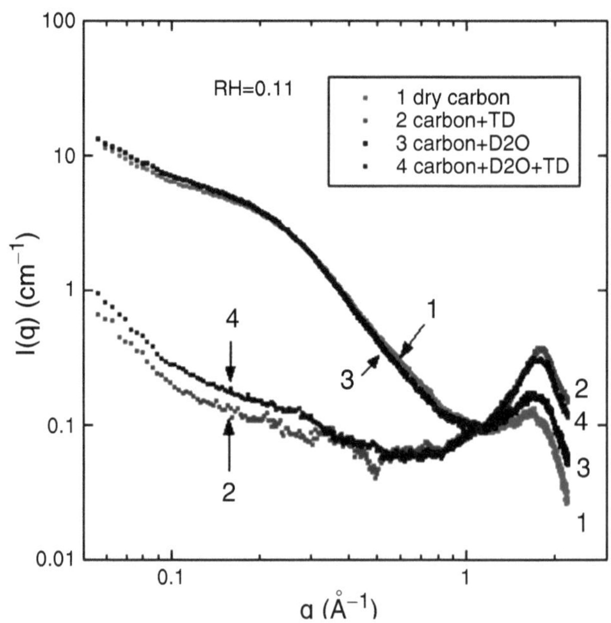

Fig. 6.2 SANS response of carbon exposed to D_2O vapour at RH = 0.11 (3), compared to dry carbon (1), carbon with TD (2) and carbon with D_2O and TD (4)

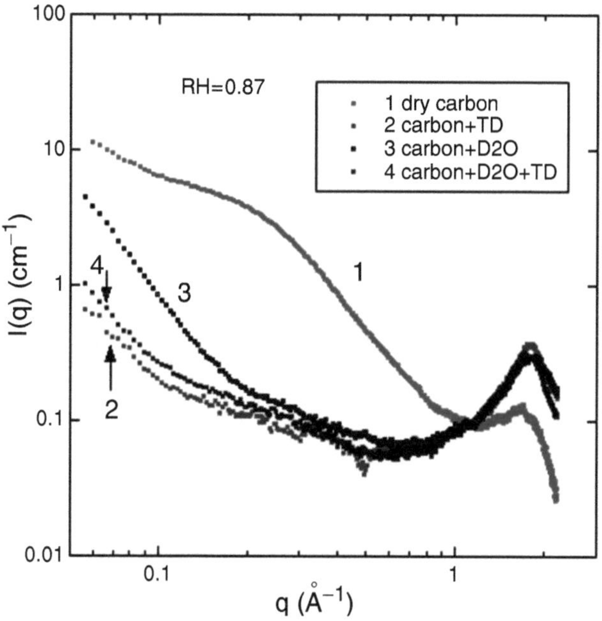

Fig. 6.3 SANS response of carbon exposed to D_2O vapour at RH=0.87 (3), compared to dry carbon (1), carbon with TD (2), and carbon with D_2O and TD (4)

the signal intensity with TD is smaller than with D_2O, even though $(\rho_C-\rho_{D2O})^2 < (\rho_C-\rho_{TD})^2$. Filling of the micropores by D_2O alone is therefore less complete than by toluene alone. When TD and D_2O are simultaneously present, the signals are almost the same as with TD alone, but at $q \leq 0.3$ Å^{-1}, masking by the contrast matching is less complete. The water appears to impede total filling of the larger pores, even, surprisingly, at RH=0.11.

When the carbon is exposed to TD and an equal mixture (v/v) of D_2O and H_2O (HDO), the signal is practically identical to that with TD and D_2O (Fig. 6.4, curves 2 and 3). Furthermore, the incoherent background signal is also identical in both (0.07 cm^{-1}), which indicates that the amount of adsorbed proton-bearing water is very small, even at this high RH=0.87. Within the error of this measurement, therefore, water does not adsorb.

In the opposite situation, when the carbon is exposed to D_2O at RH=0.87 in association with a 1:1 (v/v) mixture of TH and TD (THD), a large difference is observed with respect to the case where the toluene is fully deuterated (Fig. 6.4, curve 4). I_{inc} shows a substantial increase, to 0.11 cm^{-1}, and the contrast factor also increases as a result of the replacement of deuterium atoms in the toluene (b_D=+0.66×10^{-12} cm) by protons (b_H= −0.37×10^{-12} cm). It is also noticeable that the accumulated intensity at the peak around 1.7 Å^{-1} is much weaker owing to the reduced scattering power of the TH molecules.

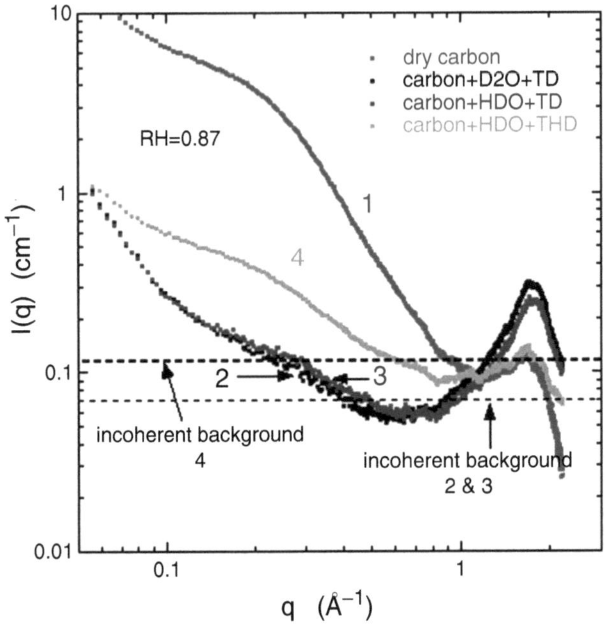

Fig. 6.4 SANS response of carbon exposed to water vapour from HDO (i.e. D_2O:H_2O = 1:1) at RH = 0.87 and TD (3) and an equal mixture of TD and TH (THD) (4), compared to that of D_2O and TD (2) and dry carbon (1). The incoherent background, 0.07 cm^{-1}, is the same for samples 2 and 3, and only slightly larger than for the dry carbon (0.06 cm^{-1}). The incoherent background due solely to the adsorbed (THD), i.e., excluding the background from the carbon (0.11–0.06 cm^{-1}), is thus approximately 5 times greater than that due to the adsorbed TD alone (0.07–0.06 cm^{-1})

6.4 Conclusions

The present results, which give a glimpse of the power of SANS in resolving multi-component systems, show that in adsorption from the vapour phase, concurrent competition for sites between water and toluene in this carbon is won overwhelmingly by the aromatic species. These findings, however, do not address the question of consecutive competition, which is the subject of separate ongoing studies. It is relevant to add that, owing to the weighting of the signal intensity that governs scattering experiments, effects that appear to be magnified at low q in SANS or SAXS observations tend to involve small amounts of material. It is likely, therefore, that the differences in Figs. 6.2 and 6.3 between the case of carbon + TD and carbon + D2O + TD, which are attributed to hindering effects of water, may be difficult to detect in direct measurements of adsorption.

Acknowledgments We are grateful to the Institut Laue-Langevin, Grenoble for access to the D16 instrument, and to Norit for providing the carbon samples. We express our gratitude to Bruno Demé, György Bosznai and Orsolya Czakkel for their technical assistance. This research was supported by the EU – Hungarian Government joint fund (GVOP – 3.2.2 – 2004 – 07 – 0006/3.0).

References

1. Lozano-Castelló D, Lillo-Ródenas MA, Cazorla-Amorós D, Linares-Solano A et al (2001) Preparation of activated carbons from Spanish anthracite: I. activation by KOH. Carbon 39(5):741–749
2. Lillo-Ródenas MA, Lozano-Castelló D, Cazorla-Amorós D, Linares-Solano A et al (2001) Preparation of activated carbons from Spanish anthracite: II. activation by NaOH. Carbon 39(5):751–759
3. Dash RK, Yushin G, Gogotsi Y et al (2005) Synthesis, structure and porosity analysis of microporous and mesoporous carbon derived from zirconium carbide. Micropor Mesopor Mater 86(1–3):50–57
4. László K, Tombácz E, Josepovits K et al (2001) Effect of activation on the surface chemistry of carbons from polymer precursors. Carbon 39(8):1217–1228
5. Dubinin MM (1980) Water vapor adsorption and microporous structures of carbonaceous adsorbents. Carbon 18:355–364
6. Mowla D, Do DD, Kaneko K et al (2003) Adsorption of Water vapour on Activated Carbon. Chemistry and Physics of Carbon, (ed.) Radovic LR, Marcel Dekker, New York 28:230–262
7. Lodewyckx P, Vansant EF (1999) Water isotherms of activated carbons with small amounts of surface oxygen. Carbon 37:1647–1649
8. Müller EA, Rull LF, Vega LF, Gubbins KE et al (1996) Adsorption of water on activated carbons: A molecular simulation study. J Phys Chem 100:1189–1196
9. Brennan JK, Bandosz TJ, Thomson KT, Gubbins KE et al (2001) Water in porous carbons. Coll Surf A 187–188:539–568
10. László K, Czakkel O, Dobos G, Lodewyckx P, Rochas C, Geissler E. (2010) Water vapour adsorption in highly porous carbons as seen by small and wide angle X-ray scattering. Carbon 48:1038–1048
11. Sandeep Agnihotri, Pyoungchung Kim, Yijing Zheng, José PB Mota, Liangcheng Yang et al (2008) Regioselective competitive adsorption of water and organic vapor mixtures on pristine single-walled carbon nanotube bundles. Langmuir 24:5746–5754
12. Nan Qi, Douglas LeVan M (2005) Coadsorption of organic compounds and water vapor on BPL Activated carbon. 5. Methyl ethyl ketone, Methyl isobutyl ketone, Toluene, and Modeling. Ind Eng Chem Res 44:3733–3741
13. Fletcher AJ, Benham MJ, Thomas KM et al (2002) Multicomponent vapor sorption on active carbon by combined microgravimetry and dynamic sampling mass spectrometry. J Phys Chem B 106:7474–7482
14. Hoinkis E (2004) Small-angle scattering studies of adsorption and of capillary condensation in porous solids. Part Part Syst Charact 21:80–100
15. Heinen AW, Peters JA, van Bekkum H et al (2000) Competitive adsorption of water and toluene on modified activated carbon supports. Appl Catal A: General 194–195:193–202
16. Ramsay JDF (1993) Applications of neutron scattering in investigations of adsorption processes in porous materials. Pure Appl Chem 65(10):2169–2174
17. László K, Rochas C, Geissler E (2008) Water vapour adsorption and contrast-modified saxs in microporous polymer-based carbons of different surface chemistry. Adsorption 14:447–455
18. S Ohe Vapor pressure Calcuations Program http://www.s-ohe.com Accessed 8 June 2009

Part II
Methods of Detection and Analysis

Chapter 7
Sensors for Breath Analysis: An Advanced Approach to Express Diagnostics and Monitoring of Human Diseases

I.G. Kushch, N.M. Korenev, L.V. Kamarchuk, A.P. Pospelov, Y.L. Alexandrov, and G.V. Kamarchuk

Abstract The study demonstrates high efficacy and expediency of the TCNQ derivatives-based point-contact multi-structure as a prospective asset for development of new sensors. Investigation of sensors' behavior in case of different duration of exposition to exhaled air showed that in case of exposition lasting longer than 30 s, the response curve of the point-contact sensors was principally different from analogous dependences of traditional and nanostructured chemical ones. Due to the complex non-homogenous structure, the obtained response curves of the point-contact sensors are much more informative than similar dependences of analog devices. The introduced phenomenological model of the response signal of the sensor under study enables application of a complex statistical analysis of its components. This may be used for exhaled air analysis with diagnostic purposes. The proposed advanced approach was successfully applied to diagnostics development and important correlations between response curve's parameters and state of human organism were discovered. High sensitivity of the point-contact multi-structure, enabling analysis of composite gas mixtures, opens up wide possibilities to apply the demonstrated approach for environment and health protection.

Keywords Chemical sensors • Point contact • Exhaled air analysis • Point-contact spectroscopy • Organic conductors • Noninvasive diagnostics • Chronic dyspepsia

---

I.G. Kushch (✉), N.M. Korenev, and L.V. Kamarchuk
Department of Pediatrics, Institute for Children and Adolescents Health Care, Academy of Medical Sciences of Ukraine, 52-A, 50 let VLKSM Avenue, Kharkiv 61153, Ukraine
e-mail: ekushch@gmail.com

A.P. Pospelov and Y.L. Alexandrov
National Technical University "Kharkiv Polytechnical Institute", 21 Frunze Str, Kharkiv 61002, Ukraine

G.V. Kamarchuk
B.Verkin Institute for Low Temperature Physics & Engineering, National Academy of Sciences of Ukraine, 47 Lenin Ave, Kharkiv 61103, Ukraine

S. Mikhalovsky and A. Khajibaev (eds.), *Biodefence*, NATO Science for Peace and Security Series A: Chemistry and Biology, DOI 10.1007/978-94-007-0217-2_7,

7.1 Introduction

Modern spheres of human activity are impossible without hi-tech approaches for reliable control and monitoring of all stages of processes involved. Sensor device systems are leading among detection methods for obtaining precise data on the real-time state of controlled objects. Development of noninvasive diagnostic approaches based on analysis of exhaled breath is among the most prospective applications of advanced sensors. It is expected that in a very near future breath analysis will take a leading position amongst new non-invasive diagnostic tools, including those applied in emergency care, in view of the great number of markers reflecting state of organism [1, 2]. New breath analysis-based diagnostic approaches offer several advantages over traditional methods. As human exhaled air is an easily accessible biological medium, the samples to be analyzed may be obtained noninvasively and as many times as needed for diagnostic purposes without causing any harm to a patient. That makes breath analysis a patient-friendly method which has a minimal risk of complications due to infection transmission and a feasible approach to monitor various physiological and pathological processes in the human body [3, 4].

Currently different techniques are applied to exhaled air analysis mostly in research settings [2, 5]. Various spectroscopic methods are widely used to record isotope markers introduced into the body [6–8]. Modified mass spectrometry techniques have been particularly successful in such applications [4, 9]. The majority of spectroscopic techniques are based on chemiluminescence. For example, the reaction of NO with ozone, which is generated by the analyzer, produces excited molecules of NO_2 that emit photons [10]. But the problem is that these techniques are rather expensive for wide utilization in clinical practice, whereas simple and inexpensive methods providing diagnostic information in a real-time mode are needed. This should be done without injecting any chemicals into the body or without any additional operations that can influence the exhaled air gas trace concentrations. It has recently become possible to fulfill these requirements by using a specifically designed new generation of gas sensors [11–18].

The field of sensors [19] has experienced rapid progress during the past years and is currently subject to world-wide research investigations combining physics, chemistry, biology and materials science. One of the perspective trends in this activity is development of sensors based on different nano-objects [20]. Undoubtedly, the breakthrough towards nano-object technologies yields new opportunities to improve considerably sensors techniques. Therefore, drastic efforts are made to improve the key parameters of these devices by a serious know-how approach combining solid state physics and materials science.

Thus we have recently proposed a novel approach in this field and have demonstrated essential advantages of the new type of sensors [21, 22]. The new sensor concept is based on the unique nonlinear properties of point contacts which provide rich physical information in many research directions [23].

A point contact is usually defined as a contact of a small size which is created between two bulk metallic electrodes touching each other on a small area. Such a probe has direct conductivity, does not contain tunneling barriers and its size is smaller or close to the mean free paths of charge carriers. As a rule, the point contact size can span from nanometers to Angströms, to the size of single molecule structures [24]. Thus, point-contact surface-to-volume ratio (~$1/d$, where d is a contact diameter) is very high, thereby significantly improving the sensitivity and response time of gas sensors. Additionally, the specific fundamental properties of point contacts considerably enhance their sensitivity parameters and predetermine fast response and short relaxation time comparatively to existing homogeneous and nanostructured sensor probes. The outstanding characteristics of point contact sensors warrant their direct use in the exhaled air analysis.

The aim of the study was to create high-sensitive point-contact type gas sensors based on derivatives of 7,7,8,8-tetracyanoquinodimethane (TCNQ) and to test them in analysis of exhaled air for diagnosis and monitoring of human organism state.

7.2 Experimental

TCNQ derivatives represent a well-known class of conductive organic compounds. The unique feature of their typical crystal structure is in the stacked packing of TCNQ molecules. The distance between the TCNQ molecules inside stacks is much shorter than that between the stacks. Thus, structurally TCNQ complexes represent a system of linear conductive chains, which are regularly packed in a three-dimensional crystal. The electrical conductivity of these compounds is due to the motion of electrons along the stacks. The probability of electron hopping between the stacks is much weaker. Such a quasi-one-dimensional type of crystal conductivity causes strong anisotropy in the electron density distribution, which, in turn, may change considerably during an adsorption process. This feature is one of the main reasons why investigation towards tailoring of sensors based on TCNQ compounds to a specific analyte is of great interest. We found that TCNQ-based sensors demonstrated high sensitivity and selectivity when they are exposed to different external agents [25]. Of particular interest is their high sensitivity to the components of breath gas exhaled by humans [11].

The design of sensitive elements (transducers) is based on the conductive principle of response registration: the output signal appears to depend on the conductive properties of the TCNQ compound as a result of its interaction with gas components. The gas-sensitive substance of the transducer has been manufactured from complex TCNQ salts with N-alkylisoquinolinium cations ([N-C_4H_9-iso-Qn] $(TCNQ)_2$) [26]. The substance of the gas sensitive layer is put in contact with copper or silver current feeding electrodes, put on the dielectric substrate manufactured from glass-cloth laminate.

To obtain a gas sensitive continuum we used a special technique for sensor manufacturing, which allowed formation of a mesoscopic point-contact multistructure of TCNQ salts (Fig. 7.1). This structure is a set of a large number of resistant elements, namely point contacts [23], formed in the points of touching of the lateral

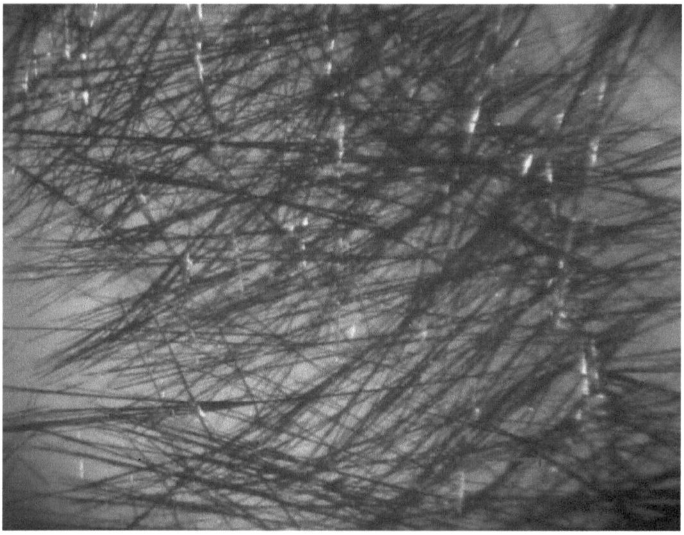

Fig. 7.1 Mesoscopic point-contact multistructure of the gas sensitive element of a TCNQ-derivative based sensor. The scale bar is 200 μm

surfaces of the needle-shaped crystals of the TCNQ salt. As it is clearly seen in Fig. 7.1, the point contacts of this structure correspond to the contacts obtained by the displacement technique [27] known to be one of the most efficient and reliable methods in point contact spectroscopy [23].

Each of these elements is able to change its resistance in the presence of gases according to the point contact gas-sensitive effect discovered by our group [21, 22]. Assemblage of point-contact sensitive elements connected with each other and located between the electric current feeding plates of a sensor forms a mesoscopic point-contact multistructure, which provides significant enhancement of an output signal and increase of selectivity to the gases under analysis.

We have manufactured active type sensors using a combination of preparative and technological approaches. The produced samples are characterized by presence of an intrinsic source of electromotive force capable of converting changes of physicochemical properties of the gas-sensitive element into an electric output signal. The process of sensor manufacturing includes polarization of the interface between the current-conducting metal and gas-sensitive substance under voltage bias on the sensor electrodes >2.0 V during formation of the point-contact multi-structure. High resistance of the gas-sensitive layer (>200 MOhm) significantly limits the rate of the active element formation. But the amount of the latter obtained during 5 min of polarization, is sufficient for over 100 h of uninterrupted work of the device.

The products formed during cathode polarization are unstable and almost entirely decompose within a few minutes. The products of anode polarization are considerably more stable as evidenced by the stability of the residual potential. The residual potential is determined as a difference between the potential of the non-polarized electrode, the solid phase of which includes the electrochemically synthesized product, and output stationary potential of the electrode before synthesis. A complex salt $Cu(TCNQ)_2$ is one of the main products of the anode process when copper is used as the current conducting material. This unstable compound dissociates almost instantaneously after its formation according to the reaction (7.1)

$$Cu(TCNQ)_2 \rightarrow Cu(TCNQ) + TCNQ \tag{7.1}$$

Its products may be considered to be the active mass of the sensor which stable potential over time.

A new portable measuring unit has been developed to provide reproducible results of medical testing. It contains a specially designed sensor holder, which simultaneously serves for breath probe taking, as an amplifier and the sensor response detector. As indicated above, there is a potential difference at the interface between copper and TCNQ compound. It generates an electric current in the circuit when the sensor contacts the atmosphere. The interaction between components of exhaled air and the active mass of the sensor leads to variation of the electric conductivity of the gas-sensitive element, causing current changes in the sensor circuit. This effect allows studying of the sensor response by means of electric measurements. During exposition to the exhaled air, the sensor is kept in a special holder. It has a removable disposable plastic mouthpiece at the top, where the sensitive element of the device is placed. During experiments the mouthpiece is put into the volunteer's mouth in order to ensure the direct contact of the gas-sensitive element with exhaled air (Fig. 7.2). The sensor holder is connected with an amplifier as well as with the system of automated recording of the response signal. The output signal

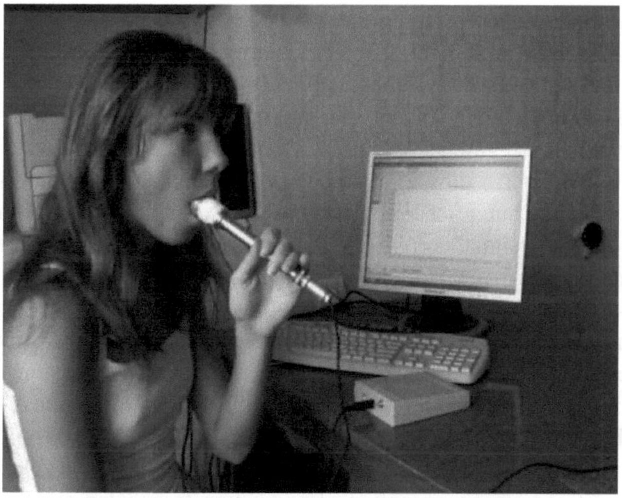

Fig. 7.2 The procedure of registration of sensor response to exhaled air

is registered by measuring the voltage drop on a standard high-precision resistor connected in series with the sensitive element. After amplification, the analogous voltage signal is transferred from the resistor to the analogue-digital transducer and registered with a computer equipped with software for registration and processing of experimental data.

The clinical part of the study was conducted with participation of 116 adolescent patients aged from 10 to18 years hospitalized by the Department of Pediatrics for examination and treatment of chronic dyspeptic complaints. The control group comprised 38 age matched healthy volunteers. The Regional Research Ethics Committee of Ukraine approved the study.

After the procedure of upper endoscopy and microscopic evaluation of gastric antral biopsy specimens, 20 patients were diagnosed with destructive changes of gastric and duodenal mucosa, among them 10 cases being duodenal and gastric ulcers and 10 cases of superficial erosions of stomach and duodenum. 96 subjects had superficial inflammatory changes of mucous membrane classified as functional dyspepsia.

Response of the sensors to exhaled air was registered after an overnight fast of the subjects in one-minute exposition mode. The measuring unit was controlled before a measurement cycle by test recording of several responses to an action of exhaled air of the investigator.

The SPSS statistical package for Windows was used [28], with level of significance was set at 5%.

7.3 Results and Discussion

Investigation of sensor response to exhaled air at different duration of exposition showed that for exposition time longer than 30 s, the response curve of the point-contact sensors was principally different from response-exposition time curves of traditional and nanostructured chemical sensors. Usually a response curve of a chemical sensor obtained in contact with gaseous media is bell-shaped, and consists of two monotonous segments: an initial segment corresponding to the period of exposition is characterized by a monotonous growth of the registered signal up to its maximal value, while after termination of gas exposition there is a monotonous decrease of response signal corresponding to the relaxation period [12, 15, 29]. The point-contact multistructure samples demonstrated a more complicated structure of the response curve. A typical dependence of a voltage drop U on a point contact sensor with time t is presented in (Fig. 7.3). Here a period of exposition is characterized by presence of the maximum on the curve $U(t)$ and area of a non-monotonous decrease and saturation of the response signal. This area of response curves may evidence that sensor sensitive matter has interacted with the exhaled air components completely. Additionally, an appearance of maximum in relaxation curve has been registered after termination of exposition to exhaled air. Such behavior pattern of the response curves has been unknown in sensor engineering so far.

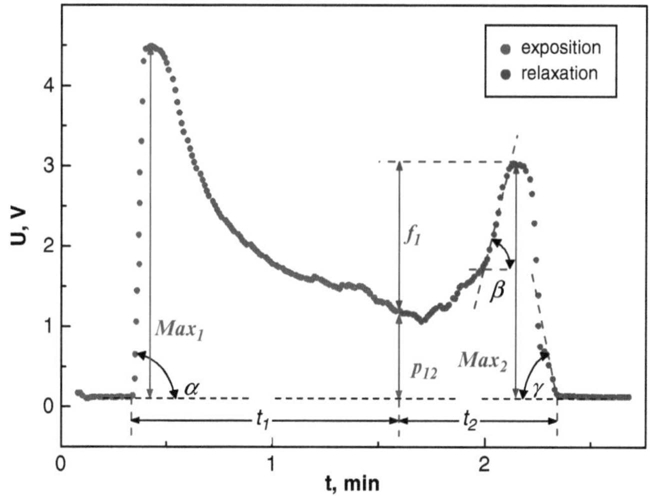

Fig. 7.3 A typical TCNQ compound-based point-contact multistructure sensor response curve. U – sensor voltage, *t* – time. Parameters of the sensor response curve: absolute value of the exposition maximum (Max_1); absolute value of the relaxation maximum (Max_2); ordinate of the final segment of the exposition phase (p_{12}); ratio between the height of relaxation maximum above the exposition signal's final level and its absolute value [$(Max_1 - p_{12})/Max_1$]; relation of the height of the relaxation maximum to the absolute value of this maximum (f_1/Max_2); slope of the initial segment of the exposition phase ($x = tg\alpha$); slope of the initial segment of the relaxation phase ($y = tg\beta$); slope of the end segment of the relaxation phase ($z = tg\gamma$); difference between the maxima of the speed of velocities change at the beginning and at the end of exposition ($g = x - z$); time of exposition (t_1); time of relaxation (t_2)

Due to a combination of the modified technique for sensor analysis of composite gas mixture with unique properties of the gas-sensitive point-contact matrix, a complex dynamic of interaction between sensitive matter and volatile compounds of exhaled air has been observed. This interaction is characterized by longer adsorption times. This behavior was not observed in our previous work on breath analysis; where film samples were used [11].

During the exposition time the sensor resistance dropped down to 2MΩ, and returned again to the initial value after the end of exposition. It is possible to conclude that during the gas-sensor contact certain components of the human exhaled air were adsorbed on the gas-sensitive point-contact matrix causing a significant improvement of its conductive properties. Exposition to exhaled air of the sensor surface shifted the adsorption-desorption equilibrium attained upon the contact of sensor with atmospheric air. Some molecules from breath mixture were adsorbed by the surface of the TCNQ compound changing its structure and respectively its electric conductivity. The rate of adsorption is directly proportional to the concentration of the gas molecules which are being adsorbed, as well as to the surface concentration of the vacant active centers. During further contact of the sensor with exhaled air, the adsorption rate decreases steadily because of the decrease of the concentration of active centers. After interruption of exposition to breath, the reverse process of gas desorption from the surface leads to the resistance increase and restores the initial potential of the gas-sensitive substance in contact with atmosphere.

Due to their complex non-monotonous structure the obtained response curves of the new type sensors are much more informative than those of traditional and nano-structured chemical sensors.

A phenomenological model based on fundamental representations of the sensor structure and intrinsic processes has been proposed to explain the mechanism of signal formation [30, 31].

The experiments have shown that all exhaled air ingredients can be divided into two groups, depending on their ability to change the current of the output signal, i.e. the stimulating and the inhibiting group. Differences between the two groups of compounds are determined by their adsorption and absorption behavior and by various chemical interactions taking place in contact with the sensitive element. Exhaled air components of one group are characterized by the ability to form current-conducting structures on the surface of gas-sensitive point-contact matrix, the so-called clusters of conductivity. Substances of the second group lead to formation of highly resistant structures, i.e., the clusters of resistivity. The dynamics of these processes is different. Increase in concentration of conductivity clusters causes a steep increase of the signal front slope. It probably indicates the dominating role of adsorption at this stage unless it is complicated by diffusion process. Growth of resistivity clusters concentration is characterized by a more moderate slope. That is apparently caused by the contribution of slow processes which accompany superficial or bulk diffusion. The concept of two types of clusters suggests that gas analytes may form structures which have an opposite impact on the conductivity.

Using this phenomenological model the sensor response may be described as follows. As mentioned above, the output signal of the sensor is registered by measuring voltage drop on a standard high precision resistor connected in series with the sensitive element. The voltage level is directly proportional to the current flowing through the sensor, and, respectively is determined by change of the sensor conductivity. During the contact with human breath the ingredients of the exhaled air are adsorbed or absorbed by the surface of the gas-sensitive element. The compounds with higher surface adsorption energy dominate the adsorption. This process causes decrease of the sensitive matter resistance and increase of the electric current in the circuit. The beginning of exposition is characterized by rapid current growth which is due to a progressive formation of conductivity clusters. Later the exposition maximum is reached as a result of competitive adsorption of exhaled air components. The competitive adsorption process is probably comprised of the following steps. At first the kinetically-controlled surface concentrations of the adsorbed compounds redistribute so that the content of components with higher adsorption energies increases. If exhaled air ingredients form less conductive surface clusters, the output signal decreases to a level which is lower than the initial level of response. Commonly it takes less than a minute for the output signal to reach a quasi-stationary state in the presence of exhaled air.

Asymmetry of the response curve to the point of the exposition end reflects the different nature of the exposition and relaxation output signals. A transition from an exposition into relaxation phase corresponds to a return of gas-sensitive matter contact with the initial atmosphere. A variety of processes take place simultaneously in that phase. They may include oxidation of adsorbed molecules by the air oxygen, desorption of the previously adsorbed molecules, competitive adsorption of the ambient atmosphere components. These circumstances cause a complicated shape of the relaxation curve. In general, its course reflects the dynamics of the surface concentration of conductivity clusters. Almost all relaxation curves are characterized by presence of a maximum. It is often more prominent that the corresponding exposition maximum. The origin of this phenomenon is determined by higher conductivity of clusters formed by the oxidized molecules of compounds adsorbed during the exposition phase.

Using the phenomenological model described above it is possible to identify characteristics of the output signal correlating with the exhaled air composition. An ordinate of the final almost stationary segment of the exposition curve can be taken as a basic integrating parameter. It corresponds to the surface concentration of conductivity clusters formed by the adsorbed components of exhaled air at given electrode potential difference. The ratio between the height of relaxation maximum above the final level of the exposition signal and its absolute value characterize behavior of those adsorbed ingredients in oxidized state which form clusters with higher conductivity.

Exposition maximum reflects the amount of adsorbed ingredients which form conductivity clusters. The ratio between the height of exposition maximum above the final level of the exposition signal and its absolute value, characterize behavior of ingredients forming clusters with higher conductivity during adsorption.

The dynamics of the output signal formation is very informative as regards the exhaled air composition. The slope of the initial segment of exposition curve is directly proportional to the concentration of the adsorbed compounds and adsorption energy. It is inversely proportional to the activation energy of the formation of conductivity clusters. The higher is the probability of surface cluster formation, the larger is the difference between the exhaled air compound adsorption energy and adsorption energy of the ambient atmosphere component which occupies active center. But the molecule has to be able to overcome an energy barrier for successful adsorption [32]. The lower is the barrier, the larger is the number of molecules that may pass it, i.e., the higher is the speed of the process, and correspondingly, the steeper the front slope of the exposition curve.

The dynamics of signal increase at the beginning of relaxation phase reflects the rate of cluster oxidation catalyzed by the gas sensitive substance. The higher is the slope of the face front of relaxation maximum, the faster is the rate of the process.

Finally, the dynamics of the back front of the relaxation maximum formation is also informative. This part of the curve characterizes the gross process of the conductivity clusters decomposition. The decomposition process comprises (1) desorption of the exhaled air components from the gas sensitive matter and (2) oxidation of these components by the atmospheric oxygen at the beginning of relaxation.

Formally, active centers are replaced by molecules of the atmospheric components. This process is to a great measure reversible at the beginning of the exposition. But there are certain differences in the nature of desorption and oxidation steps. They arise from two major factors influencing the desorption energy. On the one hand, there are temporary structural transformations of the adsorbed complexes which involve the atmospheric and exhaled air components and on the other hand the transformations are due to interaction (oxidation) of the adsorbed species with the atmospheric oxygen. The difference in the speed of signal change between the initial and final segments of the output signal may allow estimation of these factors.

Time parameters of response curve may also contain important information concerning the behavior of the components of the "gas-sensitive point-contact multistructure-analyte" system. The time required for signal stabilization in the exposition phase is directly proportional to the concentration of molecules with higher adsorption energy. The relaxation time characterizes integral value of the adsorption energy of all ingredients of the gas medium under study.

The proposed phenomenological model of the nature of the response signal of the TCNQ derivatives-based point-contact multistructure sensor enables an application of a complex statistical analysis of its components. It can be applied to exhaled air analysis for diagnostic purposes. The complex response of TCNQ compound-based point-contact multistructure sensor to the exhaled air of human breath can be considered as a kind of point-contact gas spectrum. It is known that the exhaled human breath contains 400–600 volatile organic compounds (VOCs) [2]. Exhaled air is a highly complex system with a large amount of equilibrium and non-equilibrium dynamic interactions among its constituents. The components of such a rich gas mixture form a certain breath profile reflecting specific organism dysfunctions and metabolic disturbances. Registration of this profile provides a simple and effective approach to the solution of complicated diagnostic problems without actual determination of individual components of exhaled air. This approach is opposite to a conventional determination of separate biomarkers. Endeavors to find correlations between the health state of human organism and concentrations of particular VOCs are coupled with an unavoidable loss of valuable information; as such an approach disregards many metabolic dynamic interactions in the biological object. To this end, registration of point-contact multistructure sensor response for the action of human breath with further statistical analysis of the obtained profile, in principle can be a fine and easy-to-use method for noninvasive medical diagnosis, which is similar to the procedure of electrocardiogram interpretation. The proposed approach provides the possibility to avoid a set of complex fundamental problems typical of conventional sensor analysis, in particular, determination of linear range of detection of the analyte, drift of sensor characteristics during longitudinal measurements and influence of the VOCs present in the air in close to their breath concentrations. The point-contact multistructure sensor method is similar to the solution of analytical problems by means of point-contact spectroscopy [23], which generates highly reliable results. Recording of breath profile spectra allows for characterization of pathological processes.

Table 7.1 Mean values (means) and standard errors of the means (SEM) of relaxation time t_2 and maxima of exposition-to-relaxation ratio Max_1/Max_2 of TCNQ sensor response curves obtained with exhaled air of patients with gastric and duodenal inflammation

Characteristics of the response curve	Patients with gastric and duodenal inflammation, degree of severity					
	Severe (ulcers and erosions) $n=20$		Mild $n=96$		Controls $n=38$	
	Mean	SEM	Mean	SEM	Mean	SEM
t_2 (min)	1.7*	0.3	1.1	0.04	1.1	0.1
Max_1/Max_2	1.3	0.2	1.4	0.1	1.3	0.3

n – number of subjects
*$p<0.05$ compared to patients with superficial inflammation and controls

This approach has been successfully applied to diagnostics development and important correlations between the parameters of the response curve and the health state of human organism have been discovered.

As an example of potential clinical application of the proposed theoretical model, preliminary results of a phase I clinical trial are described below. We estimated the values of relaxation time t_2 and ratio Max_1/Max_2 in adolescents with different results of endoscopy. We found that the mean relaxation time was significantly longer in subjects with a severe gastric and duodenal inflammation, namely, with ulcers and erosions compared to a healthy control group ($p<0.05$). The exhaled air of patients with milder forms of the disease and of the control group caused faster sensor relaxation after their interaction (Table 7.1).

It is known that chronic active inflammation in the gastric mucosa involves several interleukins (IL-8, IL-10 and IFN-gamma) known as immunological markers of the blood serum [33]. Hence it is possible that extensive gastric inflammation would lead to an increased release of some of the volatile inflammatory biomarkers in breath causing differences in the sensor response.

7.4 Conclusions

This study demonstrates high efficacy and expediency of the TCNQ derivative-based point-contact multistructure as a prospective asset for development of new sensors. The complex character of the sensors response curve and correlation of some response characteristics with different pathological manifestations in human breath, may be further used as a noninvasive diagnostic method alternative to some invasive approaches currently routinely used in clinic. The need for reliable and feasible gas analysis methods functional in presence of atmospheric air, opens opportunities for application of the proposed sensor technique in other spheres of human activity. High sensitivity of the point-contact multistructure enabling analysis of composite gas mixtures, opens up wide possibilities to apply the demonstrated approach for environment and health protection, such as detection of trace amounts of pollutants in atmosphere and presence of dangerous explosives and toxic substances in the air.

Acknowledgments We acknowledge V. Gudimenko for assistance in assessment of the results.

References

1. Dweik RA, Amann A (2008) Exhaled breath analysis: the new frontier in medical testing. J Breath Res 2(3):030301, 3 pp
2. Amann A, Smith D (eds) (2005) Breath analysis for medical diagnosis and therapeutic monitoring. World Scientific Publ, New Jersey-London-Singapore, p 536
3. Kushch I, Arendacka B, Stolc S et al (2008) Breath isoprene - aspects of normal physiology related to age, gender and cholesterol profile as determined in a proton transfer reaction mass spectrometry study. Clin Chem Lab Med 46(7):1011–1018
4. Kushch I, Schwarz K, Schwentner L et al (2008) Compounds enhanced in a mass spectrometric profile of smokers' exhaled breath versus non-smokers as determined in a pilot study using PTR-MS. J Breath Res 2(2):026002, 26 pp
5. Smith D, Španel P (2007) The challenge of breath analysis for clinical diagnosis and therapeutic monitoring. Analyst 132(5):390–396
6. Kharitonov SA, Barnes PJ (2001) Exhaled markers of pulmonary disease. Am J Respir Crit Care Med 163(7):1693–1722
7. Braden B, Haisch M, Duan LP et al (1994) Clinically feasible stable-isotope technique at a reasonable price - analysis of 13CO2/12CO2-abundance in breath samples with a new isotope selective nondispersive infrared spectrometer. Zeitschrift fur Gastroenterologie 32(12):675–678
8. Corradi M, Montuschi P, Donnelly LE et al (2001) Increased nitrosothiols in exhaled breath condensate in inflammatory airway diseases. Am J Respir Crit Care Med 163(4):854–858
9. Smith D, Španel P (2005) Selected ion flow tube mass spectrometry (SIFT-MS) for on-line trace gas analysis. Mass Spectrom Rev 24(5):661–700
10. Voznesensky NA, Chuchalin AG, Antonov NS (1998) Nitric oxide and lungs. Pulmonology N2:6–10
11. Kamarchuk GV, Pospyelov OP, Alexandrov YL et al (2005) TCNQ derivatives-based sensors for breath gas analysis. In: Amann A, Smith D (eds) Breath analysis for medical diagnosis and therapeutic monitoring. World Scientific Publ, New Jersey-London-Singapore, pp 85–99
12. Kuzmych O, Allen BL, Star A (2007) Carbon nanotube sensors for exhaled breath components. Nanotechnology 18:375502, 7 pp
13. de Lacy Costello BPJ, Ewen RJ, Ratcliffe NM (2008) A sensor system for monitoring the simple gases hydrogen, carbon monoxide, hydrogen sulfide, ammonia and ethanol in exhaled breath. J Breath Res 2(3):037011, 19 pp
14. Burke CS, Moore JP, Wencel D, MacCraith BD (2008) Development of a compact optical sensor for real-time, breath-by-breath detection of oxygen. J Breath Res 2:037012, 7 pp
15. Gelperin A, Johnson ATC (2008) Nanotube-based sensor arrays for clinical breath analysis. J Breath Res 2:037015, 6 pp
16. Higgins C, Wencel D, Burke S et al (2008) Novel hybrid optical sensor materials for in-breath O2 analysis. Analyst 133(2):241–247
17. Ishida H, Satou T, Tsuji K et al (2008) The breath ammonia measurement of the hemodialysis with a QCM-NH3 sensor. Biomed Mater Eng 18(2):99–106
18. Haick H, Hakim M, Patrascu M et al (2009) Sniffing chronic renal failure in rat model by an array of random networks of single-walled carbon nanotubes. ACS NANO 3(5):1258–1266
19. Fraden J (2004) Handbook of modern sensors. physics, designs, and applications. Springer Verlag, New York

20. Huang XJ, Choi YK (2007) Chemical sensors based on nanostructured materials. Sensor Actuat B 122(2):659–671
21. Kamarchuk GV, Pospelov OP, Yeremenko AV et al (2006) Point-contact sensors: New prospects for a nanoscale-sensitive technique. Europhys Lett 76(4):575–581
22. Kamarchuk GV, Kolobov IG, Khotkevich AV et al (2008) New chemical sensors based on point heterocontact between single wall carbon nanotubes and gold wires. Sensor Actuat B 134(2):1022–1026
23. Naidyuk YuG, Yanson IK (2004) Point-contact spectroscopy. Springer Verlag, New York
24. Krans JM, Ruitenbeek JM, Fisun VV et al (1995) The signature of conductance quantization in metallic point contacts. Nature 375:767–769
25. Pospelov AP, Ved MV, Sakhnenko ND et al (2002) High-conductivity organic metals as electrode materials. Mater Sci 20(3):65–72
26. Starodub VA, Gluzman EM, Pokhodnya KI, MYa V (1994) Thermophysical and electrophysical properties of conductive organic composites based on salts of TCNQ and methyl-TCNQ. Theor Exp Chem 29(4):240–244
27. Chubov PN, Yanson IK, Akimenko AI (1982) Electron-phonon interaction in aluminum point contacts. Fizika Nizkikh Temperatur (Sov Low Temp Phys) 8(1):64–80
28. Norušis MJ (2008) SPSS 16.0 advanced statistical procedures companion. Prentice Hall, Upper Saddle River, NJ
29. Kim YS, Ha SC, Kim K et al (2005) Room-temperature semiconductor gas sensor based on nonstoichiometric tungsten oxide nanorod film. Appl Phys Lett 86(21):213105-1–213105-3
30. Cattrall RW (1997) Chemical sensors. Oxford University Press, Oxford, New York-Melbourne
31. Salem RR (2003) Theory of double layer. FIZMATLIT Publ, Moscow, Russia
32. Thomas JM, Thomas WJ (1967) Introduction to the principles of heterogeneous catalysis. Academic, London-New York
33. Andersen LP, Holck S, Janulaityte-Gunther D et al (2005) Gastric inflammatory markers and interleukins in patients with functional dyspepsia, with and without Helicobacter pylori infection. FEMS Immunol Med Microbiol 44(2):233–238

Chapter 8
Express Instrumental Diagnostics of Diseases Caused by Retroviral Infections

N.F. Starodub

Abstract A surface plasmon resonance (SPR) based immune biosensor for rapid diagnostics of bovine leucosis (BL) caused by retroviruses, is described. BL was detected through the specific antibody (Ab) to the antigen (Ag) of the virus in blood and milk serum. Sensitivity of the analysis achieved by this biosensor is similar to that of the ELISA method and much higher than the radial immunodiffusion test. The optimal dilutions of the blood and milk serum were 1:500 and 1:20 respectively. The turnaround time of the analysis was less than 30 min including the time for the Ag immobilization on the transducer surface, blocking free binding sites, Ag-Ab interaction and all washing procedures. This time may be further shortened to 5 min if the transducer surface is prepared in advance. Pre-treatment of the gold surface with dodecanethiol increases sensitivity of the analysis in comparison with the untreated surface. In contrast to the ELISA method, the immune biosensor technique allows analysis without additional labelled molecules.

Keywords Express diagnostics • Instrumental diagnostics • Retroviral infections

8.1 Introduction

Viral leucosis is the tumour disease of the hemolymphopoietic system which is characterized by the malignant expansions of the blood-derived tissues and abnormalities of the process of cell maturation, mainly with the formation of young cells. All mammalian species, birds and fish may be infected by this virus.

N.F. Starodub (✉)
National University of Life and Environmental Sciences of Ukraine, 15 Herojev Oboroni Str, Kiev 03041, Ukraine
e-mail: nikstarodub@yahoo.com

S. Mikhalovsky and A. Khajibaev (eds.), *Biodefence*, NATO Science for Peace and Security Series A: Chemistry and Biology, DOI 10.1007/978-94-007-0217-2_8,

In particular this disease is widespread among bovine species, and it is registered in many countries on every continent. There are data suggesting that humans are sensitive to the animal leucosis. The existing data testify that humans and especially men may be affected by leucosis through drinking milk [1]. This disease has a long incubation period without any visible changes in the animal health, which is one of its peculiarities. The main cause of bovine leucosis (BL) is a V-type virus from the retrovirus family and the genus of oncoviruses. These viruses contain six proteins and the most important among them are the surface glycoprotein *gp51* and the internal *p24* polypeptide [2, 3]. The prophylaxis and treatment of BL are complicated due to its wide spread infection. The main source of this disease is the infected animals that are introduced into healthy herds. Improvement of the diagnostic methods, that are capable of revealing sick animals in the early stages of the disease, is a very important and urgent step. At present, radial immunodiffusion (RID) and ELISA are the main methods of the laboratory diagnosis of BL [4–6]. Blood samples from the jugular vein are used for the analysis. The mass observations of the animals should be carried out every 4 months. In cases where the disease is discovered, it is necessary to perform analysis every 10 days for the duration of 6 months. It is not possible to assess the entire epizootic situation by the existing analytical methods due to their high costs and invasiveness leading to high rates of animal trauma. There is a high demand for the development of a new sensitive and specific, simple and rapid diagnostic method for BL detection in the early stages. A device based on the principles of biosensorics can be a viable alternative to RID and ELISA.

The use of optical immune biosensors based on surface plasmon resonance (SPR) for the diagnostics of human and animal diseases as well as for environmental pollution monitoring, is one of prospective directions in biosensorics. The sensitivity of immune biosensors is similar to the ELISA-method but the simplicity of obtaining results in the real time regime and the speed of the analysis are the main advantages of the biosensor approach. Performance of optical biosensors based on SPR depends on the state of the metallic surface as well as on the density, structure and the space volume of the immobilized molecules. It was demonstrated that the application of intermediate layers between the transducer surface and the sensitive biological molecules can optimize the working characteristics of the immune biosensor [7–14].

The search for new approaches which can give increasing sensitivity to SPR-based biosensors is associated with the optimization of immobilization of the biological components on the transducer surface.

Our investigation was aimed at the development of the instrumental method for the diagnostics of BL with the help of the immune SPR-based biosensor which is able to determine viral specific Ab in the blood and milk serum. Such a biosensor should provide: (1) direct analysis without any additional reagents; (2) obtaining results within 3–5 min; (3) use of milk samples instead of blood and (4) low cost analysis (less than ELISA).

8.2 Experimental

The immune biosensor analysis was carried out in the SPR-4 M device produced by the Institute of Physics of Semiconductors of the Ukrainian National Academy of Sciences. SPR spectroscopy was carried out in the Kretschmann configuration using He-Ne laser ($\lambda = 632.8$ nm), goniometer (G-5 M), glass prism (the angle at the basis 68°) and photodiode (FD 263). The optical contact between the prism and the metallic layer was achieved by the application of polyphenyl ether (refractive index $n = 1.62$).

It is well known that the SPR may be registered as the sharp minimum of the reflection coefficient for the plane-parallel light which depends on the incidence angle. The position of the resonance angle and the minimum depth of the incidence are determined by the parameters of the metal layer, and the optical constants of the external medium. As molecules adsorb and interact at the gold surface, the dielectric properties of the formed layer change, which leads to the transformation of the resonance curve and to the displacement of the resonance angle [7, 9, 15].

For the modification of the gold surface different chemical and biological substances (dodecanethiol, lectins, dextran sulfate DS, with the mass of 5 kDa and polyelectrolytes) were used. The mercaptane layer was formed in ethanol at10^{-3} M concentration of thiol. Polyaniline hydrochloride (PAH), "Aldrich", USA, was used to cover the transducer surface by a water insoluble polymer. Lectins from *Phaseolus vulgaris* (PLA), *Solanum tuberosum* (STA), *Helix pomatia* (HPA) and *Tuberosum vulgaris* (WGA) were immobilized on the surface pre-treated with dodecanethiol or PAH. These lectins were used for the immobilization of glycoproteins. Blocking of the free binding sites was carried out with 1% bovine serum albumin (BSA).

A purified viral Ag was obtained from "Leiconad" company (Poltava, Ukraine). For the procedure of the immobilization, Ag was dissolved at the concentration of 2 mg/mL in 0.01 M phosphate buffer (pH 8.2) containing 0.14 M sodium chloride (PBS).

The blood and milk serum from Poltava and Lugansk regions of Ukraine were supplied by "Leiconad". Serum dilutions from 1:50 to 1:20000 were prepared in PBS (pH 7.4). The blood serum of the immunized animals was obtained from 6 to 12 months old calves after their vaccination with the medication developed by "Leiconad". To prepare milk serum the fresh sample was acidified with 5% acetic acid and then centrifuged for 15 min at 400 g.

Both RID and ELISA were used as the control tests for detection of the specific anti-viral Ab. Anti-bovine Ab labeled with the horse radish peroxidase ("Sigma", USA) was used in the ELISA assays. IDEX system (USA) served as the control.

The standard stocks of the positive and negative serum were obtained from the State Research Institute of Biotechnology and Strains of Microorganisms Control of the Ministry of Agroindustrial Policy of Ukraine as well as from the National Reference Laboratory for EBI (Federal Research Institute for Animal Health, Germany).

8.3 Results and Discussion

Initially, the possibility to use the preparations of the viral Ag's commercially produced by the "Leiconad" company (Ukraine) and by the Kursk Pharmaceutical Plant (Russian Federation) for the RID test were tested. It was stated by the manufacturers that these preparations require additional purification to increase the concentration of the Ag markers which should be immobilized on the transducer surface. We used the antigen after the extra purification by chromatography on porous glass for our following experiments.

The retention of the Ag physically adsorbed by the transducer surface is strong and the adsorbed molecules were not desorbed by washing with a buffer solution. The Ag immobilization was accompanied by a change of the resonance angle within 1,000–1,200 angular seconds (arcseconds). After the treatment of the transducer surface with BSA the resonance angle did not change. It means that the number of the free binding sites was minimal and the Ag concentration was enough for the formation of a dense layer. At the introduction of the specific antiserum of infected cows into the measuring SPR cell the value of the biosensor response correlated with the degree of its dilution. Thus it was confirmed that the purified viral Ag allows detection of the antigen specific Ab in the blood serum at 1:16,000 dilution. At the same time the Ab titer in the RID was 1:256 (Fig. 8.1).

As the next step of investigation, 10 RID-positive (with the titer of 1:64–1:128), 18 RID-negative and 15 RID-dubious (which formed the precipitation line at 1:4 dilution) samples were identified. It was found that the immune biosensor is sensitive to Ab diluted in the serum up to 16,000 times. The change of the resonance angle varied from 700 to 1,000 angular seconds. In the samples which were identified as RID-dubious, the presence of the specific Ab was detected at the serum diluted up to 500–1,000 times.

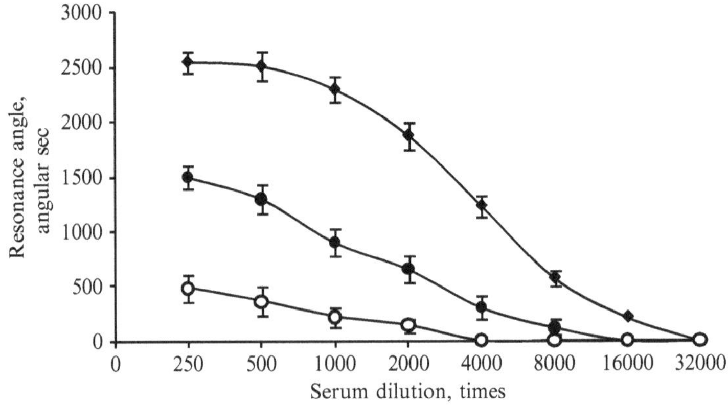

Fig. 8.1 The change of the resonance angle of the immune biosensor in bovine blood serum tests: 1–3 – RID-positive, RID-dubious and RID-negative, respectively

The largest differences in the results were obtained in the analysis of RID-negative samples. The sera of the vaccinated animals induced the Ab-specific signal of the immune biosensor.

8.3.1 Optimization of the Viral Ag Immobilization on the Transducer Surface

Since the sensitivity of the immune biosensor is very high, we chose the most simple and highly efficient Ag immobilization approaches (Fig. 8.2).

8.3.1.1 Modification of the Surface by Dodecanethiol and PAH

Pre-treatment of the transducer surface with PAH increased the amount of the immobilized Ag and the response of the immune biosensor was much more stable in comparison with the bare gold surface. The sensor with Ag immobilized after pre-treatment with PAH served for 2 months versus 2–3 weeks for Ag deposited on the bare surface. Ag immobilization on the PAH layer increased the sensitivity of the immune biosensor by 15–20% in comparison with Ag immobilized on the bare surface. At the same time dodecanethiol did not affect the biosensor sensitivity but increased its service life.

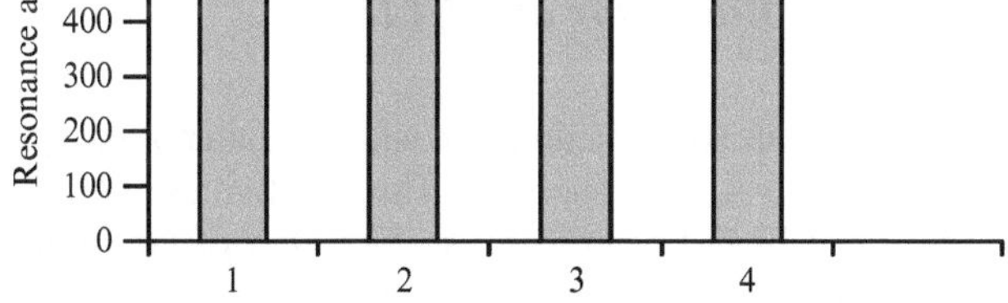

Fig. 8.2 Response of SPR immune biosensor to the introduction of the blood serum at the dilution of 1:500 in the measuring cell which has a different transducer surface: 1 – bare gold, 2 – dodecanethiol, 3 – PAH, 4 – dextran sulfate

8.3.1.2 Modification of the Transducer Surface by Dextran Sulfate

Modification with dextran sulfate increased the signal by 20% in comparison with the bare surface. Unfortunately, this approach has the disadvantage of a relatively high cost of dextran sulfate.

Ten blood serum samples from sick cows were investigated, for which the extinction coefficient in the ELISA assays was 2.0–2.5 at 1:500 dilution. PAH, dodecanethiol and dextran sulfate were used for the intermediate layer formation. The maximal sensitivity was observed when the transducer surface was pre-treated with PAH and this method was used in further experiments.

8.3.1.3 Application of Lectins for the Detection of Ab to Viral Glycoproteins in the Blood Serum

The preliminary results showed that the blood serum of healthy animals and the vaccinated ones both contained a high titer of the virus specific Ab. It is necessary therefore to resolve the question of how to distinguish sick from vaccinated animals.

The main viral Ag proteins are *gp51* and *p24*. The vaccine from the "Leiconad" company contains inner proteins, in particular, *p24*. To differentiate the sick from vaccinated cows the glycolated protein *gp51* can be used. It can be immobilized on the transducer surface through the intermediate layer created from various lectins. It was found that among all the lectins tested (PLA, STA, HPA and WGA), PLA and WGA were the most suitable lectins, especially the latter. The application of WGA generates the maximal response of the immune biosensor.

We studied the response of the immune biosensor with WGA-treated transducer surface in the analysis of the blood serum of vaccinated animals, which had Ab titer 1:128–1:256 according to the data obtained from RID test. It was found that the response of the immune biosensor to the blood serum of the sick and vaccinated animals was considerably different. In case of the non-modified transducer surface no difference was observed.

8.3.2 Comparison of the Results Obtained Using the Immune Biosensor and ELISA

Blood serum samples from 10 sick animals in which the titer of the specific Ab was 1:256 according to RID test, were analyzed. The sensitivities of both methods (the immune biosensor and ELISA) were similar. The limit of the serum dilution for detection of the specific antibodies was 1:15,000.

In a separate experiment, 20 samples of the blood serum provided by the State Research Institute of Biotechnology and Strains of Microorganisms Control of the Ministry of Agroindustrial Policy of Ukraine, were studied. These samples were

Table 8.1 Comparison of the results obtained by the immune biosensor, ELISA and PCR methods

	SPR immune biosensor		ELISA		
Sample N	Resonance angle, angular sec	Characteristic reaction	Extinction, r.u.	Characteristic reaction	PCR
1	0	–	0.028	–	–
2	1,330	+	3.456	+	+/–
3	30	–	0.00	–	–
4	1,120	+	2.504	+	+/–
5	20	–	0.00	–	–
6	980	+	2.512	+	+
7	0	–	0.00	–	–
8	120	+	0.02	–	+/–
9	60	–	2.444	+	–
10	140	+	0.014	–	–
11	0	–	0.01	–	–
12	800	+	2.444	+	–
13	50	–	0.01	–	–
14	1,420	+	3.262	+	+
15	980	+	2.860	+	+
16	1,190	+	3.252	+	+
17	1,300	+	3.892	+	+
18	250	+	0.00	–	+/–
19	890	+	3.173	+	+
20	0	–	0.00	–	–

analyzed by the immune biosensor, ELISA and by the polymerase chain reaction (PCR) method. For the immune biosensor analysis the serum samples were diluted 1:500. In 90% of experiments the results obtained by all three methods were in good agreement (Table 8.1).

Similar tests were carried out with the blood serum obtained from the National Reference Laboratory for EBI (Federal Research Institute for Animal Health, Germany). In this case a pool of 21 serum samples was analyzed. The results of three methods were in agreement except for two samples for which ELISA tests were low positive, whereas the immune biosensor analysis results were negative.

8.3.3 Detection of the Viral Specific Ab in the Milk Serum

The detection of viral specific Ab in milk serum is very important since the use of milk serum for the analysis rather than blood avoids physical injuries to the animals and extends the potential of the analytical method. We examined 15 samples of milk from RID-positive cows in the blood serum of which the titer of the viral specific Ab was 1:64–1:256. Simultaneously 10 samples of the milk from RID-negative cows

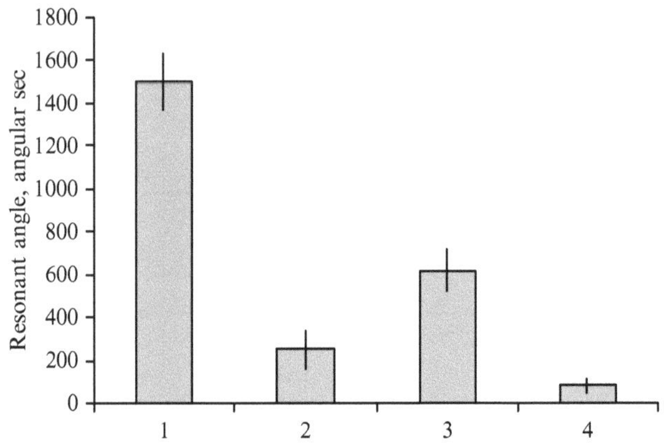

Fig. 8.3 The resonance angle of the immune biosensor in the analysis of the blood and milk serum.1,2 – blood serum, dilution 1:500, from RID-positive and RID-negative cows, respectively; 3,4 – milk serum, dilution 1:20, from RID-positive and RID-negative cows, respectively

were analyzed. The response of the immune biosensor was within 1,500–1,600 and 600–650 angular seconds in the analysis of blood and milk serum from the RID-positive cows, respectively. The optimal milk dilution was 1:20 (Fig. 8.3). It is worth mentioning that the milk serum from the RID-negative cows gave a very low signal within 60–90 angular seconds.

8.4 Conclusions

Use of the developed immune biosensor in serological diagnostics meets the practical requirements, since it is sensitive, selective, quick and inexpensive. It allows for a reduction in real time analysis and can be performed directly in field conditions such as at a cattle-breeding farm. The sensitivity of the immune biosensor is similar to ELISA and much higher than the sensitivity of a conventional RID test. Overall, the immune biosensor analysis including the immobilization of the viral Ag, blocking of the residual binding sites, serum introduction and all washing procedures takes about 40 min. This time may be shortened up to 5–10 min if the transducer surface is prepared in advance. The optimal dilution of the blood and milk serum should be 1:500 and 1:20 respectively. The results of the immune biosensor analysis are in good agreement (up to 90% of tests) with those obtained by RID and ELISA. The registration part of the biosensor could be made portable and the transducer may be provided with removable plates containing the immobilized antigen. All these features of the immune biosensor analysis make it an efficient tool for use in veterinary medicine.

References

1. Donham KJ, Berg JW, Sawin RS (1980) Epidemiologic relationships of the bovine population and human leukemia in Iowa. Am J Epidemiol 112:80–92
2. Kukajn RA, Nagajeva LI (1983) Bovine leucosis virus. Znanije Publ, Riga, Latvia
3. Starodub NF, Starodub VM (2003) Infectious bovine leucosis and its diagnostics. Biopolym Cell 19:307–316
4. Nguyen VK, Maes RF (1993) Evaluation of an enzyme-linked immunosorbent assays for detection of antibodies to bovine leukemia virus in serum and milk. Clin Microbiol N4:979–981
5. Llames L, Goyache J, Domenech A et al (1999) Rapid detection of specific polyclonal and monoclonal antibodies against bovine leukemia virus. J Virol Methods 82:129–136
6. Carli KT, Sen A, Batmaz H, Minbay A (1999) Detection of IgG antibody to bovine leukaemia virus in urine and serum by two enzyme immunoassays. Lett Appl Microbiol 28:416–418
7. Kooyman RPH, DeBruijn HE, Eenink RG et al (1990) Surface plasmon resonance as a bioanalytical tool. Mol Structure 218:345–350
8. Liedberg B, Nylander C, Lundstrom I (1983) Surface plasmon resonance for gas detection and biosensing. Sensor Actuat B N4:299–304
9. Starodub NF, Dibrova TM, Shirshov YM, Kostyukevych KV (1999) Ukr Biochem J 41:33–37
10. Starodub NF, Starodub VM (2000) Immune sensors: origin, achievements and perspectives. Ukr Biochem J 72:147–163
11. Starodub NF, Nabok AV, Starodub VM et al (2001) Immobilization of biocomponents for immune optical sensors. Ukr Biochem J 73:16–24
12. Starodub NF, Starodub VM (2001) Electrochemical and optical biosensors: origin of development, achievements and perspectives of practical application. In: Bozoglu F (ed) NATO Proc "Novel Processes and Control Technologies in the Food Industry". Cluwer Acad Publ, Turkey, pp 1–246
13. Starodub NF, Starodub VM (2003) Structuring of the recognizing elements of the biosensors. Genetic constructions for the direct immobilization and combination of the structures which are able to recognize the analyzed substances and to generate the specific signals. Ukr Biochim J 75:37–44
14. Starodub NF, Pirogova LV, Demchenko A, Nabok AV (2005) Antibody immobilization on the metal and silicon surface. The use of self-assembled layer and specific receptors. Bioelectrochem 66:111–115
15. Homola J, Yee SS, Gauglitz G (1999) Surface plasmon resonance sensor: review. Sensor Actuat B 54:3–15

Chapter 9
Nanostructured Silicon and its Application as the Transducer in Immune Biosensors

N.F. Starodub, L.M. Shulyak, O.M. Shmyryeva, I.V. Pylipenko, L.N. Pylipenko, and M.M. Mel'nichenko

Abstract New biosensors based on detection of the formation of specific antibody-antigen (Ab-Ag) immune complexes using the structured nanoporous silicon (sNPS) are proposed. We used boron doped single-crystal silicon with square wafers of 0.3 mm thickness and resistance of 1 Ohm*cm. sNPS layers with thickness of 3–60 nm were prepared. Electrical contacts were formed by magnetron sputtering of Al. The formation of the immune complex (specific antibody-T2 mycotoxin) was detected by the 2–5-fold increase of current depending on the antigen concentration in the sample. At the same time the sNPS photoluminescence sharply decreased. These biosensors may be applied for measuring the concentration of different substances which are capable of forming a specific complex. The proposed method may provide a simple and cost effective procedure for express control of toxic substances in field conditions.

Keywords Nanostructured silicon • Photoluminescence • Electro-conductivity • Immune biosensors • T2 mycotoxin

---

N.F. Starodub (✉) and L.M. Shulyak
National University of Life and Environmental Sciences, 15 Herojev Oboroni Str., Kyiv 03041, Ukraine
e-mail: nikstarodub@yahoo.com

O.M. Shmyryeva
National Technical University of Ukraine "KPI", 37 Prospect Peremogy, Kyiv 03056, Ukraine

I.V. Pylipenko and L.N. Pylipenko
National Academy of Food Technology, Odessa, Ukraine

M.M. Mel'nichenko
Taras Shevchenko Kiev National University, 2 Prospect Glushkova, Kyiv 03127, Ukraine

S. Mikhalovsky and A. Khajibaev (eds.), *Biodefence*, NATO Science for Peace and Security Series A: Chemistry and Biology, DOI 10.1007/978-94-007-0217-2_9,

9.1 Introduction

Currently, great attention is given to the study of nanostructured materials and their application in different areas including biosensors. Structured nanoporous silicon (sNPS) is one of such materials. Its geometrical, chemical, electronic and surface adsorptive properties are strongly dependent on the porosity, pore diameter and penetration depth into the monocrystalline silicon (mono-cSi). Creation of new types of electronic devices on the basis of sNPS requires developing preparation methods of sNPS with long-term stability of its properties. sNPS properties are determined by the quantum-dimensional effects but the complete understanding of the microstructure, its relation with the luminescence, transport and other properties have not been studied. Recently, a number of investigations have demonstrated a high stability of sNPS obtained by the chemical method [1–3].

9.2 Methods for sNPS Preparation

The technology of sNPS preparation in the form of so-called holes and strings is very complicated. Previously porous silicon was prepared by the electrochemical etching and chemical etching with nitric acid [3, 4]. A number of other methods were developed, in particular, re-crystallization of the amorphous silicon as a result of thermal annealing and chemical precipitation from the gas phase, thermal or laser evaporation and the high-frequency dispersion, precipitation by the voltaic arc and ionic synthesis in the SiO_2 matrix [3, 5–12]. As most of these methods require the use of complicated and expensive equipment, as well as high temperatures, for instance in thermal annealing, the electrochemical anode and chemical etchings are commonly used.

9.2.1 Preparation of sNPS by Chemical Etching

Chemical etching is simpler than the galvanic anodization and it forms a thin (less than 1 μm) homogeneous layer of sNPS. Chemical etching is carried out by immersing a silicon plate in a hydrofluoric acid based electrolyte containing and oxidizing agent. Dissolution of silicon occurs without any external voltage. The electrolyte usually contains HNO_3 (70%) or $NaNO_2$ as oxidants, with different concentrations of hydrofluoric acid: $HF:HNO_3:H_2O$ =1:5:10, or 1:3:5, or 4:1:5, or $HF:NaNO_2$ = 100 ml:2 g. The cathode reaction occurs through the oxidant reduction by electrons from the anode:

$$HNO_3 + 3H^+ \rightarrow NO + 2H_2O + 3h^+. \tag{9.1}$$

The complete chemical reaction on the Si surface may be presented as:

$$3Si + 4HNO_3 + 18HF \rightarrow 3H_2SiF_6 + 4NO + 8H_2O + 3(4-n)h^+ + 3(4-n)e^- \quad (9.2)$$

Unlike the electrochemical process chemical etching is a self regulated process which strongly depends on the initial solution content. The oxidant plays the same role in the etching as the anode current density in the electrochemical method. It means that a higher HNO_3 concentration corresponds to the higher electric current density. The content of HNO_3 is the most important parameter in chemical etching.

The position of the maximum in the photoluminescence spectra is independent of the oxidant type and appears at $\lambda \sim 625$ nm. The method of chemical etching is most adapted to mass manufacturing and it is currently used for the preparation of thin homogeneous luminescent layers of sNPS for sensor devices.

9.2.2 *Properties of sNPS*

By controlling the structural and electronic properties of sNPS which are related to the nanocrystallite dimensions and porosity, their surface selectivity and sensitivity to different gases (nitrogen and carbon oxide, vapors of water and organic substances) can be adjusted. This approach for the effective detection of acetone, methanol and water vapor in air was described in [13–15].The minimal detectable acetone concentration was reported to be 12 μg/mL. Silicon sensors for detection of SO_2 and some medicines such as penicillin were created [16–18]. sNPS were used for the development of a number of immune biosensors, particularly using the photoluminescence detection. Earlier we developed similar immune biosensors for the control of the myoglobin level in blood and for monitoring of bacterial proteins in air [19–23].

9.3 Experimental

9.3.1 *Some Characteristics of sNPS*

Our investigation of sNPS showed that the samples prepared by the chemical etching method described above have consistent photoluminescence, conductivity and photoconductivity properties, which have remained unchanged over 5 years. sNPS structure was investigated by scanning electronic microscopy (Fig. 9.1).

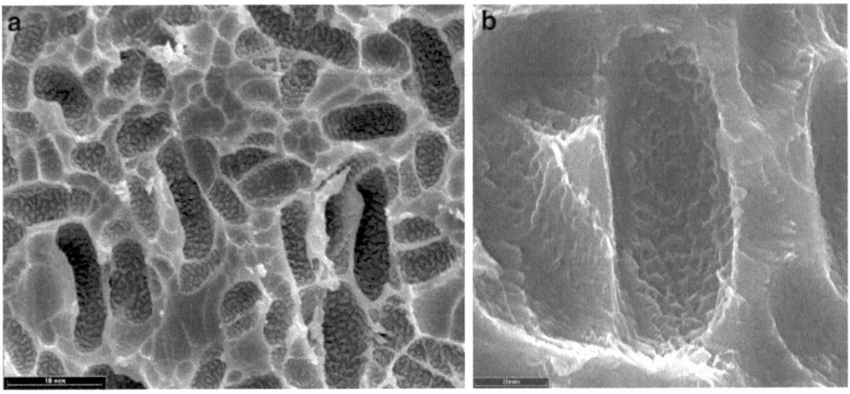

Fig. 9.1 SEM images of the sNPS surface: general view (**a**) and its fragment (**b**). The scale bar is 10 μm

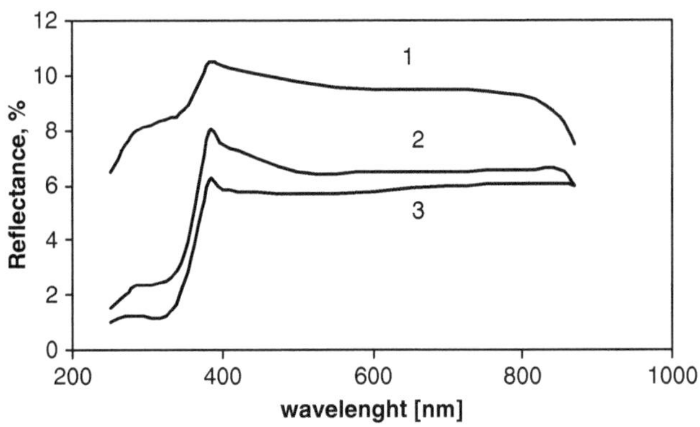

Fig. 9.2 Optical reflectance spectra of the sNPS layer depend on the nanocrystallite dimensions: *1* – 5 nm, *2* – 15 nm, *3* – 30 nm

The optical reflectance spectra were dependent on the nanocrystallite structure and dimensions, porosity and the layer thickness (Fig. 9.2). The maximal photosensitivity in the visible wavelength range of the spectra (30–35 mA/Lm) was typical of the sNPS layers with the nanocrystallite dimensions of 15 nm, and it decreased with increasing size of the nanocrystallites. The maximal sensitivity to the ultraviolet irradiation was obtained for sNPS layers with nanocrystallite dimensions of 20–25 nm. sNPS layers obtained by electrochemical etching as well as by chemical etching showed the photoluminescence typical of this material: a broad peak in the visible spectrum with the intensity sufficient for observation of the photoluminescence with a naked eye. sNPS samples obtained by chemical or electrochemical etching had intensive emission with the maximum at $\lambda \sim 640$ nm and 700 nm, respectively. The optimal chemical treatment conditions and duration of the etching were chosen to maximize the photoluminescence and the photoconductivity of the sNPS films.

The sNPS chemical composition was analyzed by the Auger spectroscopy. The results are shown in Fig. 9.3.

9.3.2 Photoconductivity of sNPS

The samples with a nanolayer of 15–18 nm thickness had the maximal photosensitivity. This result is in agreement with the results of the photoluminescence experiments (Fig. 9.4).

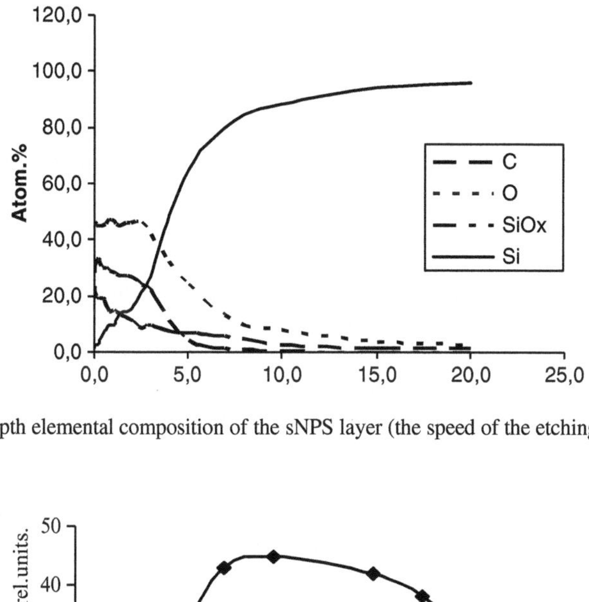

Fig. 9.3 In-depth elemental composition of the sNPS layer (the speed of the etching – 3 nm/min)

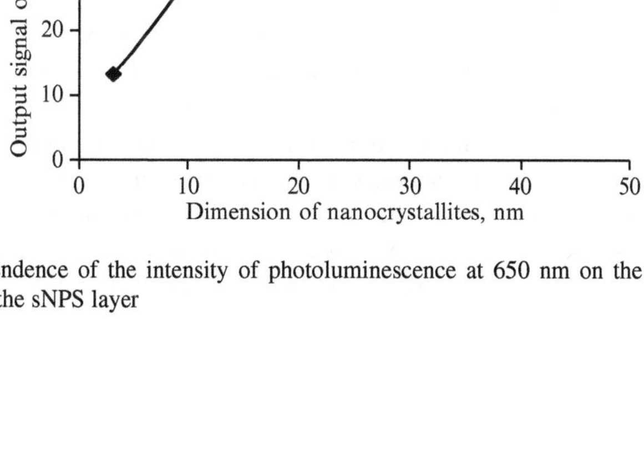

Fig. 9.4 Dependence of the intensity of photoluminescence at 650 nm on the nanocrystallite dimensions in the sNPS layer

9.3.3 Materials and Chemicals for the Immunochemical Analysis

The electrical (ohmic) contacts on the sNPS surface were made from aluminum by magnetron sputtering technique. It was found previously that the electrical contacts made from indium were unstable due to its mechanical softness. Their integrity was destroyed during measurements because of the porous surface underneath the contacts. In our investigations Al contacts with the thickness of about 3 μm were formed.

T2 mycotoxin was used as the antigen. *Fusarium tricinctum* during cultivation may form about 9 g of T2 toxin per 1 kg of the solid or liquid substrate with the final output of the crystalline product about 2–3 g/kg [24–26]. T2 mycotoxin is sometimes referred to as the biological weapon of omnicide [27–29] since its toxicity is more than 400 times higher than most other biological warfare agents [30].

The existing methods of mycotoxin analysis may be divided into two groups: biological and physicochemical methods. In biological methods different biological objects ranging from living vertebrate organisms to cell cultures are used. Unfortunately biotests have a lot of disadvantages as they are time consuming and require use of special laboratory techniques. Moreover, they are able to detect only some specific mycotoxin types. Physicochemical methods are based on thin-layer chromatography (the sensitivity is 2–2.5 μg/mL), gas-liquid chromatography (10 ng/mL), radioimmune analysis (2–5 ng/mL), immunochemical analysis (2–50 ng/mL), mass spectroscopy with gas liquid chromatography (1 ng/mL), and mass spectroscopy with high performance liquid chromatography (0.01 ng/mL) [31–34]. Although these methods are sensitive, they also require a large input of time and special laboratory conditions. It is necessary to develop detection techniques that can complete analysis in a very short time, and do it in field conditions or in an on-line regime.

For the express detection of some biochemical analytes we have developed biosensors based on surface plasmon resonance (SPR) and total internal reflection ellipsometry (TIRE) [28, 29, 35–40]. These biosensors are highly sensitive, easy to use and allow for rapid analysis [41]. However, they have some disadvantages, mainly the high cost of the chips and the necessity to use a complicated procedure for the preliminary treatment of the transducer surface. Moreover SPR and, in particular, TIRE recorders are very expensive and do not provide for a sufficient number of repeat analyses. Because of that other types of optical biosensors have been applied for express detection of toxins. Biosensors based on sNPS have attracted particular attention. Earlier we developed sNPS biosensors for the control of the myoglobin level in blood and for the monitoring of bacterial protein in the air [19–23]. The analyte specific signal was registered by measuring changes in the intensity of photoluminescence. This approach has met the practical requirements regarding the simplicity, sensitivity, selectivity and time of the analysis, but the stability of the sNPS biosensors was very low and the signal registration required a complicated device. In continuation of this work a new version of the immune biosensor based on sNPS has been proposed.

The semi-lethal dose of T2 mycotoxin is considered to be 5 mg/kg, although at a dose of 0.1 mg/kg vital changes in a number of biochemical indexes are observed. The maximal permitted concentration of this toxin in corn is 100 μg/kg [32, 34]. Taking into account this value we chose appropriate T2 mycotoxin concentrations for the experiments. Initially it was dissolved in ethanol and then diluted with 0.05 M Tris–HCl buffer (pH 7.3) to make a series of solutions with different concentrations. T2 mycotoxin was kindly provided by Dr. Kotik from the Institute of Poultry Farming (Ukraine). Specific antibodies (Ab) against T2 were purchased from Sigma (USA).

9.3.4 Detection of the Specific Immune Complex Using the sNPS Photoconductivity

Specific Ab against T2 (1 μL) were placed on the photo-resistor surface between the contacts (Fig. 9.5) and the solvent was evaporated at room temperature or in an air flow.

The direct voltage (5 V) from a stabilized power supply was applied to the ohmic contacts and the baseline current was measured by a digital voltmeter in the dark and the photocurrent was measured upon exposure of the sensitive surface to the white spectrum light source with illuminance of 7,000 lx. The difference between the light and dark currents was registered. The measurements of the dark and light currents were repeated after adding an Ab layer on the sensitive plate and after its drying. The time required for cleaning the sensor to its initial state was face by a buffer solution. A single analysis including loading of all biological materials, washing and drying takes only 30–40 min and it may be reduced by half, if the antibodies were immobilized on the surface in advance.

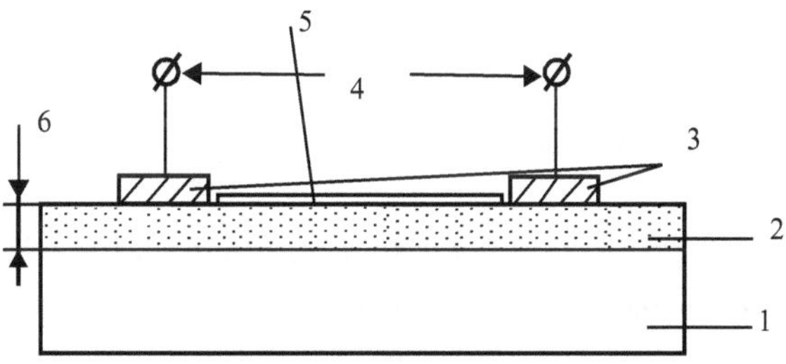

Fig. 9.5 Sketch of the sNPS based photoresistor for the analysis of biochemical solutes. *1* – crystalline silicon, *2* – sNPS, *3* – electrical contacts (Al with the thickness of ~3 μm), *4* – the applied voltage, *5* – the bioligand (Ab against T2), *6* – the thickness of the sNPS layer (10–40 nm)

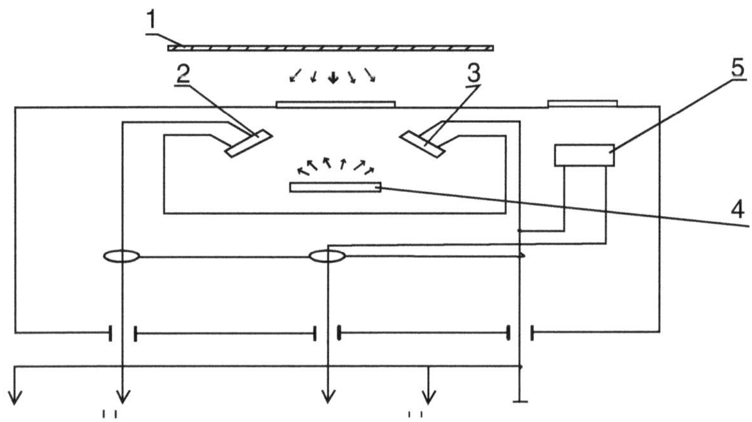

Fig. 9.6 Design of a photoluminescence biosensor (see explanation in the text)

9.3.5 Detection of the Specific Immune Complexes Using Photoluminescence of sNPS

The developed prototype includes a source of ultraviolet (UV) radiation (1) with the wavelength of 350 nm, two photodiodes (2 and 3) based on a silicon monocrystal and placed at the angle of 20–25° relative to the plate with sNPS layer (4) and a photodiode (5) for detection of the incident UV light (Fig. 9.6). Upon adsorption of biomolecules the level of the sNPS photoluminescence and the output of the voltage of the consecutively connected photo detectors decrease. Use of two photodetectors of photoluminescence increases the biosensor sensitivity.

To account for the possible changes in the incident UV light the photodiode 5 is used. The output signal is defined as the ratio between the output signal from the photodiodes 2 and 3 and the output signal from the photodiode 5. Such a construction is characteristic of the differential type systems.

9.4 Results and Discussion

9.4.1 Determination of the T2 Mycotoxin Level by the sNPS Photoconductivity Measurement

The sNPS photosensitivity increased after the immobilization of antibodies but it rose sharply following the addition of T2 mycotoxin at the concentration of 100 ng/mL (Fig. 9.7).

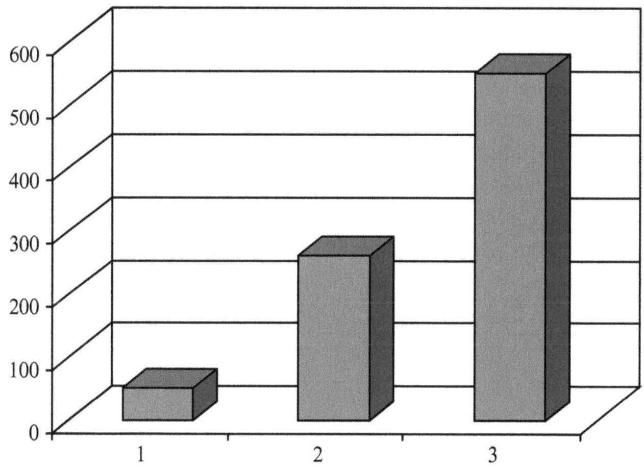

Fig. 9.7 The photocurrent values on the sPNS surface: *1* – bare; *2* – with antibodies against T2; *3* – with Ab and mycotoxin T2 (antigen)

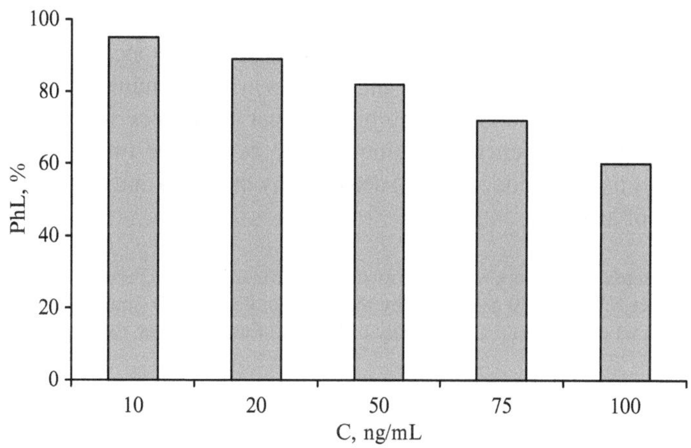

Fig. 9.8 The dependence of the sNPS immune sensor photoluminescence (PhL) signal on the concentration of T2 mycotoxin in solution

9.4.2 Determination of the T2 Mycotoxin Level Using the sNPS Photoluminescence Method

The deposition of the specific Ab on sNPS increases the photoluminescence level, but upon formation of the specific immune complex it decreases. The level of photoluminescence decrease depends on the concentration of T2 mycotoxin in the solution (Fig. 9.8). If a non-specific antibody is used or serum bovine albumin is used as an antigen the photoluminescence level does not change.

In our opinion, the red photoluminescence may be related to the tunnel mechanism of the recombination of the charge carriers, following their excitation in the nanocrystallites of the oxide or at the interface. The role of hydrogen in the photoluminescence quenching cannot be excluded. These are several possible reasons for the decrease of photoluminescence in case of the immune complex formation on the sNPS surface: (a) change in the absorbance of the solution, or (b) the effect of the immune complex components or their interaction on the recombination process of the photocurrent charge in the sNPS. It is known that there is no light absorption at the wavelength of the excitation ($\lambda = 350$ nm) and in the wide field of the sNPS photoluminescence in the solutions of Ab, Ag and their complexes.

9.5 Conclusions

The experimental data presented show that sNPS can be used as transducers, which are stable for a long time after the construction of an immune biosensor. The specific immune complex formed on the sNPS surface may be registered by measuring its photoluminescence or photoconductivity. Such immune biosensors can be applied for control of T2 mycotoxin. The biosensors developed are sensitive and simple; and allows for rapid analysis and analysis in field conditions. This approach may be applied for detection of any biochemical substances which can form an immune complex. Further investigations should be directed towards studying the mechanism of the biochemical signal detection by the sNPS and characterization of all the steps of analysis.

Acknowledgments This work was supported by the State Fund of Fundamental Research of Ukraine, project N F28.7/020 as well as by the Collaborative NATO grant (CBR.NUKR.CLG-983381) and grant of the National University of Life and Environmental Science of Ukraine.

References

1. Luchenko AI, Melnichenko MM, Svezhentsova KV, Shmyryeva OM (2006) Complex studies of properties of nanostructured silicon. Proc of SPIE 6327:1–11
2. Starodub NF, Starodub VM (2002) Porous silicon: some theoretical aspects and practical application as transducer for immune sensor. In: Extended abstracts of the 3rd international conference porous semiconductors science and technology, Puerto de la Cruz, Tenerife, Spain, pp 155–157, 10–15 Mar 2002
3. Starodub NF, Starodub VM (2004) Biosensors based on the photoluminescence of porous silicon: overall characteristics and application for the medical diagnostics. Sensors Electronics and Microsystem Technol 2:63–83
4. Uhlir JrA (1956) Electrolytic shaping of Ge and Si. Bell Syst Tech J N35:333–347
5. Fauchet PM (1998) Porous silicon: photoluminescence and electroluminescent devices. In: Semiconductors and semimetals, vol 49. Academic, San Diego, pp 206–252
6. Bsiesy A, Vial JC, Gaspard F et al (1991) Photoluminescence of high porosity and of electrochemicaly oxidized p-Si layers. Surf Sci N254:195–200

7. Canham LT (1997) Porous semiconductors: a tutorial review. Proc Mat Res Soc Symp 452:29–42
8. Canham LT (1990) Silicon quantum wire array fabrication by electrochemical and chemical dissolution of wafers. Appl Phys Lett N57:1046–1048
9. Gardelis S, Rimmer JS, Dawson P et al (1991) Evidence for quantum confinemenr in the photoluminesce of p-Si and SiGe. Appl Phys Lett 59:2128–2120
10. Koshida N, Koyama H (1991) Efficient visible photoluminescence from p-Si. Jpn J Appl Phys N30:L1221–L1223
11. Lackwood DJ (1998) Light emission in silicon. In: Semiconductors and semimetals, vol 49. Academic, San Diego, pp 1–35
12. Svechnikov SV, Sachenko AV, Sukach GA et al (1994) Light emitted layers of the porous silicon: preparation, abilities and application (review). Optoelectronics and Semiconductor Technique N27:3–28
13. Kim SJ, Jeon BH, Choi KS (1999) Improvement of the sensitivity by UV light in alcohol sensors using porous silicon layer. In: CAS'99 Proceedings of the international semiconductor conference, Sinaia, Romania, 2:475–478
14. Rittersma ZM, Benecke W (1999) A novel capacitive porous silicon humidity sensor with integrated thermo- and refresh resistors gas sensors. In: Proceedings of 13th European conference on solid-state transducers "Eurosensors XIII", The Hague, Netherlands, pp 371–374, 12–15 Sept 1999
15. Sorli B, Garcia M, Benhida A et al (1999) Porous silicon layer used as a humidity sensor. In: Proceedings of the european matter conference E-MRS spring meeting. Symposium I: microcrystalline and nanocrystalline semiconductors, I–8
16. Thust M, Schoening MJ, Frohnhoff S et al (1996) Porous silicon as a substrate material for potentiometric biosensors. Meas Sci Technol N7:26–29
17. Bogue RW (1997) Novel porous silicon biosensor. BIOSENS BIOELECTRON 12:xxvii–xxix
18. Schoening MJ, Ronkel F, Crott M et al (1997) Miniaturization of potentiometric sensors using porous silicon microtechnology. Electrochim Acta 42:3185–3193
19. Starodub NF, Fedorenko LL, Starodub VM et al (1996) Extinguishing of visible photoluminescence of porous silicon – stimulated by antigen-antibody immunocomplecx formation. In: Optical organic and semiconductor inorganic materials, Riga, Latvia, pp 73–76, 26–29 Aug 1996
20. Starodub VM, Fedorenko LL, Starodub NF (1998) Control of a myoglobin level in solution by the bioaffine sensor based on the photoluminescence of porous silicon. In: Proceedings of the european conference on solid-state transducers and 9th UK conference on sensors and their applications, Southampton, UK, 2:817–820, 13–16 Sept 1998
21. Starodub VM, Fedorenko LL, Sisetskiy AP, Starodub NF (1999) Control of myoglobin level in an immune sensor based on the photoluminescence of porous silicon. Sensors and Actuator B58:409–414
22. Starodub VM, Starodub NF (1999) Optical immune sensors for the monitoring protein substances in the air. In: Eurosensor XII and 13th european conference on solid-state transducers. The Hague, Netherlands, pp 181–184, 12–15 Sept 1999
23. Starodub VM, Fedorenko LL, Starodub NF (2000) Optical immune sensor for the monitoring protein substances in the air. Sensors and Actuator B68:40–47
24. Burmeister HR (1971) T-2 toxin production by Fusarium tricinctum on solid substrate. Appl Microbiol 21:739–742
25. Cole RJ, Cox RH (1981) The trichothecenes. In: Cole RJ, Cox RH (eds) Handbook of toxic fungal metabolites. Academic, New York, NY, pp 152–263
26. Miller JD, Taylor A, Greenhalgh R (1983) Production of deoxynivalenol and related compounds in liquid culture by Fusarium graminearum. Can J Microbiol 29:1171–1178
27. Madsen JM (2001) Toxins as weapons of mass destruction. A comparison and contrast with biological-warfare and chemical-warfare agents. Clin Lab Med 21:593–605
28. Starodub NF (2009) Biosensors in a system of instrumental tools to prevent effects of bioterrorism and automotive control of water process purification. In: Jones JAA et al (eds)

Proceedings of NATO science for peace and security, series C: environmental security, Threats to global water security, Springer Sci+Business Media BV, 59–71
29. Starodub NF (2009) Biosensors in the system of express control of chemicals regularly used as terrorist means to prevent non diserable consequences. In: The role of ecological chemistry in pollution research and sustainable development. Springer Sci+Business Media BV, 275–384
30. Bunner DL, Upshall DG, Bhatti AR (1985) Toxicology data on T-2 toxin. In: Report of focus officers meeting on mycotoxin toxicity, Defense research establishment at Suffield Alta, Canada, 23–24 Sept 1985
31. Artjuch VP, Gojster OS, Khmelnitsky GA, Starodub NF (2003) Trichtezene mycotoxins: determination in environmental objects. Biopolym Cell 19:216–223
32. Starodub NF, Pylipenko LN, Egorova AV et al (2008) Analysis of mycotoxins: preparations of samples. Biotechnology 1:106–115
33. Starodub NF, Pylipenko LN, Egorova AV, Pylipenko IV (2008) Mycotoxin patulin: producers, biological effects, indication in foods. Mod Probl Toxicol 3:50–57
34. Starodub NF, Kanjuk MI, Ivashkevich SP et al (2009) Determination of patulin toxicity and its control in environment by optical biosensor system. In: Proceedings of OPTO 2009&IRS2, Nurenberg, Germany, pp 151–156, 26–28 May 2009
35. Starodub NF, Dibrova TI, Shirshov YuM, Kostiukevich KV (1997) Development of sensor based on the surface plasmon resonance for control of biospecific interaction. In: Proceedings of eurosensors 12 and 11th european conference on solid-state transducers, Warsaw, Poland, 3:1429–1432, 21–24 Sept
36. Starodub NF, Dibrova TL, Shirshov YuM, Kostjukevich KV (1999) Development of myoglobin sensor based on the surface plasmon resonance. Ukr Biochem J 71:33–37
37. Starodub VM, Starodub NF (2001) Electrochemical and optical biosensors: origin of development, achievements and perspectives of practical application. In: Bozoglu F et al (eds) NATO series novel processes and control technologies in the food industry, Amsterdam, 63–94
38. Nabok AV, Tsargorodskaya A, Hassan AK, Starodub NF (2005) Total internal reflection ellipsometry and SPR detection of low molecular weight environmental toxins. Appl Surf Sci 246:381–386
39. Starodub NF, Nabok AV, Tsargorodskaya A et al (2005) Optical biosensors for the registration of some pesticides, mycotoxins and endocrine disrupting substances in environmental objects. 84 ICB seminar on biochemical sensing – Utilization of micro- and nanotechnologies, Warsaw, p 30
40. Starodub NF, Pylipeko LN, Pylipenko IV, Egorova AV (2008) Mycotoxins and other low weight toxins as instrument of bioterrorists: express instrumental control and some ways to decontaminate polluted environmental objects. Timisoara Medical J 58:9–18
41. Starodub MF, Romanov VO, Kochan RV et al (2006) Implementation of SPR-biosensors for express-diagnostics of acute viral infection and mycotoxicosis. Bull Khmelnitski Nat Univ N6:223–226

Chapter 10
A New Method of Testing Blood Cells in Native Smears in Reflected Light

A.A. Paiziev, V.A. Krakhmalev, R. Djabbarganov, and M.S. Abdullakhodjaeva

Abstract A new method of colour visualisation of red blood cells without using any chemical staining has been developed. The method is based on a physical phenomenon, the white light interference on thin transparent films. It is shown that in the case of thin human blood smears, colour interference contrast occurs on solid polished substrates. The best contrast was determined on substrates with maximal refractive index (Mo, W, Si). These materials have been selected as the substrate, in place of ordinary microscopic slides used in reflected light microscopy. It has been shown that reflection of incident white light from the blood cell surface and cell-substrate interface, generates two coherent lights. The object signal after passing through the red blood cell gathers additional phase and after interference interaction with reference signal (light reflected from outer cell surface) enables cell imaging in colour. A number of blood smears of healthy persons (control) and patients who were diagnosed with cancer have been analysed. It is concluded that the proposed method may be used as an effective diagnostic tool for detection of early stage blood cell lesions, by examining their interference colour in white light. This method can be used in research laboratories, hospitals, diagnostic centres and for emergency medicine as a diagnostic tool complementary to existing conventional optical and electron microscopy techniques.

Keywords Light interference • Reflected interference microscopy • Erythrocytes

---

A.A. Paiziev (✉), V.A. Krakhmalev, and R. Djabbarganov
Institute of Electronics, Uzbek Academy of Science, Republic of Uzbekistan, Durmon Yuli 33, Academgorodok, Tashkent 100125, Uzbekistan
e-mail: adxam_payziev@rambler.ru

M.S. Abdullakhodjaeva
Institute of Pathology, Ministry of Public Health, Republic of Uzbekistan, A. Khodjaeva 11, Tashkent 100109, Uzbekistan

S. Mikhalovsky and A. Khajibaev (eds.), *Biodefence*, NATO Science for Peace and Security Series A: Chemistry and Biology, DOI 10.1007/978-94-007-0217-2_10,

10.1 Introduction

Tests which allow rapid diagnosis of victims of suspected biological terrorism are of crucial significance for urgent medical treatment. Unfortunately, clinical diagnostics using laboratory methods is time consuming and not always available, as it requires time for sample preparation and performing tests. Obtaining accurate authentic information about the form and micro relief of the elements of blood cells in normal and pathological status patients is of particular practical interest. However, the majority of clinical blood analyses are related to chemical or physical treatment of the sample under investigation resulting in the occurrence of various artifacts and loss of these valuable parameters. For blood analysis expensive electronic and optical equipment is often required, such as an electron microscope, phase-contrast, interferometer and luminescent microscopes [1, 2]. In the case of electron microscopy the sample needs to be transported to an electron microscopy laboratory and undergo specimen preparation before being tested. This preparation may take several days before the sample is ready for examination. Rapid embedding protocols can reduce the time to approximately one day but with a loss in specimen quality. Besides, under the electron beam and pumping of vacuum chamber, the specimen undergoes additional destruction. As a result, the native intact pattern of biomedical specimens cannot be seen and a loss of many important specimen morphological features occurs [3].

Optical microscopy techniques are more readily available and less destructive to test cell and tissue cultures, but sample preparation requires chemical fixation, cutting ultra thin sections, staining and other pre-treatment. However, optical microscopy is a very suitable tool which allows rapid morphological identification and early differential diagnosis of different agents contained within the specimen [4, 5]. Thus optical morphology diagnosis in many cases is sufficient to permit a provisional diagnosis and to initiate treatment without waiting for other laboratory test results.

Conventional optical microscopy is based on image amplitude contrast "peek-a-boo" [6]. This method usually generates black and white images dependent on the optical properties of sample (light absorption). It allows amplitude contrasting of the sample, clearly distinguishing between separate morphological elements of cells (nucleus, cytoplasm, cell shell), which have different absorption index. The objects, however, have to be stained using dyes. Interaction of chemicals with the sample destroys native structure of tissues and cells, which can result in false information about their morphology caused by the specimen preparation and viewing conditions at the very start [6]. These difficulties could be avoided with application of light transmission interference microscopy based on visualisation of phase gradients within unstained specimens [7] and differential interference contrast microscopy [8]. The interference microscopy techniques require special additional optical units that significantly raise the price of diagnostic equipment. For this reason they are not used in routine screening [12,13].

In the present paper a new optical nondestructive method for visualisation of native cells in their natural colours without need for staining is described. A specially designed substrate for deposition of biological samples and observation of their native structure in reflected light has been used [9].

10.2 Experimental

The setup for colour reflected interference microscopy is based on an ordinary optical microscope (Neophot-2, Carl Zeiss, Germany) equipped with a digital photo camera (Sony) and substrate which serves as the object-plate for a sample and a source of coherent light for scattering of morphological structures of the sample (object signal). Light from a 100 watt Xenon source was directed onto the specimen. Microscopic images were obtained with Zeiss lens and digital camera and recorded on a personal computer using commercially available software.

The polished surfaces of polycrystalline Al, Cu, Ni and Si(p) and monocrystalline samples of Mo, Si(m) and W were tested to choose the best substrate providing maximal colour contrast. The surface of the substrate was chemically polished to provide mirror reflection. Thin blood smears of the same patient were deposited under the same experimental conditions. After air drying for 10 min, blood samples were placed on the microscope holder. The images were taken by a digital camera.

10.3 Results and Discussion

10.3.1 Interference Contrast in Reflected Light

In phase contrast [7] or differential interference contrast [8] microscopy we have an interference picture for two light rays passing through the sample and transparent object-plate. In the present work, two coherent rays are generated as a result of incident light reflection from cell surface (reference signal) and cell-substrate interface respectively (object signal). This allows conversion of previously invisible gradients of refractive index within the specimen, into intensity gradients of the image at the image plane. A colour interference contrast image was created due to a combination of special experimental conditions such as the choice of incidental light angle, wavelength of the reflected light ray, chemical composition, thickness and refractive index of the sample, and chemical composition and refractive index of the substrate.

The human red blood cell (erythrocyte) has a shape of biconcave disc with minimal (D_{min}) and maximal (D_{max}) thickness and radius R (Fig. 10.1a). The optical scheme of a reflected microscope with deposited red blood cells is shown in Fig. 10.1b. The light scattering process takes place at the interface of three media: air-erythrocyte-substrate with refractive index n_0, n_1 and n_2, respectively. Since the erythrocyte thickness is of the same order of magnitude as the wavelength of incidental light, the interference phenomena take place on these blood cells. The reflective capacity of an interface between two media with refractive indices n_0 and n_1 is described by Eq. 10.1 [10]:

$$p = \frac{I_{ref}}{I_0} = \left(\frac{n_0 - n_1}{n_0 + n_1}\right)^2 \tag{10.1}$$

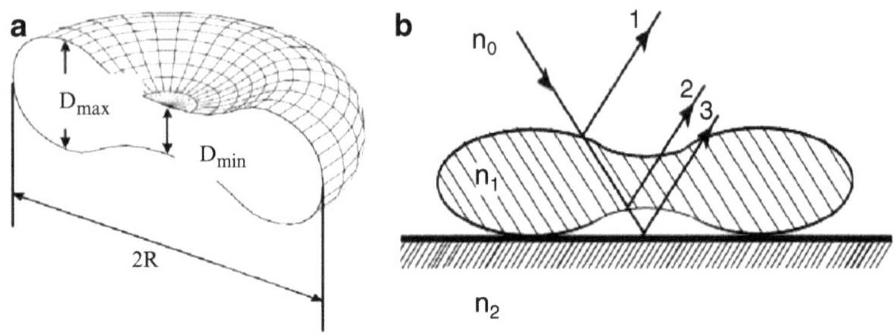

Fig. 10.1 (**a**) Geometrical model of human erythrocyte. D_{max} and D_{min} are maximal and minimal thickness of erythrocyte, respectively. *R* is erythrocyte radius. (**b**) Schematic drawing of erythrocyte gross-section and light ray part reflected on interface air-cell, cell-air and air-substrate

where I_0 and I_{ref} are the intensity of incident and reflected light accordingly. Hereby the higher the difference between n_0 and n_1, the higher is the refractive capacity of the interface and contrast of its image. In the case of an erythrocyte on a substrate (Fig. 10.1b) the light is reflected from three interfaces, air-erythrocyte (ray 1), erythrocyte-air (ray 2) and air-substrate (ray 3). In addition to the above mentioned cases, the light reflection on the interface erythrocyte-substrate takes place. It is known that refractive index of human erythrocyte $n_1 = 1.34$, air refractive index $n_0 = 1$ and refractive index of silicon substrate $n_2 = 4.24$ [11]. According to Eq. 1 the maximal refractive capacity occurs in the area of tight contact of an erythrocyte with a substrate and near the cell centre where the air is in contact with the substrate. Because of little difference of reflective capacity in the above mentioned areas this interface will not have considerable contrast.

10.3.2 Optical Scheme of Reflected Interference Microscope

In this section colour visualisation of biomedical samples transparent to visible light is described using the reflected interference microscope scheme. Contrary to previously mentioned interference microscope types [7, 8] the proposed method is based on using light reflective properties of the substrate, which at the same time serves as the microscope object slide. The method is based on generating two coherent light signals (object and reference signals) resulting in visible light reflection from the object surface (reference signal) and from the substrate after passing of incident light through the erythrocyte. The light ray reflected from the substrate in turn passes through the cell, and makes a phase shift (object signal). Interaction of object and reference coherence light rays leads to the formation of an interference pattern in the focus of the microscope objective, which is a colour image of the phase object. It should be noted that in conventional optical microscopes the image is generated as the object's shadow due to light absorption by the object. In the case of conventional interference microscopy (transition light mode) the light from the source adds to reference and object signal generating unit.

Then, from this unit two coherent light rays are formed; one of them (object signal) generated by passing through the sample and the other one (reference signal) after interference interaction with the second coherent light. The two rays form the interference pattern of the phase contrast object. In this case the object signal is formed as a result of light passing through the sample deposited on the transparent microscope glass. In our scheme which uses reflected light interference microscopy, the interference microscope is set up in transferred light mode. A refractive non-transparent substrate serves as a support for sample deposition and as a unit to form the second coherent object signal. The reflected light interference microscopy allows the use of standard units of conventional optical reflected microscopy which has the integrated unit for sample deposition and generation of two coherent rays.

The diagram of a reflected interference microscope is presented in Fig. 10.2. The light ray from white light source (1) passes through a heat reflecting filter (2), collimating lens (3) and diaphragm (4). The optical filter (5) is used to observe a cell pattern in monochromatic light. Next the light falls on a semi-transparent silvered mirror (8) oriented at 45° and perpendicularly reflects from a sample surface (12). A part of the light is falling through the cell and reflecting from boundary cell-substrate (13). This ray gathers additional phase against the ray which reflects from the cell surface (12). Both reflected coherent rays travel in a reverse direction and after passing through the silvered mirror they form an interference image of the object on the photo film or the ocular of the microscope.

As a result of light interference at different parts of the sample its colouration can be seen. The colour depends on the sample thickness at the interference point and sample refractive index.

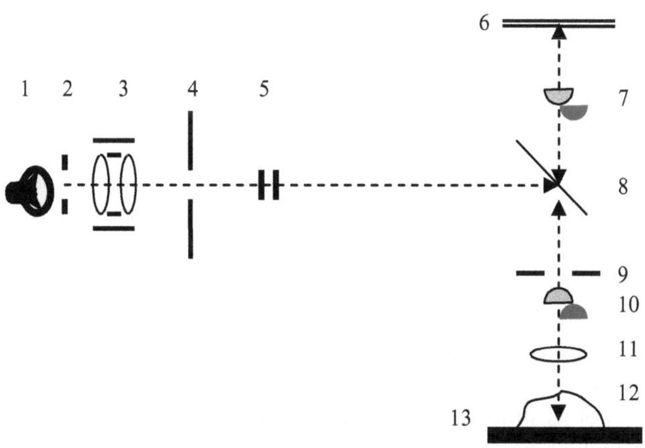

Fig. 10.2 Schematic diagram of a reflected interference microscope: *1* – light source, *2* – heat reflecting filter, *3* – collimator, *4* – diaphragm, *5* – light filter, *6* – photo film, *7* – projection ocular, *8* – semi-transparent silvered mirror, *9* – aperture diaphragm, *10* – auxiliary lens, *11* – immersion lens, *12* – sample under investigation, *13* – substrate

10.3.3 Choice of Substrate Material to Reach Maximal Interference Contrast

As the colour contrast depends on substrate refractive index, to ensure maximal reflectivity of the cell-substrate interface the maximal difference between their refractive indices for the visible light wavelength range should be obtained. Among the substrate materials, refractory metals Mo ($n = 3.15$) and W ($n = 3.31$) and Si ($n = 4.24$) have the maximal reflectivity [11]. These materials also provide the maximal interference contrast for blood cells. The polished surfaces of polycrystalline Al, Cu, Ni and Si(p) and monocrystalline Mo, Si(m) and W have been tested to find the best substrate for maximal colour contrast as described in Section 2. The substrate surface was chemically polished to achieve mirror reflection. As can be seen from Fig. 10.3, the background colour (substrate) corresponds to its refractive index for visible wavelength range. The best colour contrast was obtained for mono- and polycrystalline silicon and for monocrystalline surfaces of refractory metals molybdenum and tungsten, which possess maximal reflectivity and provide the best colour contrast of red blood cells.

10.3.4 Comparison between Optical Microscopy Techniques for Red Blood Cell Imaging

Conventional bright-field microscopy generates black and white images of separate morphological elements of blood smears only (Fig. 10.4a). To demonstrate the potential of the reflected interference microscopy, colour images of human blood cells obtained by conventional light microscopy (Fig. 10.4a) were compared with images generated by new colour contrasting method in reflected light (Fig. 10.4b). The blood cell surface is clearly visible in colour images of separately located erythrocytes (Fig. 10.4a–g) obtained on solid substrates. In addition to its own colour, every red corpuscle is surrounded by white-yellow shell that gives additional information about the cell status and its environment. The organic shells around blood cells are clearly seen and easily detected. Time consuming processing operations of smear fixing and colouring commonly used in conventional microscopy are not needed in this case. The optical setup requires neither phase-contrast nor interference microscope, nor special light source of a short wavelength light beam, because interferometric colouring of blood elements occurs on the surface of a specially selected substrate.

The colour of blood elements or other transparent biological objects placed on a substrate depends on their optical properties, chemical structure of blood elements, refraction index of its structural components, thickness, angle of light incidence on an object, wavelength of incident light. The resulting colour images of blood elements are formed due to interferometric phenomena occurring under interaction of light rays reflected from the front and back surfaces of blood elements smeared on a substrate.

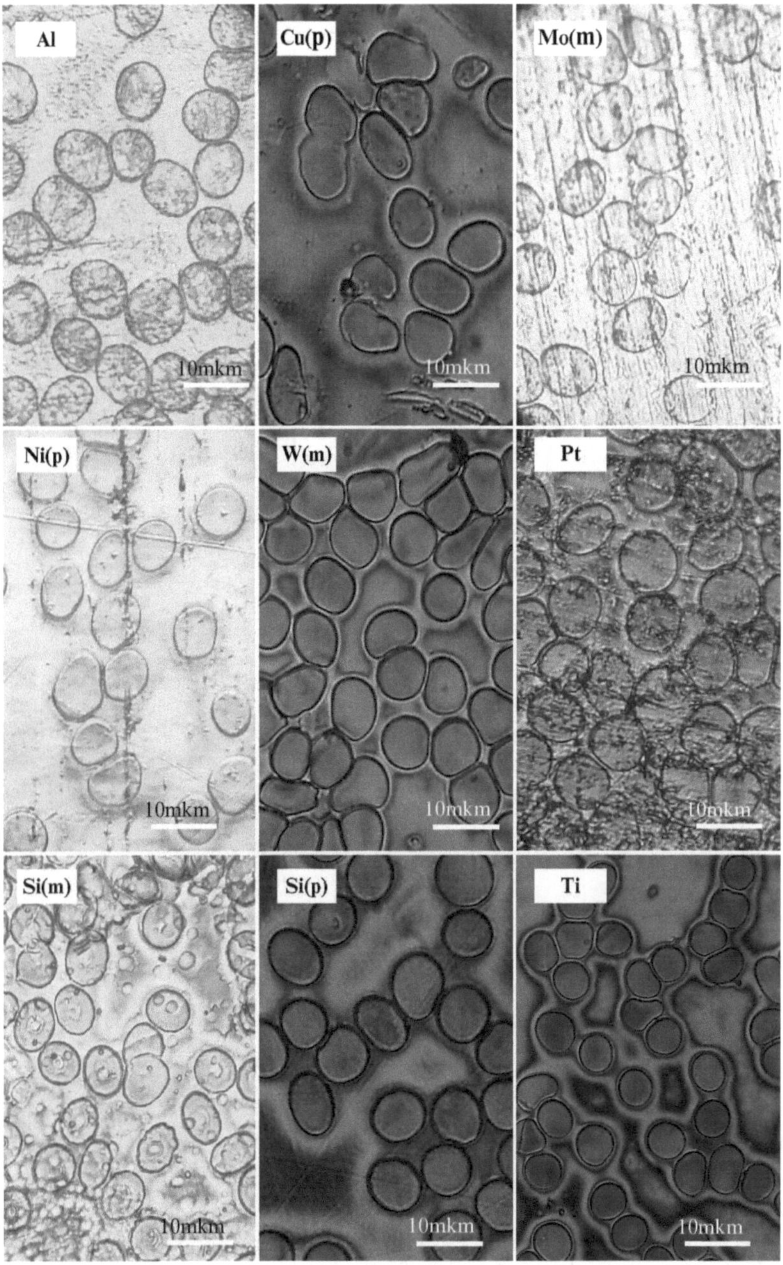

Fig. 10.3 Colour contrast of human erythrocytes on different solid reflective substrates: *Al* – polycrystalline aluminum; *Cu* – polycrystalline copper; *Mo* – monocrystalline molybdenum; *Ni* – polycrystalline nickel; *Pt* – chemically polished platinum; *Si(m)* – monocrystalline silicon; *Si(p)* – polycrystalline silicon; *Ti* – chemically polished titanium; *W* – monocrystalline tungsten

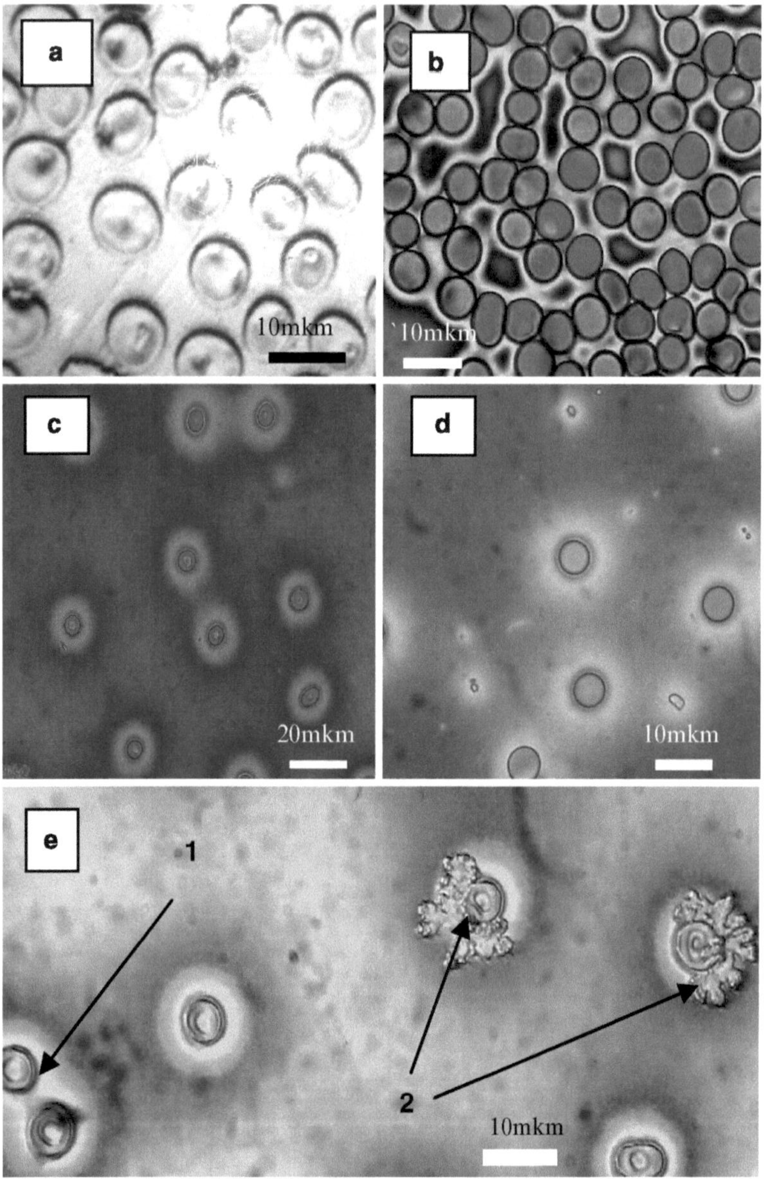

Fig. 10.4 Interference 'staining' of normal and pathological human blood cells: (**a**) control: erythrocytes of a conditionally healthy person under conventional microscope without any staining, (**b**) the same sample deposited on the silicon substrate, (**c**) and (**d**) multilayer structure of interference pattern, (**e**) live erythrocytes of a patient diagnosed with colorectal cancer

Taking into account the simplicity of obtaining optical patterns of erythrocytes and the ability to detect the structures of pathological precipitation of substances, which are not characteristic of a normal blood plasma sample, the proposed method has significant diagnostic importance and advantages summarised below:

- Special sample preparation not required
- Samples can be measured immediately
- It is a non-destructive test
- Ability to see a native pattern of a live cell
- Ability to get a native colour image without using any chemicals that can damage the cell and are often expensive
- Ability to perform chemical analysis of a sample by using colour scale map of standard (calibrated) specimen
- Analysis can be performed outdoors
- Possibility to organise a mobile microscopy laboratory and carry out measurements in field conditions
- Cost of equipment is lower in comparison with conventional microscopic methods
- Potential for elaboration of new clinical tests
- Possibility of computer processing of digital images

10.4 Conclusions

A new optical microscopy method which enables interference contrast imaging of biological cells has been developed. The method is based on a well known physical phenomenon, white light interference on a thin transparent film.

It has been shown that the colour interference image of blood cells is a result of interaction of two coherent rays, one reflected from the cell surface (reference signal) and the other reflected from the cell-substrate interface (object signal).

- The colour interference contrast image is achieved via special experimental conditions, which comprise the angle of the incident light, wavelength of the light of the reflected ray, chemical composition, thickness and refractive index of a sample, and refractive index and chemical composition of a substrate.
- The best colour contrast of red blood cells is achieved on mono- and polycrystalline silicon, and monocrystalline surfaces of refractory metals molybdenum and tungsten, which possess maximal reflectivity.
- Integration of a reflective solid substrate into conventional light microscopy provides a unit that generates two coherent rays in a reflected mode.
- These features provide for a less expensive and accessible method capable of revealing effect of biological agents suitable for both laboratory and field conditions.

References

1. Hafez ESS, Kenemans P (eds) (1982) Atlas of human reproduction by scanning electron microscopy. MTP Press, Boston
2. Andrews PM (1981) Characteristic surface topography of cells living the respiratory tracts. Biomed Res 2(Suppl):28–288

3. Chang L-P, Wang T-L, Chang H (2003) Applicability of bioterrorism preparedness in SARS: focus on laboratory examination. Ann Disaster Med 2(1):32–38
4. Lane HC, LaMontagne J, Fauci AS (2001) Bioterrorism: a clear and present danger. Nat Med 7:1271–1273
5. Hazelton PR, Gelderblom HR (2003) Electron microscopy for rapid diagnosis of infectious agents in emergent situations. Emerg Infect Dis 9(3):294–303
6. Kozlovskaya LV, Nikolaev AYu (1984) Textbook on clinical laboratory methods of investigations. Medicine, Moscow, p 288
7. Zernike F (1942) Phase contrast: a new method for the observation of transparent objects. Physica 9:686–693
8. Nomarski G (1955) Microinterferometric differential a on des palarisees. J Phys Radium 16:S9
9. Krakhmalev V, Paiziev A (2006) Non-invasive color visualization of blood cells. Online J Nondestr Test 11:6, http://www.ndt.net/article/v11n06/paiziev1/paiziev1.htm
10. Curtis ASG (1964) The mechanism of adhesion of cells to glass: a study by interference reflection microscopy. J Cell Biol 20:199–215
11. Kikoin IA (ed) (1976) Handbook of physical magnitudes. Atomizdat, Moscow, p 1006
12. Finko DI (1994) Etiopathogenesis of malignant tumors: red corpuscular theory of cancer origination. Joint-Stock Company AKME, Moscow, p 176
13. Abdullakhodjaeva MS (1997) Essential principles of human pathology. Part I. Ibn Sino Publ House of Medical Literature, Tashkent, p 560

Chapter 11
The Crystallographic Method of Identification of Microorganisms

L.G. Bajenov

Abstract A simple, accessible and cost effective method of crystallographic identification of microorganisms has been developed. It allows rapid and sufficiently reliable identification of many clinically significant pathogens based on their crystallogenic properties. The use of the crystallographic method substantially accelerated and simplified the identification of *Candida spp.* when compared with traditional methods of identification of microorganisms.

Keywords Crystallogram • Bacterial pathogen • *Candida spp.*

11.1 Introduction

Recently a number of more sophisticated methods for identification of microorganisms have been developed. However, alongside their increase in accuracy and complexity their cost has also risen. Widespread biochemical methods of identification are rather labour intensive and the results obtained are not always reliable due to the high variability of microbial species.

In this paper a new crystallographic method of identification of microorganisms is described. We investigated a method of crystal coating [1] used as an auxiliary diagnostic criterion to determine the nature of the pathological process in rhinitis and stomach diseases. Our preliminary work showed that the original method [2] cannot be used for microbiological identification, therefore it has been modified. Briefly, pure cultures were isolated, cultivated in test tubes with slope nutrient agar, and washed with saline solution. The prepared microbial suspension was

L.G. Bajenov (✉)
V.Vakhidov Republican Specialised Center of Surgery, Tashkent, Uzbekistan
e-mail: leobaj@tps.uz

S. Mikhalovsky and A. Khajibaev (eds.), *Biodefence*, NATO Science for Peace and Security Series A: Chemistry and Biology, DOI 10.1007/978-94-007-0217-2_11,

dried in a desiccator with silica gel at 37°C till its full desiccation (within 16–18 h). The received crystal image (crystallogram) was examined under the microscope (magnification × 16–32) and was compared with crystallograms of the known microorganisms (reference-cultures).

The modified method of crystal coating was used to assess *Candida spp*. The choice of the pathogen was stipulated by the growing importance of this microorganism in the development and maintenance of various pathological conditions, and the lack of quick and reliable methods to identify *Candida spp*. in practical laboratories.

11.2 Experimental

Twenty-one strains of *Candida spp*. isolated from the gastric juice of the patients with gastroduodenal diseases were studied. According to their cultural, physiological and biochemical features pathogens were identified as following species: *C. tropicalis* ($n=10$), *C. krusei* and *C. stellatoidea* ($n=4$), *Candida albicans* ($n=3$). Crystallograms, obtained as described earlier, were analyzed under the microscope (magnification × 16–32) and were compared with crystallograms of the known microorganisms (reference-cultures) [1, 3].

11.3 Results and Discussion

The crystallograms of *Candida spp*. showed characteristic structures in the form of a complex of crystals, in which axial lines with the lateral branches diverged from the corners, and differed for different species. Other differences were also revealed (see below), allowing the determination of a specific structure belonging to the investigated strain.

The representative crystallograms of the studied species of *Candida spp*. (Fig. 11.1) were as following:

C. albicans: formed crystals of the regular shape, tri- and tetrahedral, lateral lines were straight and parallel to each other. There were either no branches or there were 1–2 short branches. The central part of the crystals was clear, background was fine-grained.

C. stellatoidea: formed quadrangular crystals with strongly indented edges. There were no lateral branches. The central part of the crystals was densely striated with the lines parallel to lateral sides, background was fine-grained.

C. tropicalis: formed crystals of the awkward shape, with shifted centers and indented edges. There were lateral branches, background was fine-grained.

C. krusei: formed large crystals of the regular shape, tri-and tetrahedral, with well-expressed centers and dense banding. Background was fine-grained.

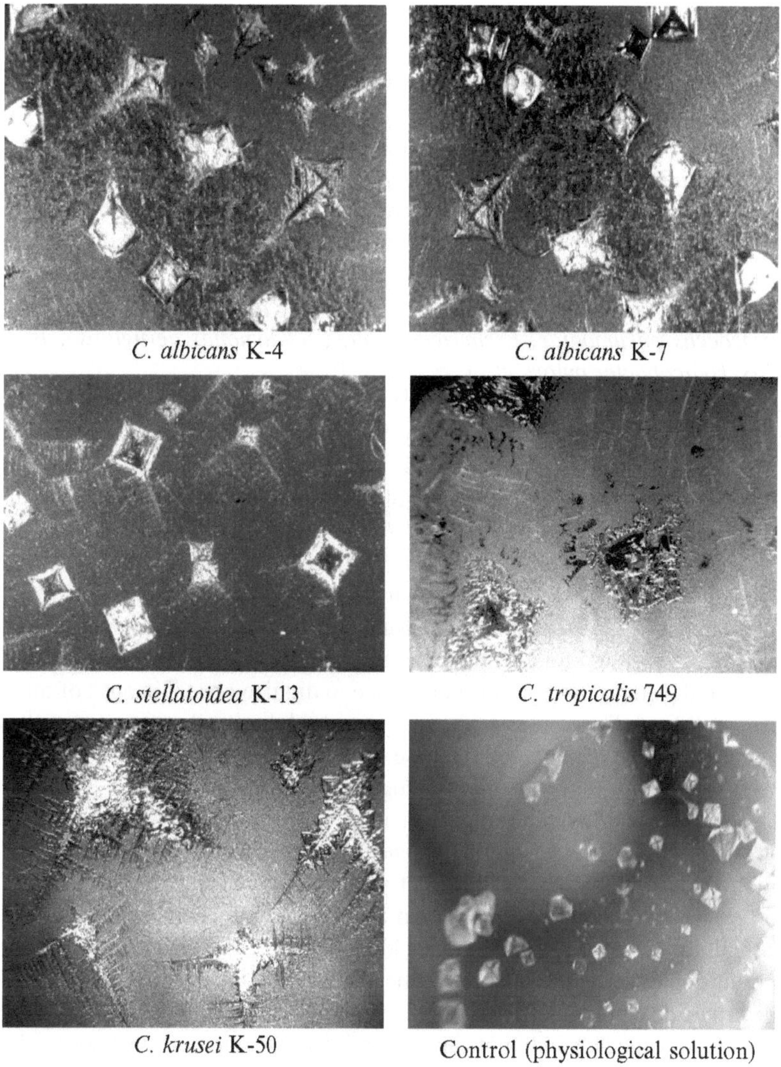

Fig. 11.1 Crystallograms of *Candida spp.*

The control (physiological solution): fine, robust crystals, mainly of the regular shape, crystal background was absent.

All studied strains of the listed species formed identical crystallograms, allowing precise differentiation. The data obtained by means of traditional and crystallographic methods was fully concordant.

Following the same procedure, the crystallograms were characterized by high reproducibility. It normally takes 16–18 h to obtain crystallograms and to identify *Candida spp.*, whereas traditional methods of identification *Candida spp.* usually take up to 2–3days. Moreover, 8–9 tests are needed for routine identification by traditional methods, often requiring the use of expensive and deficient reagents. The use of the crystallographic method requires one test based on application of inexpensive physiological solution.

The use of the crystallographic method allows significantly acceleration and simplification in the identification of *Candida spp.* when compared with traditional methods of recognition of the given microorganisms.

We also created a bank of crystallograms of many other clinically significant microorganisms (*Staphylococcus spp.*, *Micrococcus spp.*, *Enterobacter spp.*, *Proteus spp.*, *Klebsiella spp.*, *Serratia spp.*, *Lactobacterium spp.*, *Bacteroides spp.*, *Streptococcus pneumoniae*, *Escherichia coli*, *Pseudomonas aeruginosa*, *Bacillus subtilis*, *Helicobacter pylori*, etc.).

Crystallograms of over 600 cultures of the various microorganisms isolated from patients with purulent and inflammatory diseases and gastroduodenal pathology, as well as cultures obtained from hospital swabs were studied and compared with known crystallograms. The presence of specific features of crystallograms of *Serratia marcescens*, *Escherichia coli*, *Pseudomonas aeruginosa*, *Brucella spp.*, *Bacillus spp.*, *Vibrio cholerae*, *Helicobacter pylori* and other microorganisms [1–6] was determined. The use of the given method allows quick, simple and reliable identification of the listed microorganisms with just one test, whereas 5–20 and more tests are required for traditional identification.

We also developed and produced a device to digitize crystal images of microorganism cultures. These electronic images could be easily e-mailed, allowing researches to create a computer database of crystallograms of microorganisms and to develop the algorithms for image recognition and assessment.

The further development of the method, investigation of crystal formation mechanisms and effects of various physical and chemical factors on this process, creation of crystallogram databases of typical cultures of microorganisms and expert systems for their recognition and assessment will considerably expand our opportunities in systematization and identification of pathogens. The use of electronic copies of crystal images for the analysis and their safe and quick transfer by electronic channels will help to solve a problem of fast and reliable identification of dangerous pathogens in remote areas of primary isolation of suspicious cultures, thus limiting the possible spread of dangerous and lethal diseases.

11.4 Conclusions

A simple, easily available and cost effective method of identification of microorganisms has been developed. It allows a fast and sufficiently reliable determination of many clinically significant pathogens.

The use of the proposed crystallographic method accelerates and simplifies the identification of the *Candida spp.* when compared with conventional methods of their identification.

A device for digitisation of crystal images of microorganism cultures has been developed to allow quick and safe transfer of images by electronic means of communication.

References

1. Bajenov LG (1994) Identification of Serratia marcescens with the modified method of crystal coating. Clin Lab Diagn N4:41–42
2. Bajenov LG (1994) Patent N1231 of the republic of Uzbekistan
3. Bajenov LG (2004) Crystallographic method of studying of microorganisms and its usage at identification of fungi of the genus Candida. In: First International Scientific Teleconference "New Technology in Medicine. Saint-Petersburg," Russia, pp 12–13
4. Bajenov LG (2008) Crystallographic properties of Helicobacter pylori. Helicobacter 13:421
5. Bajenov L, Artemova E (1999) Identification of Candida species by using a crystallographic method. In: Abstracts of the IXth Congresses of Bacteriology and Applied Microbiology and Mycology. 16–20 August 1999. Sydney, Australia, p 111
6. Bajenov LG, Ruzimurodov MA, Artemova EV, Ten RM (2008) Study and application of crystallogenic properties of Brucella for their identification and differentiation. Bull Int Sci Surgl Assoc N1:21–22

Part III
Biological and Chemical Methods of Protection

Chapter 12
Drug Delivery Systems and Their Potential for Use in Battlefield Situations

J.D. Smart

Abstract Different types of medication and drug delivery systems that could be used in battlefield situations are compared and discussed. Rapidly acting therapies that are easy to administer are required for acute injuries, while prolonged therapy would be needed for prophylactic treatments, for example with antimicrobial therapies when exposed to microbiological weapons, or health maintenance after the acute phase of treatment of a battlefield injury. To give prolonged therapy, depot injections, implants and transdermal patches (the latter having the advantage of allowing rapid discontinuation of therapy) could be used. The development of biological products from advances in biotechnology and the advanced drug delivery systems required to deliver them using the emerging nano- and targeting technology, provide new opportunities for therapies that could find use in a conflict situation.

Keywords Drug delivery systems • Battlefields • Medical support

12.1 Introduction

The aim of this review is to consider the types of medications/drug delivery systems that could be developed for administration in battlefield situations, current systems and possible future developments. It will consider battlefield situations, the medical aid provided, current drug delivery technologies and those employed at the front line, followed by a consideration of some future possible developments.

J.D. Smart (✉)
School of Pharmacy and Biomolecular Sciences, University of Brighton,
Brighton BN2 4GJ, United Kingdom
e-mail: john.smart@brighton.ac.uk

S. Mikhalovsky and A. Khajibaev (eds.), *Biodefence*, NATO Science for Peace and Security Series A: Chemistry and Biology, DOI 10.1007/978-94-007-0217-2_12,

12.2 Modern Battlefields

It has been recognised for many years that 'modern' warfare is less often that of conventional 'army versus army' confrontations [1], but now more often army versus semi-military (guerrilla) forces, street battles (urban terrain environments) [2] and insurgencies involving civilians. It can also involve challenging terrains such as deserts, jungles or mountains [3].

Threats posed to military personnel include wounding (by bullets and shrapnel), chemical and biological weapons, infection and disease, and other hazards (accidents, altitude, terrain etc.). Medical treatments are therefore required for acute traumas arising in the battlefield, to prevent illness e.g. diseases associated with the country or conditions encountered during military action along with those resulting from chemical or biological weapons.

Trauma arising during combat is of particular concern. In an operation by American army forces involving an assault on a Central American airfield the following injuries were reported: two wounds to the head (with one mortality), four to the thorax (two mortalities), four to the abdomen (one mortality) and three to the extremities [4]. A study of wounding patterns for US Marines and sailors during operation the major combat phase of the Iraqi war, revealed that wounding arising from explosive munitions and small arms were the major cause of injury [5] (Tables 12.1 and 12.2).

In addition to battlefield trauma, there is also the risk of exposure to chemical weapons such as the 'nerve' agents, notably the organophosphorus gases (soman, sarin, VX, tabun) [6]. Organophosphorus toxicity arises largely from their ability to irreversibly inhibit acetyl-cholinesterases, leading to effects associated with peripheral acetyl-choline accumulation (muscarinic syndrome) such as meiosis, profuse sweating, bradychardia, bronchioconstriction, hypotension, and diarrhoea. Central nervous system effects include anxiety, restlessness, confusion, ataxia, tremors,

Table 12.1 Wounding patterns for US Marines and sailors during operation 'Iraqi Freedom', - Major combat phase [5]

Diagnosis	Number (%)
Open wounds	259 (42)
Fractures	109 (18)
Other wounds	92 (15)
Burns	22 (4)
Sprains and strains	20 (3)
Amputations	15 (2)
Contusions	15 (2)
Post haemorrhagic anaemias	14 (2)
Bacterial infections	12 (2)
Superficial injuries	12 (2)
Intracranial injuries	10 (2)
Others (hearing, nerve, visual, crushing)	39 (6)

Table 12.2 Causes of wounding of US Marines and sailors during operation 'Iraqi Freedom' - Major combat phase [5]

Primary causative agent	Number (%)
Explosive munitions	130 (46)
• Shrapnel	40 (14)
• RPG	39 (14)
• IED/blasts	20 (7)
• Mortar	20 (7)
• Landmines	11 (4)
Small arms	70 (25)
Motor vehicle accidents	26 (9)
Falls	18 (6)
Weaponry accidents (in the battlefield)	10 (4)
Other	14 (5)

seizures, cardiorespiratory paralysis and eventually death. Strategies to treat exposure to these agents include protective measures to prevent exposure (clothing, masks etc.), the administration of atropine to reduce muscarinic syndrome, oximes to reactivate acetylcholinesterases, benzodiazepines to treat seizures, organophosphate scavengers (e.g. butyrylcholinesterase), and pyridostigmine, a reversible inhibitor of acetylcholinesterase [6, 7].

Biological warfare is now a potential threat, with the use of micro-biological agents such as anthrax, Ebola virus, pneumonic plague, cholera, tularaemia, smallpox, or other biological materials such as botulism toxin, ricin, mycotoxins [8]. An ideal biological weapon material would have high potency, target humans, not have a vaccine, and be capable of forming an aerosol. Anthrax, which forms spores that are easily aerosolised, would appear to have many advantages in this respect. The use of biological weapons has been prohibited by the Geneva Protocol and Biological Weapons Convention.

Battlefield tactical nuclear weapons also pose a potential threat, but to date have not been used.

12.3 Medical Support

For battlefield trauma, the concept of the 'golden hour', where a patient must be treated within 60 min of multiple traumas, was identified in data gathered by the French during the First World War. In order to achieve rapid treatment, trauma therapies must be administered directly by the combatants themselves (or their colleagues), trained military medical officers or by a mobile army surgical hospital (MASH) unit located close to the combat zone.

To this end soldiers are given basic first aid training to deal with themselves and colleagues, while specialist medical trained solders are embedded in the forward units, with additional first aid supplies [9, 10]. How medical services align behind this will depend on the proximity of the war zone to full medical services, and the terrain. For the United States army, in close proximity to the battlefield front are often easily deployable battalion aid station/forward support medical company [2, 11]. Behind these may be a field hospital (MASH), and finally, in areas away from the war zones, full military hospitals. For the United States army (along with other western armies) Critical Care Air Transport Teams have been added to military teams to allow ongoing treatment of casualties when transported from battlefield treatment centres to hospital intensive care units [10, 12].

12.4 Drug Delivery Systems

The area of modern drug delivery systems is well reviewed in many texts [13, 14], and a brief summary is given below.

The requirements of a drug delivery system depend on the nature of the drug to be administered. A drug can be defined as chemical agent that interacts with a specific pharmacological target to produce the required therapeutic effect. The nature of what constitutes a drug has widened from referring to relatively small stable molecules to include modern biopharmaceuticals (proteins, peptides, oligonucleotides), products of the developments in molecular biology, and these provide specific challenges in terms of their size, stability and mode of action.

There are few occasions where a drug is delivered alone in a pure form into the body, but it is usually combined with other materials (called excipients) to form 'drug delivery systems' ('medicines', 'formulations' or 'dosage forms'). These promote accurate dosing, therapeutic effectiveness, stability and patient acceptability. By far the most common route for delivering drugs into the body is by the oral route, swallowing a tablet or capsule.

Drug delivery systems can be classified in terms of the route into the body in which they are administered. For 'systemic' delivery to the whole body these include:

1. The oral route (through the mouth and into the gastrointestinal tract), and can be solid systems (tablets, capsules) or liquids (mixtures, linctuses, syrups).
2. The parenteral route (injected into the body), which can be subdivided into:

   • Intravenous: Liquids injected directly into the veins in the systemic circulation;
   • Intramuscular: Liquids (or solids) injected into larger muscles;
   • Subcutaneous: Liquids or semisolids placed under the skin;
   • Others: Intraocular, intraarterial, intrathecal (into the spinal canal).

3. The transdermal route (drug delivered through the skin into the systemic circulation), using trandermal patches, creams, ointments, gels.
4. Inhalation route (drugs inhaled into the lungs, and absorbed systemically, using inhalers and nebulisers).

5. The rectal route/vaginal route (drug administered locally to give a systemic effect),
   - Solid formulations: Pessaries, suppositories, tablets;
   - Liquids/semisolids: Foams, enemas, ointments and gels;
6. Other routes: Buccal/sublingual (drug absorbed through the oral cavity membranes); nasal (drug absorbed through the nose).

These routes can also be classified in terms of:

- The speed of onset of action, with the fastest typically being parenteral and the slowest transdermal;
- The barriers to drug absorption into the blood; injections having the least and transdermal being the greatest;
- Patient acceptability; oral being the most acceptable and injection the least.

Targeting a drug to its site of action is useful to enhance its effectiveness and reduce toxicity. If accessible this can be achieved by direct local application, e.g. eye drops to treat ophthalmic conditions, inhalers to treat respiratory conditions, but currently strategies such as the development of targeting agents such as monoclonal antibodies or the use of the more permeable nature of tumour capillaries to allow accumulation of macromolecular carriers have also been employed.

12.5 Medication Needs in the Battlefield Situation

In the battlefield situation, the selection of a delivery system would depend on whether a rapid or prolonged response is needed. In acute situations (trauma or sudden exposure to nerve agents), there is a need for a rapid onset of action, and this would usually favour (single dose) injections. Under the stress of a conflict situation, ease and simplicity of administration is vital, and delivery system that involves coordination (e.g. inhalation therapy) is unlikely to be successful for all but the most experienced users. For acute injuries a rapid onset of action is needed for pain relief, along with rehydration solutions when there is extensive loss of body fluids. The preferred route for drug administration tends to be parenteral, notably intramuscular, into the larger readily accessible muscles of the thigh or buttock. The injection device must be quick and easy to use, robust and stable. Autoinjectors, which are simple to use and allow administration of a precise dose, are widely used. These are sterile solutions in a single use device, which when placed onto the injection site, activates a spring or compressed air to force a needle into the skin (and through clothing) and then the solution out of the device through the needle [15, 16]. A safety device to prevent inadvertent activation may also be included. In the U.S. army assault operation soldiers carried two autoinjectors containing 10 mg morphine for pain relieve after a severe trauma [4]. Autoinjectors are also available for administration of antidotes to organophosphorus nerve agents. An issued item, the Mark 1 NAAK (Nerve agent antidote kit), provides separate doses of the drugs atropine (Atropen®) and pralidoximine chloride for use as first aid. Later versions combine these in one autoinjector, and further autoinjectors of diazepam are provided to prevent seizures [17].

U.S. airbase soldiers also carried battle dressings and 500 mL lactated Ringer's solution (for fluid replacement) [4]. Specialist medical trained soldiers (corpsmen) carried standard trauma packs, first aid kits and antibiotics, with the expectation that the seriously injured would be evacuated directly to a military facility by helicopter.

Prolonged therapy would be required for prophylactic (preventative) treatments, for example with antimicrobial therapies when exposed to microbiological weapons, or health maintenance after the acute phase of treatment of a battlefield injury. To give prolonged therapy depot injections, implants and transdermal patches (the latter having the advantage of allowing rapid discontinuation of therapy) could be used. Some suggestions for selection of a drug delivery system appropriate for use in the battlefield situation are given in Table 12.3.

12.6 The Future

It is clear that the nature of modern warfare will continue to change. Fighting is more likely to be amongst civilian populations and in difficult terrains rather than on conventional battlefields. The need to treat casualties as soon as possible means that there will continue to need to be medications available for immediate administration by soldiers with only basic medical training. Although explosive munitions pose a real current threat, the effects of nerve, biological and nuclear weapons, perhaps delivered by terrorist groups rather than governments, may become more important in future. To address these, new battlefield formulations will be required, along with the technology to deliver them. For acute effects the autoinjector should continue to provide an appropriate rapid first line treatment, and the drugs delivered by this route could be expanded to address these new threats. If such a rapid response is not essential, then conventional tablets provide an alternative, although fast-melt technology [18] that does not require water for the formulation to be swallowed, might be appropriate. Expecting someone in a combat situation to remember to regularly take their medication is impractical, and oral controlled release technology, for potent drugs would be appropriate. In the future, the development of biological products from advances in biotechnology (therapeutic proteins, peptides and oligonucleotides), and the advanced drug delivery systems required to deliver them using the emerging nano- and targeting technology [19, 20], will invariably provide new opportunities for therapies that could find use in a conflict situation.

Table 12.3 Some modern drug delivery systems and suggestions as to their potential use in battlefield situations

Requirement	Delivery system	Comment
Rapid response (seconds) (e.g. severe pain relief, acute exposure nerve agents)	Parenteral route (autoinjectors)	Sterile solutions for injection, in single dose prefilled syringes. Easy to use in stressed environment. 1–2 doses only, needs an easily accessed site for administration (intramuscular)
	Nasal sprays	Aqueous solutions aerosolised into the nasal cavity. Easy to apply under stress but require potent drugs that are absorbed from the nasal cavity (small and stable)
Rapid response (minutes) (e.g. less severe pain relief)	Unit/small dose oral liquids	Single dose drug dissolved in an aqueous solution. Needs to be robust, easy to open and swallow. One dose only (in most cases)
	Sublingual Tablets	Compressed tablets that dissolve under the tongue. Needs to dissolve quickly. Limited to drugs that are permeable to buccal mucosa (small, lipophilic) and have an acceptable flavour
	Rapidly dissolving tablets or films	Films or compressed powders that contain drugs that are rapidly released in the mouth. Limited to drugs with an acceptable flavour and well absorbed in the GI tract
Response within circa half hour (e.g. antibiotics, antimalerials)	Oral tablets and capsules	Powder compacts, or fills in gelatin capsules, that are swallowed. Must be easy to swallow Drugs must be stable and absorbed in the GI environment; delay in onset of action
Prolonged action (circa 12 h) (e.g. protection from nerve agents)	Oral controlled release tablets/ capsules	Tablets or capsules containing an excipient that regulates drug release. Must be easy to swallow. Potent drug easily absorbed throughout GI tract; delay in onset of action
	Buccal tablets	Tablets containing a bioadhesive for locating between the upper gingival and buccal mucosal tissue. Must be sufficiently adhesive to avoid dislodgement. Limited to drugs that permeate buccal mucosa (small lipophilic)
Prolonged action (days) e.g. protection from nerve agents	Transdermal patches	An adhesive formulation where the drug release is regulated (typically by a rate limiting membrane. Apply in advance under clothing or to accessible skin. Limited to potent drugs that readily cross skin (small and lipophilic): delay in onset of action
Prolonged action (days to weeks) (e.g. Protection from nerve agents)	Depot injections and implants	Typically a sparingly soluble drug as a solid or dispersed in an oil. Easier to administer in advance. Limited to high potency drugs only

References

1. Hawley PR (1951) Medical planning for modern war. J Med Education 26:266–268
2. Earwood JS, Brooks DE (2006) The Seven P's in battalion level combat health support in the military operations in urban terrain environment: the Fallujah experience, Summer 2003 to Spring 2004. Mil Med 171:272–277
3. Truesdell AG (2006) Training for medical support in mountain operations. Mil Med 171:463–467
4. Mucciarone MC, Llewellyn CH (2006) Tactical combat casualty care in the assault on Punta Paitilla Airfield. Mil Med 171:687–690
5. Zouris JM, Walker J, Dye J, Galarneau M (2006) Wounding patterns of US Marines and sailors during operation Iraqi freedom, Major combat phase. Mil Med 171:246–252
6. Albuquerque EX, Pereira EFR, Aracava Y et al (2006) Effective countermeasure against poisoning by organophosphorous insecticides and nerve. PNAS 103:13220–13225
7. Bajgar J (2004) Organophosphates/nerve agent poisoning: mechanism of action, diagnosis, prophylaxis, and treatment. Adv Clin Chem 38:151–216
8. Dire DJ (2005) Biological warfare. www.emedicinehealth.com/ biological_warfare/article_em.htm
9. Skinner AM (2006) Management of unconscious casualties in far forward deployed special forces. Mil Med 171:2–4
10. Gulland A (2008) Lessons from the battlefield. Brit Med J 336:1098–1100
11. Stinger H (2006) The army forward surgical team: update and lessons learned 1997/2004. Mil Med 171:269–272
12. Brewer TL, Ryan-Wenger NA (2009) Critical care air transport team (CCATT) nurses' deployed experience. Mil Med 174:408–514
13. Aulton MJ (2007) Aulton's pharmaceutics, 3rd edn, The design and manufacture of medicines. Churchill Livingstone, London
14. Touitou E, Barry BW (2007) Enhancement in drug delivery. CRC, Boca Raton, Florida
15. Bergens T, Åmark M (2001) Autoinjector. US Patent 6270479
16. Scherer B (2006) Autoinjector comprising a resettable releasing safety device. US Patent 7118553
17. Meridian Medical Technologies (2009) US Armed services products. www.meridianmeds.com/us_armed_forces.html
18. Hamilton EL, Lutz EM (2005) Orally disintegrating tablets. Drug Deliv Technol 5(1):34–37
19. Srinivas G, Harikrishna D, Aliasgar S, Mansoor A (2008) A review of stimuli-responsive nanocarriers for drug and gene delivery. J Control Rel 126:187–204
20. Torchilin VP (2006) Multifunctional nanocarriers. Adv Drug Deliv Revs 58:1532–1555

Chapter 13
Biological Means Against Bio-Terrorism: Phage Therapy and Prophylaxis Against Pathogenic Bacteria

N. Chanishvili

Abstract This review describes the use of bacteriophages against bacterial infections in the battlefield and protection of the civilian population. High therapeutic and protective potential of bacteriophages suggests that they could be an efficient means against bio-terrorist attacks.

Keywords Bacteriophage therapy • Bioterrorism • Biological warfare

13.1 Introduction

It is well known that biological weapons can be used to kill or disable people, to poison foods, or to contaminate pharmaceutical products, kill livestock, destroy crops, and thus harm a nation's economy [1]. Vulnerability of the target victims and capability of the aggressors are two prerequisites of bio-terrorism. Limiting our vulnerability is the most promising way to prevent or mitigate biological terror attempts. With this regard researchers have been actively seeking novel effective means of protection against potential biological weapons and neutralization of their action. The use of biological means against bio-terrorism seems to be rather logical. One of most promising approaches which provides therapy, prophylaxis and identification of bacterial infection is application of bacterial viruses – bacteriophages.

A bacteriophage (from 'bacteria' and Greek φαγεῖν, phagein "to eat") is a bacterial virus able to infect and kill (lyse) bacteria. The first reports about bacteriophage were published by F. Twort [2] and F. d'Herelle [3] but it was d'Herelle who proposed that bacteriophage might be applied to control bacterial diseases.

N. Chanishvili (✉)
Eliava Institute of Bacteriophage, Microbiology and Virology (IBMV), 3 Gotua street, Tbilisi 0160, Georgia
e-mail: n_chanish.ibmv@caucasus.net.

S. Mikhalovsky and A. Khajibaev (eds.), *Biodefence*, NATO Science for Peace and Security Series A: Chemistry and Biology, DOI 10.1007/978-94-007-0217-2_13,

Within the former Soviet Union (FSU), bacteriophage therapy was researched and extensively applied for the treatment and prophylaxis of a wide range of bacterial infections. In the West however, it was not explored with the same enthusiasm and was eventually discarded with the arrival of antibiotics.

From the review of the Soviet literature it is apparent that phage therapy and prophylaxis were widely used especially in war times, since the desperate need for therapeutic drugs inspired the Soviet doctors to perform new trials with phages and develop novel methods for their administration. Later phage therapy became very popular all over the Soviet Union. Our analysis of the literature indicates that phage therapy was used extensively in medicine to treat a wide range of bacterial infections in the areas of dermatology [4–11], ophthalmology [12–14], pediatrics [15–18], surgery (especially against wound infections) [19, 20], urology [21], pulmonology [22–24], otolaryngology [25] and stomatology [26].

Here some examples of phage therapy and prophylaxis are presented to stimulate further interest in its application to protect military and civilian populations in cases of bio-terrorist attacks. It is also important that phage therapy may be considered as an alternative to antibiotic and other therapies in combating the increasing range of multi-drug resistant bacteria against which phages still remain active.

13.2 Phage Therapy in Military Surgery

The application of phage therapy in surgery and for wound treatment began during the Soviet war with Finland in 1939–1940 with the first review of this work published by Kokin [cited in 27], who described the application of mixtures of bacteriophages (produced by the Eliava IBMV) to infect anaerobes, Staphylococci and Streptococci for the treatment of gas gangrene. The mixture was applied in 767 infected soldiers with lethality of 18.8% compared with 42.2% in the control group of soldiers treated by alternative methods. Using the same mixture of bacteriophages other authors observed lethal outcomes of 19.2% in a group of soldiers treated with phage compared with 54.2% in a group treated with other medications [Lvov & Pasternak, cited in 27].

In addition to its therapeutic use, this phage preparation was also used by mobile sanitary brigades as an emergency aid for treatment of wounds (prophylaxis of gas gangrene). Krestovnikova [27] summarized the observations of three mobile sanitary brigades carried out over periods of 2–6 weeks following evacuation to frontline hospitals.

The first brigade treated 2,500 soldiers with phages. Only 35 soldiers (1.4%) in this group showed symptoms of gas gangrene while in the control group of 7,918 wounded soldiers symptoms were observed in 342 (4.3%). The second brigade applied phage therapy in 941 soldiers, of which only 14 (1.4%) suffered from gas gangrene, in contrast to 6.8% of the control group who were treated by other methods. The third brigade treated 2,584 soldiers and observed the development of the disease in 18 soldiers (0.7%), whilst in the control group gas gangrene emerged in 2.3% of cases. Data comparison and observations described by the three independent brigades showed a 3-fold decrease in the incidence of gas gangrene as a direct consequence of the prophylactic treatment of wounds through the application of the phage mixtures [27].

A book written in 1941 by Professor Tsulukidze [28] which summarizes the results obtained after the Finnish Campaign is particularly interesting for military surgeons.

The majority of patients arriving from the front line with wounds were bedridden and in a severe condition; 38.3% of them had soft tissue injuries and 61.7% – bone injuries. Prior to obtaining the results of bacteriological analysis, Pio-bacteriophage preparation (a broad spectrum phage preparation effective against species related to *Staphylococcus, Streptococcus, E. coli, Proteus* and *Pseudomonas* infections that are the main causes of purulent infections) or a mixture of Strepto- and Staphylo- bacteriophages was applied topically or directly to the accessible part of the wound. Initially the application of phage therapy was only used in the most severe cases when the lethal outcome was very likely. Later a wider range of patients were involved in the study. The patients that arrived to the hospital did not undergo any selection. These patients often had major tissue damage with the wounds going through the tissues from one side to the other. The patients were divided into two major groups: those with closed sites of infection such as tendovaginitis, phlegmon, abscesses, etc. and those with open wounds. In the first group of 39 patients, 19 suffered from phlegmon, 14 from tendovaginitis, three were with abscesses and three with furunculosis. The open wounds were characterized by abundant pus, complicated infections and inflammation around the wound, sometimes with necrotic loci. The treatment of such patients was performed by decontaminating wounds with iodine and alcohol, then washing with 2% sodium chloride solution followed by spraying with phages. Simultaneously, 5–10 mL of phage preparation was injected remotely from the wound into the front wall of the abdomen, shoulder or hip. Subcutaneous injections of phages were performed 3–4 times every second day to avoid the development of anti-phage antibodies, and the spraying of phages over the wound was carried out each time dressings were changed. The wound was dressed with the gauze soaked with phage. Tampons and drainages were not applied. None of the patients treated with this method required additional surgical wound revisions or any other surgery. Only 3–4 phage-associated manipulations were normally applied to achieve a complete cure and the blood test results were also improved. Since recovery from traumatic injuries and numerous lesions requires rather a long time, the wounds were stitched after the infection was eliminated by phage therapy on the 6th–8th day of treatment, so that the wounds became inaccessible to additional infectious agents. In general, the treatment by phage therapy took a few days whereas in the control group treated with chloramines, rivanol, Vishnevsky ointment, etc., the same successful results could be achieved only in several weeks.

Summarizing the data Tsulukidze [28] indicated that no side effects were observed with the topical application of phages, however if phage preparations were injected into the infected site a pain could emerge and continue over the next 1–2 hours. This pain could be explained by the tissue pressure developing after

24.8% of patients showed no evidence of bleeding after 4–10 days of phage therapy with only 19.5% showing no relief of symptoms. Overall 74.4% of patients out of the 219 patients treated with bacteriophages showed an improvement or were completely cured, with only 25.6% showing no improvement.

Lurie [34] underlined the difficulty in drawing objective conclusions from the results described since the majority of patients were already receiving a variety of emergency treatments at home including cleansing enemas, change of diet, and relief of dehydration or receiving a purgative treatment. This mixed background made it difficult to conclude that the therapeutic effect was due solely to phage therapy.

13.4 Phage Prophylaxis

Phages have also been used extensively in the USSR for prophylaxis, especially in communities where the rapid spread of infections may occur, such as kindergartens, schools, and military accommodation. An experiment on the prophylactic use of phages was successfully carried out in 1935 on thousands of people in the regions with a high incidence of dysentery [25]. The results were reported at scientific conferences in 1934 and 1936 in Kiev and in 1939 in Moscow after which the dysenteric phage preparation was finally approved as a preventive measure for mass application. It was recommended that repeated seasonal prophylactic "phaging" be carried out in areas where it was endemic. Later modifications included the supply of the dysenteric phages in dry tablet forms which also began to be included in clinical studies.

One of the later studies described the results of preventive treatment carried out with the phage tablets having an acid-resistant coating [38]. Experimental and control groups were selected at random, and one soldier provided an "observation unit". The populations in the experimental and control groups were located in different geographical zones, however they were all placed in similar types of endemic area. Bacteriophage and placebo were coded and were given when there was a rise in morbidity threatening to become an epidemic, particularly in June-July and September-October. Two tablets of the coded preparations were given to the people in the experimental and control groups 1.5 hours prior to meals. One group was given the tablets once every 3 days, while another group of the same size received the preparation once every 5 days. Calcium gluconate was used in placebo experiments. The efficiency of prevention using phage prophylactics given once every 3 days was 75%, and 67% when given every 5 days leading to a recommended use of the phage tablets once every 3 days. During the course of this study coincidental outbreaks of dysentery related to water contamination with *Sh. dysenteriae* were observed in two separate communities. Analysis of morbidity showed great differences between the experimental and control groups with morbidity in the control group appearing to be 5.7 to 9.5 times higher than in the experimental group receiving phage tablets once every 3 or 5 days. The phage tablets therefore provided a high level of prophylactic action [38].

For the prevention of typhoid epidemics specific phages were also used with two tablets administered once every 5–7 days during the outbreak season [35, 36]. Intestinal colonization and overgrowth with *Pseudomonas aeruginosa* in young hospitalized children was prevented successfully by phage administration [39].

Phage preparations have also been found to be very useful in the disinfection of surfaces and facilities in hospitals. Walls in wards, different surfaces, and even instruments and wounds (the source of some pathogens) have also been treated, with a considerable effect in children's clinics [41]. Recent studies demonstrated a high eradicating effect of *P. aeruginosa* and *S. aureus* phages in a laboratory environmental model [42, 43].

13.5 Conclusions

From the experiments described above, the therapeutic and protective potential of bacteriophages is apparent and they may be recommended as a potential means against bio-terrorist attacks.

Acknowledgments This review was supported by the ISTC Partner Program Grant G-1467 and the UK Global Threat Reduction Programme.

References

1. Siegrist DW (1999) The threat of biological attack: Why concern now? Emerg Infect Dis 5:505–508
2. Twort FW (1915) An investigation on the nature of the ultra-microscopic viruses. Lancet 1241–1243
3. d'Herelle F (1917) Sur un microbe invisible antagoniste des bacilles dysentériques. C R Acad Sci Se 165:373–375
4. Beridze MA (1938) Role of bacteriophage therapy in combating of purulent skin infections. Tbilisi, Georgia
5. Ukelis II (1946) Treatment of furunculosis and other purulent skin infections with di-phage. Sovetskaia Meditsina (Russian "Soviet Medicine") 3:11–12
6. Vartapetov LI (1941) Predictive significance of correspondence of the results of in vivo and in vitro lysis in case of treatment of piodermatitis, Selected Papers. Institute of Dermatology and Venereal Diseases, Tbilisi, Georgia, pp 93–97
7. Vartapetov LI (1947) Results of phage therapy of deep forms of piodermitis. Selected Papers. Institute of Dermatology and Venereal Diseases, Tbilisi, Georgia, pp 205–207
8. Vartapetov LI (1957) Phage therapy of deep forms of piodermitis caused by Staphylococcus, In "Bacteriophages", Tbilisi, Georgia, pp 411–422
9. Khuskivadze ZF (1954) On the issue of phage therapy of deep forms of piodermitis. CandSci Diss, Tbilisi, Georgia
10. Gvazava AI (1957) Results of therapy of deep forms of piodermitis with the expired phage preparations. CandSci Diss, Tbilisi, Georgia

11. Shvelidze KD (1970) Treatment of deep forms of dermatitis of Staphylococcus etiology performed with the specific bacteriophage and some immune reactions of the organism. CandSci Diss, Tbilisi, Georgia
12. Rodigina AM (1938) Pneumococcal bacteriophage: Its application for treatment of the ulcerous corneal serpens. Perm, USSR
13. Cherkasskaja RS (1984) Application of bacteriophages for treatment of purulent conjunctivitis among newborns. Materials of the Symposium dedicated to 60th anniversary of the Tbilisi Scientific-Research Institute of Vaccine and Sera. Tbilisi, Georgia, pp 264–266
14. Protopopov SV (1974) Treatment of the experimental corneal ulcer caused by Staphylococcus aureus. Materials of the Scientific Symposium dedicated to the 50th anniversary of the Tbilisi Scientific Research Institute of Vaccine and Sera. Tbilisi, Georgia, pp 422–424
15. Samsygina GA (1985) Festering inflammatory infections among newborns (Etiology, risk factors, clinic and immune diagnostic criteria and strategy of treatment). DSc Diss, Moscow, Russia
16. Tsistishvili GI (1940) On the issue of phage application for puerperial infectious diseases. Akusherstvo i ginekologia (Russian "Obstetrics and Gynecology") 12:20–22
17. Purtseladze MD (1941) Treatment of purulent forms of mastititis. Akusherstvo i ginekologia (Russian "Obstetrics and Gynecology") 11–12:22–24.
18. Bochorishvili EV (1988) Method of treatment of tube infertility of the inflammatory genesis. SU Patent N 1395331
19. Tsulukidze AP (1940) Phage treatment in surgery. Khirurgiia (Russian "Surgery") 12:132–133
20. Tsulukidze AP (1957) Results of phage application for treatment of surgical infections. In: Bacteriophages. Tbilisi, Georgia, pp 99–108
21. Tsulukidze AP (1938) Application of phages in urology. Urologiia (Russian "Urology") 15:10–13
22. Ioseliani GG, Meladze GD, Chkhetiia NSh et al (1980) Use of bacteriophage and antibiotics for prevention of acute postoperative empyema in chronic suppurative lung diseases. Grudnaia Khirurgiia (Russian Breast Surgery) 1:63–67
23. Meladze GD, Mebuke MG, Chkhetiia NSh et al (1982) Efficacy of staphylococcal bacteriophage in the treatment of purulent lung and pleural diseases. Grudnaia Khirurgiia (Russian Breast Surgery) 1:53–56
24. Chkhetia NSh (1984) Treatment of lung diseases. CandSci Diss, Tbilisi, Georgia
25. Ermolieva VV (1939) About bacteriophage and its application. J Microbiol Epidemiol Immunol 9:9–17
26. Ruchko I (1936) Therapeutic effect of Staphylococcus phage for oral and dental infections. Sovetskaya Stomatologia (Russian "Soviet Stomatology") 1:11–20
27. Krestovnikova VA (1947) Phage treatment and phage prophylactics and their approval in the works of the Soviet researchers. J Microbiol Epidemiol Immunol 3:56–65
28. Tsulukidze AP (1941) Experience of Use of Bacteriophages in the Conditions of War traumatism. Tbilisi, Georgia, pp 418
29. Tucker JB (1999) Historical trends related to biorerrorism: An empirical analysis. Emerg Infect Dis 5:498–504
30. Palvin JA (1999) Epidemiology of bio-terrorism. Emerg Infect Dis 5:528–530
31. Moores LE (2002) Threat credibility and weapons of mass destruction. Neurosurg Focus 12(3):E4
32. Blendon RJ, Benson JM, DesRoches CM et al (2002) The impact of anthrax attacks on the American public. Medscape Gen Med 4(2):1
33. Relman DA, Olson JE (2001) Bioterrorism preparedness: what practitioners need to know. Infect Med 18:497–514
34. Alexandrova MB (1935) Phage therapy against dysentery. J Microbiol Epidemiol Immunol 11:860–868
35. Lurie MN (1938) Treatment of dysentery and haemolytic intestinal diseases among children and adults. Selected Papers of Azerbaijani Institute of Epidemiology and Microbiology 6:31–34

36. Vlasov KF, Artemenko EA (1946) Treatment of chronic dysentery. Sovetskaia Meditsina (Russian "Soviet Medicine") 10:22–28
37. Gnutenko MP (1951) Treatment of S. typi and paratyphi bacterial carriers with bacteriophages. J Microbiol Epidemiol Immunol 5:56–60
38. Anpilov LI, Prokudin AA (1984) Preventive effectiveness of dried polyvalent Shigella bacteriophage in organized collective farms. Voenno-Meditsinskii Zhurnal (Russian "Military-Med J") 5:39–40
39. Agafonov VI, Liashenko NI, Novikov NL (1984) Epidemiology of typhoid-paratyphoid infections and their prophylactics. Voenno-Meditsinskii Zhurnal (Russian "Military-Med J") 6:36–40
40. Kurochka VK, Karniz AF, Khodyrev AP (1987) Experience in conducting epidemic-control measures in a focus of intestinal infections with a water mechanism of transmission. Russian "Military-Med J" 7:36–37
41. Pavlenishvili I (1988) Method of selective decontamination in newborns clinic. Certificate of Invention №269
42. Glonti T (2004) Study of the biological properties of bacteriophages active against P. aeruginosa and evaluation of their potential use for sanitation of the environment. CandSci dissertation, Tbilisi, Georgia
43. Chanishvili N, Glonti T (2007) Method of disinfection or decontamination of infected pen or building interior using bacteriophages. Patent AU 2007 9051U, Official Bulletin of Industrial Property 15:22

Chapter 14
Enzyme Stabilization in Nanostructured Materials, for Use in Organophosphorus Nerve Agent Detoxification and Prophylaxis

R.J. Kernchen

Abstract Enzyme immobilization and encapsulation in various nanostructures has drawn great interest as it offers both increased stability and reusability without significant loss in activity. Although we are still at the beginning of exploring the use of these materials for biocatalysis, by now several nanostructures have been tested as hosts for enzyme immobilization. The beneficial application of enzyme stabilization in nanostructured materials for use in nerve agent detoxification and pre-treatment is reviewed and discussed in this article. Enzymes hydrolyzing organophosphorus compounds (e.g. OPAA, OPH, Paraoxonase) are capable of detoxifying neurotoxic chemical warfare (CW) agents, i.e. G-type, V-type, and related organophosphorus (OP)-based industrial materials. The nano-encapsulation of OP-hydrolyzing enzymes with mesoporous materials or dendritic polymers can provide a very stable and convenient formulation for use in chemical agent detoxification. Nano-encapsulated enzymes demonstrated the ability to retain their activity in the presence of a number of organic solvents, commercial disinfectants and anti-microbial agents and foams, making them suitable for personnel decontamination and individual protection applications. OP-hydrolyzing enzymes also show great promise as catalytic bioscavengers to be used as safe and effective medical countermeasures to OP intoxication. Novel enzyme-complexed nano-delivery systems, particularly polymeric nanocapsules and sterically stabilized liposomes, can be used to carry these metabolizing enzymes to the circulation. Thus, it is possible to avoid the physiological disposition and potential immunological reactions of these bacterial derived enzymes. Nanostructured delivery systems, consequently, allows for increasing the enzymes efficacy by extending their circulatory life and in some cases also their specific activity.

R.J. Kernchen (✉)
Fraunhofer Institute for Technological Trend Analysis (INT),
Appelsgarten 2, 53879 Euskirchen, Germany
e-mail: roman.kernchen@int.fraunhofer.de

S. Mikhalovsky and A. Khajibaev (eds.), *Biodefence*, NATO Science for Peace and Security Series A: Chemistry and Biology, DOI 10.1007/978-94-007-0217-2_14,

Keywords Enzymes • Nanostructured materials • Organophosphorus • Detoxification

14.1 Introduction

Organophosphorus (OP) compounds are a broad class of neurotoxic chemicals which may be used as pesticides or chemical warfare agents (CWAs). OP-based chemical warfare agents are the nerve agents of the G-type, i.e. tabun (GA), sarin (GB), cyclosarin (GF), soman (GD) and of the V-type, i.e. forms of VX. Organophosphorus nerve agents were designed specifically to cause incapacitation or death in military use and are particularly effective because of their extremely high toxicity [1]. The acute toxicity is three to four orders of magnitude greater than most of the chemically similar OP pesticides [2]. The toxicity of OPs is due primarily to the practically irreversible inhibition of acetylcholine esterase (AChE), the enzyme responsible for hydrolysis of the neurotransmitter acetylcholine. The accumulation of acetylcholine in synapses effectively prevents the transmission of nerve signals and results in the characteristic symptoms.

OP nerve agents are a serious threat to military and civilian personnel [3]. In case of an attack with nerve agents widespread areas may become contaminated [4]. In such an incident both environmental decontamination and personal detoxification are essential for survival. Furthermore, medical countermeasures, such as emergency treatment of acute intoxication and supportive therapy of OP intoxication, are required. Since post-exposure therapy has its limitations, research has also been focused on the possibility of pre-treatment in order to limit the toxicity of nerve warfare agents if exposed afterwards. Enzymes have considerable potential for each of these application areas. The use of enzymes for the decontamination and detoxification of nerve agents has been a subject of study for over 50 years. The toxicity of OP compounds is strongly reduced by enzymatic hydrolysis [5]. Several organophosphate degrading enzymes have been identified which accomplish the hydrolysis of specific classes of organophosphorus compounds. OP compound hydrolyzing enzymes are capable of detoxifying neurotoxic chemical warfare agents, and related organophosphorus-based industrial materials. The best characterized enzymes among them against CW agents are phosphotriesterase (PTE), organophosphorus acid anhydrolase (OPAA), organophosphorus hydrolase (OPH), and di-isopropylfluorophosphatase (DFPase), which hydrolyze nerve agents to their respective, stable methylphosphonate alkyl ester products.

OP-hydrolyzing enzymes also show great promise as catalytic bioscavengers to be used as safe and effective medical countermeasures to OP intoxication [6]. Current antidotal regimens for organophosphorus compound poisoning consist of a combination of pre-treatment with carbamates (pyridostigmine bromide), to protect acetylcholinesterase (AChE) from irreversible inhibition by OP compounds, and a post-exposure therapy with anticholinergic drugs such as atropine sulphate to reactivate OP-inhibited AChE and oximes such as 2-PAM chloride to reactivate OP-inhibited AChE [7]. These antidotes are effective in preventing lethality from OP intoxication but do not prevent post-exposure incapacitation (i.e. convulsions, seizure, brain damage, etc.). Whereas enzyme bioscavengers as a pretreatment are able to sequester highly toxic Ops, before they reach their physiologic targets and prevent the in vivo toxicity OPs and post-exposure incapacitation. If an effective bioscavenger is present in the blood before exposure, reduction of the nerve agent concentration to toxicologically irrelevant level will be very rapid. Enzyme candidates for catalytic scavengers against OP compounds currently are; Paraoxonase (PON1), mutants of butyrylcholinesterase (BChE) and acetylcholinesterase, bacterial and eukaryotic OPH, OPAA and DFPase.

However, enzymes used for decontamination/detoxification of OP nerve agents or as nerve agent bioscavengers are required to operate under harsh conditions such as extreme pH and temperature, organic solvents, adverse physiological disposition factors, etc, that often lead to enzyme deactivation. The stability of enzymes generally is a critical issue in biotechnology [8, 9]. Both storage and operational stabilities affect the usefulness of enzyme-based products. Storage stability refers to an enzyme maintaining its catalytic abilities in the period between manufacture and eventual use. Operational stability describes the persistence of enzyme activity under conditions of use. An effective way to overcome limitations caused by insufficient stability to some extent is enzyme immobilization. Moreover, immobilization might improve enzyme properties because substrate specificity might be enhanced and the effect of inhibitors might be reduced [10]. It further provides a convenient means to separate and reuse the biocatalyst to improve process economics. An immobilized enzyme is an enzyme that is physically attached to a solid support (carrier). The stability of an immobilised enzyme is determined by many factors such as the number of bonds formed between the enzyme and carrier, the nature of the bonds, the degree of confinement of enzyme molecules in the carrier, the microenvironment of the enzyme and carrier, and the immobilization conditions [11]. The immobilization or encapsulation of enzymes has attracted continuous attention in the fields of fine chemistry, biomedicine and biosensors and has also been proposed for enzyme-based methods of environmental decontamination and personal detoxification as well as for catalytic scavengers.

The success of immobilization, including the performance of immobilized enzymes, strongly depends on the properties of supports, which are usually referred to particularly as material type, composition and structure. Substantial R&D efforts have been conducted to optimize the structure of the carrier materials in order to obtain better catalytic stability and efficiency [12, 13]. In this regard, nanotechnology provides opportunities to formulate desirable features in balancing key factors that determine the efficiency of biocatalysts, including specific surface area, mass transfer resistance, and effective enzyme loading. Nanotechnology can be defined as the science and engineering involved in the design, synthesis, characterization and application of materials and devices whose functional organization in at least one dimension is within the range of 1–100 nm [14]. The incorporation of enzymes in polymer nanostructures provides diverse opportunities for chemically re-engineering enzymes for a wide range of applications. Nanostructured supports are believed to be able to retain the catalytic activity as well as ensure the immobilization efficiency of enzymes to a high extent [15, 16]. Hitherto different nanostructured materials have been used as supports, such as mesoporous silica, nanotubes, nanoparticles, nanofibres and crosslinked enzyme crystals or aggregates [17]. Compared to other supports their surface area-to-volume ratios are very high, which can provide large specific surface areas for enzyme immobilization as well as stabilization. The other essential advantage offered by their chemical structures, is the immense possibilities to establish a suitable microenvironment for a chosen enzyme. In terms of controlled porosity and flexibility, tailored balance between hydrophobicity and hydrophilicity, and the high degree of structural availability and functionality, respective nanostructures are particularly attractive for fabricating effective enzyme supports.

In recent times the incorporation of enzymes into nanostructured materials is commonly referred to as nanobiocatalysis. Nanobiocatalysis has emerged as a rapidly growing research and development area. Lately, nanobiocatalytic approaches have evolved beyond simple enzyme immobilization strategies to include also topics like artificial enzymes and cells, nanofabrication, and nanopatterning [18]. A recent bibliometric analysis [19] of nanobiocatalysis publications shows a strong increase within the last decade (Fig. 14.1). The analysis has been compiled from

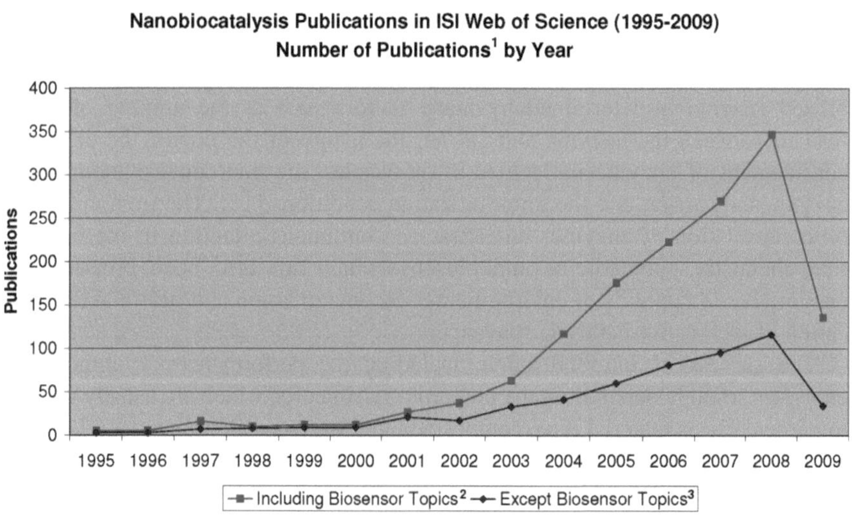

Fig. 14.1 Nanobiocatalysis publications in ISI Web of Science by year (1995–2009). [1] Research articles, proceedings and reviews, [2] Search in title, abstract and keywords for: enzyme* or biocatalysts* and nanostructured or nanosized or nanoscale or nanoporous or nanoencapsulation or nanoparticle or nanotube or nanocluster or nanofibre or nanotechnolog* or nanocolloid* or nanocapsule* or nanoreactor* or nanoliposome*, [3] Search like in [2] excluding: biosens* or sensor* or electrode* or detect* or electrochem* or chemiluminescence* or assay* in title, abstract and keywords

searches in the ISI Web of Science (expanded Science Citation Index, Thomson Reuters) conducted during May 2009.

A substantial part of the total nanobiocatalysis publications is concerning enzyme immobilization on nanostructured supports for enzymatic biosensor applications (Fig. 14.1). Furthermore, areas of applied research in nanobiocatalysis are particularly fine chemistry, medicine and pharmacology, as well as food technology (Fig. 14.2). However, at the present stage R&D activities in nanobiocatalysis are still primarily focused on basic research topics (Fig. 14.2). These include questions regarding interactions of enzymes with the microenvironment and their impact on catalysis of a given substrate, confinement effects of immobilized enzymes, new fabrication methods of biocatalysts, e.g. via in situ growth of polymer chains from the enzyme surface.

Research and development activities in nanobiocatalysis are currently conducted in particular in the USA and in Asian countries (PR of China, Japan, South Korea and India) (Fig. 14.3).

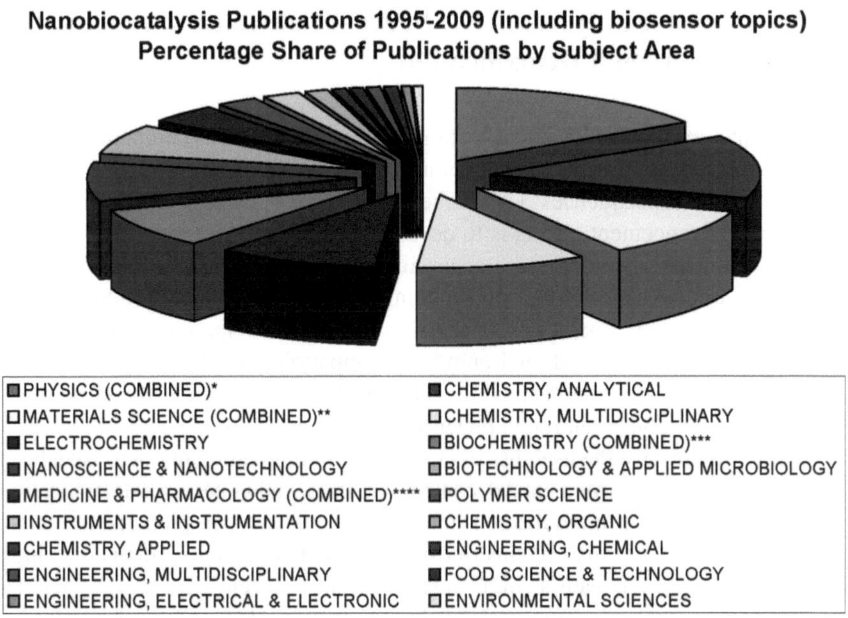

Fig. 14.2 Nanobiocatalysis publications by subject area (1995–2009). * Physics (combined): physics, applied; physics, condensed matter, ** Materials science (combined): materials science, multidisciplinary; materials science, biomaterials, *** Biochemistry (combined): biochemistry & molecular biology; biochemical research methods, ****Medicine & pharmacology (combined): pharmacology & pharmacy; engineering, biomedical; medicine, research & experimental; chemistry, medicinal

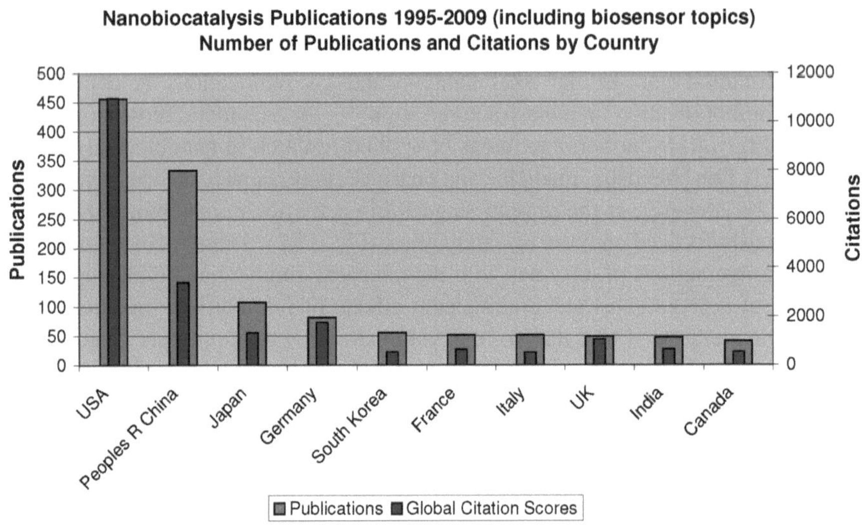

Fig. 14.3 Nanobiocatalysis publications by country (1995–2009)

14.2 Nanobiocatalysis for OP Nerve Agent Decontamination and Personal Detoxification

The current methods for the detoxification of organophosphorus compounds, which rely on bleach treatment or incineration, are harmful and possess serious environmental consequences [20]. The objective of current decontamination technology advancement efforts is to develop systems that are rapid and effective in detoxifying OP nerve agents, environmentally safe, have no impact on the operational effectiveness of the subject being decontaminated, and minimizing the logistical impact on operations. Enzyme mediated decontamination, which is non-toxic, noncorrosive and environmental compatible, could widely fulfil these aims. Enzyme-based approaches for OP agent detoxification therefore have received considerable attention in recent years.

In order to improve the usability of enzymes, immobilization matrices have been proposed with both environmental decontamination as well as personal detoxification in mind. Effective immobilization methods allow for the preparation of an immobilized enzyme that retains most of its native activity, maintains high operational stability as well as high storage stability. Recent advances in material synthesis using enzymes have allowed the preparation of a variety of bioplastics and enzyme-polymer composites, which involve the incorporation of the enzyme material directly into the polymer. Enzymes stabilized in this way maintain considerable stability under normally denaturing conditions [21]. A number of methods have been used to prepare bioplastic or enzyme-polymer composite materials with OP-degrading enzymes. Drevon & Russel described the incorporation of the OP-degrading enzyme DFPase into polyurethane foams [22]. In a buffered media, the recovered enzyme activity was approximately 67% of the activity of the soluble enzyme. The loss in activity was attributed to the harsh polymerization conditions, such as elevated temperature and use of organic solvent. Also organophosphorus hydrolase has been incorporated within polyurethane foams during polymer synthesis as a means of reducing the environmental sensitivity of enzymes to alterations in pH and bleach-induced enzyme denaturation [23].

One of the most widely used methods for immobilizing enzymes is encapsulation inside sol-gel silica [24]. However, the specific activity of immobilized enzymes using conventional immobilization supports such as sol-gel-silica is usually lower, or much lower than that of the free enzyme in solution because of small pore sizes, non open pore structures and harsh immobilization conditions [25]. Recently, many research groups have immobilized enzymes on mesoporous silica (MPS) which showed improvement on enzyme stability, catalytic activity, products specifity, and resistance to extreme environmental conditions [12, 26]. MPS materials provide tunable and uniform pore systems, functionalizable surfaces, and restricted nanospaces for enzyme immobilization. Mesoporous silica can facilitate mass transport of the enzyme substrate and product and allow the enzyme to be spontaneously entrapped inside the mesopores under neutral mild conditions. The enzyme confinements in the nanochannel of MPS materials generate synergistic effects that enhance enzyme stability and improve selectivity [25]. The effect of microenvironment on enzyme activity was demonstrated by immobilization of OPH on different mesoporous silicas, bearing different binding functionalities such as negatively charged MPS (HCOOH-CH_2-CH_2), positively charged MPS (-NH_2) and unfunctionalized mesoporous silica UMPS (native negatively charged surface) [11, 27]. It was found that with UMPS only a protein loading of 3.1% (w/w) and a specific activity of 935 units/mg of adsorbed protein were achieved, whereas a higher protein loading of 4.7% (w/w) with significantly enhanced specific activity of 4,182 units/mg was obtained with the negatively charged silica as carrier. Unexpectedly, the specific acitivity with 2% NH_2-MPS was as high as 2,691 units/mg with a protein loading of 3.8% (w/w), while 20% NH_2-MPS retained almost zero activity and 0.25% (w/w) enzyme load. This result clearly suggests that the microenvironment of the binding functionalities is of vital importance for the activity expression. The outlook of using OP-degrading enzymes encapsulated in mesopores for decontamination from CW is promising. The encapsulation procedure is relatively simple and inexpensive to perform with standard laboratory equipment. It has been shown that respective enzymes such as OPAA, exhibit good activity not only in aqueous but also in mixed aqueous-organic solvent-base media that are commonly found in military field environments. Furthermore, the reuse of encapsulated OPAA for as many as eight times has been demonstrated [28]. Cheng, Rastogi et al. observed stabilization of the OP-degrading enzymes OPH and OPAA through nanoencapsulation of the enzyme by use of non-toxic water soluble dendritic polymers [29]. The dendritic polymers were used in a series of experiments to test for the compatibility of OPH and OPAA with a commercial disinfectant/ anti-microbial agent. Activities of both enzymes were reduced in the presence of the disinfectant by >85%. OPAA and OPH encapsulated under the same conditions (in the presence of the disinfectant and ammonium carbonate) with the C18-dendritic polymer retained a 70–80% higher enzymatic activity.

14.3 Nanobiocatalysis for OP Nerve Agent Medical Therapy and Prophylaxes

The use of enzyme bioscavengers is a relatively new approach to reduce the in vivo toxicity of chemical warfare nerve agents. As a pre-treatment, bioscavengers demonstrated efficacy to sequester highly toxic OPs before they reach their physiological targets and prevent the *in vivo* toxicity of OPs and post-exposure incapacitation [7]. A critical prerequisite for any bioscavenger is a prolonged circulatory residence time of the enzyme. To achieve maximal hydrolysis rates, sufficient concentrations of enzyme must be available for the hydrolysis of the OP molecules in the body. Further requirements for an effective OPs scavenger *in vivo* are high reaction rate with OP molecules, immunotolerance, and no adverse effects on physiological processes, like e.g. behavioural effects [6]. The injection of purified free enzyme preparations directly into the blood stream, however, has serious limitations because of possible immunologic reactions and unfavourable physiological factors. These disadvantages can be partly overcome by encapsulating the enzyme. Biodegradable enzyme carriers, which are permeable to the toxin molecules, can provide sufficiently large amounts of metabolizing enzymes to remain protected in the circulation for a long period of time with minimal leakage and few immunologic reactions [30]. Injectable nanocarriers generally represent an emerging strategy for managing intoxications [31]. Nanosized carriers can take the form of liposomes, nanoemulsions, dendrimers, nanoparticles and macromolecules. As carriers for OP bioscavengers, in particular liposomes and dendritic polymers have been extensively studied [31–34].

Liposomes are spherical lipid vesicles that consist of an aqueous core entrapped by one or more bilayers composed of natural or synthetic lipids. Drug delivery technology utilizing liposomes has made considerable progress, several important formulations for the treatment of different diseases are now available or in advanced clinical trials. In the last years research and development in liposome technology has progressed from conventional vesicles to long-circulating liposomes, which are obtained by modulating the lipid composition, size, and charge of the vesicle [35]. A significant step in the development of long-circulating liposomes came with the inclusion of the synthetic polymer poly-(ethylene glycol) (PEG). PEG is a linear polyether diol with many useful properties, such as biocompatibility, solubility in aqueous and organic media, lack of toxicity, very low immunogenicity and antigenicity. Surface modification of liposomes with PEG has demonstrated several biological and technological advantages. The most important properties of PEGylated vesicles are their strongly reduced uptake by the mononuclear phagocyte system (MPS), prolonged blood circulation, improved distribution in perfused tissue, and improved stability, especially due to avoidance of vesicle aggregation.

Such sterically stabilized PEG-coated liposomes, also referred to as stealth liposomes, were demonstrated to be effective as a carrier system for recombinant OPAA or OPH in an OP scavenger [36, 37]. The liposomal carrier system provided an enhanced protective effect against the applied OP compound paraoxon. Administered with 2-PAM and/or atropine, it showed a dramatic enhancement of protection. The optimal lipid composition for the liposomal carrier offering a relatively high encapsulation efficiency and a stable preparation, was found to be 1-palmitoyl-2-oleol-sn-3-phosphocholin (POPC)/cholesterol (CHOL)/1,2-dipalmitoyl-sn-glycero-3-phosphoethanolamine-N-[methoxy(polyethylene glycol)-2000 (PEG-PE-2000) = 56.9/38.0/5.1. The average diameter of the unilamellar vesicles was ~140 nm, hence the carrier system fulfils the requirement for i.v. application (<200 nm). The vesicles did not exhibit any leakage resulting in loss of encapsulated enzyme after one week of storage. Thus, it can be concluded that the PEG-coated liposomes are stable against fusion and/or aggregation, and that *in vitro* stability of liposomes is not influenced by the presence of the loaded enzyme.

Furthermore, the usability of polyoxazoline based hyperbranched polymers as nanosized delivery system for enzyme bioscavengers was demonstrated [34]. Hyperbranched polymers are a class of highly branched macromolecules belonging to the dendritic polymer family. The size of hyperbranched polymers is typically larger than that of dendrimers, ranging from 10 nm to a few hundred nanometers. The three-dimensional, tree-like spherical macromolecule can encapsulate proteins in its void space. The enzymes OPH and OPAA were encapsulated within the dendritic nanocapsule. Compared with the free enzyme, the carrier system provided only a slightly enhanced protective effect against the applied OP compounds DFP and paraoxon. In contrast, the co-administration of 2-PAM and atropine with the nanoencapsulated bioscavenger provided a significantly more effective antidotal system. Compared with the sterically stabilized liposomes, neither encapsulation technology demonstrated a clear advantage when considering *in vivo* efficacy.

The application of dendritic polymers as drug delivery systems has gained interest mainly due to their inertness relative to temperature, solvent, and pH extremes [38]. However, dendritic polymers require further improvements in biocompability and biodistribution profiles. The cytotoxicity of dendrimers currently has been primarily studied *in vitro*.

References

1. Munro NB, Ambrose KR et al (1994) Toxicity of the organophosphate chemical warfare agents GA, GB, and VX: implications for public protection. Environ Health Perspect 102(1):18–38
2. Karpouzas DG, Sing BK (2006) Microbial degradation of organophosphorus xenobiotics: Metabolic pathways and molecular basis. Adv Microb Physiol 51:119–185
3. Gordon RK, Clarkson ED et al (2009) Rapid decontamination of chemical warfare agents. In: Handbook of toxicology of chemical warfare agents. Academic Press, San Diego, pp 1069–1081

4. Yair S, Ofer B et al (2008) Organophosphate degrading microorganisms and enzymes as biocatalysts in environmental and personal decontamination applications. Crit Rev Biotechnol 28(4):265–275
5. Richardt A, Blum MM (eds) (2008) Decontamination of warfare agents. Enzymatic methods for the removal of B/C weapons. Wiley-VCH Verlag GmbH & Co. KgaA, Weinheim
6. Rochu D, Chabriere E et al (2007) Human paraoxonase: A promising approach for pre-treatment and therapy of organophosphorus poisoning. Toxicology 233(1–3):47–59
7. Doctor BP, Saxena A (2005) Bioscavengers for the protection of humans against organophosphate toxicity. Chem-Biol Interact 157–158; 167–171
8. Ó'Fágáin C (2003) Enzyme stabilization - recent experimental progress. Enzyme Microb Technol 33(2–3):137–149
9. Polizzi KM, Bommarius AS et al (2007) Stability of biocatalysts. Curr Opin Chem Biol 11(2):220–225
10. Betancor L, Luckarift HR (2008) Bioinspired enzyme encapsulation for biocatalysis. Trends Biotechnol 26(10):566–572
11. Cao L (2005) Immobilised enzymes: Science or art? Curr Opin Chem Biol 9(2):217–226
12. Zhao XS, Bao XY et al (2006) Immobilizing catalysts on porous materials. Mater Today 9(3):32–39
13. Wang P (2009) Multi-scale features in recent development of enzymatic biocatalyst systems. Appl Biochem Biotechnol 152(2):343–352
14. Sahoo SK, Parveen S et al (2007) The present and future of nanotechnology in human health care. Nanomed Nanotechnol Biol Med 3(1):20–31
15. Wang P (2006) Nanoscale biocatalyst systems. Curr Opin Biotechnol 17(6):574–579
16. Wang Z-G, Wan L-S et al (2009) Enzyme immobilization on electrospun polymer nanofibers: An overview. J Mol Catal B Enzym 56(4):189–195
17. Ge J, Lu D et al (2009) Recent advances in nanostructured biocatalysts. Biochem Eng J 44(1):53–59
18. Kim J, Grate JW et al (2008) Nanobiocatalysis and its potential applications. Trends Biotechnol 26(11):639–646
19. Kernchen RJ, Jovanovic M (2009). Nanobiokatalyse. Bibliometrische Analyse des F&E-Gebietes, Arbeitsbericht 27-09. Euskirchen, Fraunhofer Institute for Technological Trend Analysis (INT): 1–9
20. Ghanem E, Raushel FM (2005) Detoxification of organophosphate nerve agents by bacterial phosphotriesterase. Toxicol Appl Pharmacol 207(2, Supplement 1):459–47
21. Russell AJ, Berberich JA et al (2003) Biomaterials for mediation of chemical and biological warfare agents. Annu Rev Biomed Eng 5(1):1–27
22. Drevon GF, Russell AJ (2000) Irreversible immobilization of diisopropylfluorophosphatase in polyurethane polymers. Biomacromolecules 1(4):571–576
23. LeJeune KE, Swers JS et al (1999) Increasing the tolerance of organophosphorus hydrolase to bleach. Biotechnol Bioeng 64(2):250–254
24. Taguchi A, Schüth F (2005) Ordered mesoporous materials in catalysis. Microporous Mesoporous Mater 77(1):1–45
25. Lei CH, Soares TA et al. (2008) Enzyme specific activity in functionalized nanoporous supports. Nanotechnology 19(12)
26. Lee C-H, Lin T-S et al (2009) Mesoporous materials for encapsulating enzymes. Nano Today 4(2):165–179
27. Lei CH, Shin YS et al (2002) Entrapping enzyme in a functionalized nanoporous support. J Am Chem Soc 124(38):11242–11243
28. Ong KK, Dong H et al. (2003) Nanoencapsulation of OPAA with mesoporous materials for chemical agent decontamination in organic solvents. DoD Joint service scientific conference on chem & bio defense research, Hunt Valley (MD)
29. Cheng TC, Rastogi VK et al. (2003). Compatibility of CW agent degrading enzymes with disinfectants and foams. Proceedings of the joint service sientific conference on chemical & biological defense research, Hunt Valley, USA

30. Petrikovics I, Papahadjopoulos D et al (2004) Comparing therapeutic and prophylactic protection against the lethal effect of paraoxon. Toxicol Sci 77(2):258–262
31. Petrikovics I, Hong K et al (1999) Antagonism of paraoxon intoxication by recombinant phosphotriesterase encapsulated within sterically stabilized liposomes. Toxicol Appl Pharmacol 156(1):56–63
32. Leroux J-C (2007) Injectable nanocarriers for biodetoxification. Nat Nano 2(11):679–684
33. Petrikovics I, McGuinn WD et al (2000) In vitro studies on sterically stabilized liposomes (SL) as enzyme carriers in organophosphorus (OP) antagonism. Drug Deliv 7(2):83–89
34. Petrikovics I, Wales ME et al (2007) Enzyme-based intravascular defense against organophosphorus neurotoxins: Synergism of dendritic-enzyme complexes with 2-PAM and atropine. Nanotoxicology 1(2):85–92
35. Immordino ML, Dosio F et al (2006) Stealth liposomes: Review of the basic science, rationale, and clinical applications, existing and potential. Int J Nanomedicine 1(3):297–315
36. Budai M, Chapela P et al (2009) Physicochemical characterization of stealth liposomes encapsulating an organophosphate hydrolyzing enzyme. J of Liposome Research 19(2):163–168
37. Petrikovics I, Cheng TC et al (2000) Long circulating liposomes encapsulating organophosphorus acid anhydrolase in diisopropylfluorophosphate antagonism. Toxicol Sci 57(1):16–21
38. Svenson S, Tomalia DA (2005) Commentary - Dendrimers in biomedical applications - reflections on the field. Adv Drug Deliv Rev 57(15):2106–2129

Chapter 15
The Investigation of Relationship between the Poly-Morphism in Exon 5 of Glutathione S-Transferase P1 (Gstp1) Gene and Breast Cancer

E. Akbas, H. Mutluhan-Senli, N. Eras-Erdogan, T. Colak, Ö. Türkmenoglu, and S. Kul

Abstract Beside environmental factors, genetic factors have an important place in the etiology of breast cancer which is one of the most common worldwide and highest mortality cancers among women. Breast cancer is associated with different types of somatic genetic alterations such as mutations in oncogenes and tumor suppressor genes. Glutathione S-transferases (GSTs) are a superfamily of enzymes that are potentially important in regulating susceptibility to cancer because of their ability to metabolize reactive electrophilic intermediates to usually less reactive and more water soluble glutathione conjugates. In GSTP1 (chromosome 11q13), an amino acid transition has been reported at codon 105 (Ile105Val), leading to expression of an active but functionally different protein. The aim of this study was to investigate the frequencies of Ile105Val polymorphism in the exon 5 of GSTP1 gene and its effect on the risk of developing breast cancer in a Mersin sample of the Turkish population. In addition, we investigated whether an association exists between breast cancer and other risk factors including age at menarche, age at menopause, smoking, BMI, and family history.

Our study group consisted of 167 individuals, of whom 99 were healthy women controls and 68 breast cancer cases. The experimental group was comprised of women who had been diagnosed with breast cancer at the Department of Medical Oncology, Mersin University, Turkey. Controls were selected by taking age and sex variable into consideration. Genomic DNA from breast cancer patients and control subjects was analyzed by PCR-RFLP.

E. Akbas (✉), H. Mutluhan-Senli, and N. Eras-Erdogan
Department of Medical Biology and Genetics, University of Mersin, Mersin, Turkey
e-mail: etem_a@yahoo.com

T. Colak and Ö. Türkmenoglu
Department of General Surgery, University of Mersin, Mersin, Turkey

S. Kul
Department of Biostatistics, University of Mersin, Mersin, Turkey

S. Mikhalovsky and A. Khajibaev (eds.), *Biodefence*, NATO Science for Peace and Security Series A: Chemistry and Biology, DOI 10.1007/978-94-007-0217-2_15,

For the exon 5 of GSTP1 gene, the distribution of AA and GG genotypes in the Mersin sample of the Turkish population were 64% and 4% in control group, whereas this genotype distribution were 58% and 7% in patients, respectively. Putative risk factors including age, body mass index or family history were found to be correlated with the developing breast cancer. However, it was determined that smoking, menarch age and menopause status were not associated with breast cancer risk.

Keywords Breast cancer • Glutathione s-transferase • Polymorphism

15.1 Introduction

Breast cancer is one of the most frequent cancers among women worldwide, but its etiology is still unclear. The incidence and the mortality rates vary between different ethnical and geographically distinct populations [1]. Along with environmental factors, genetic factors have an important place in the etiology of breast cancer. Also, advanced age, age at menarche, age at menopause, nutritional habits, Body Mass Index (BMI), and family history of breast cancer are among the other factors that are thought to play a role in breast cancer [2, 3]. GSTs are ubiquitous multifunctional proteins involved in the detoxication of all of these products, i.e., catechol estrogen metabolites, polycyclic aromatic hydrocarbon diol epoxides and ROS [4]. In humans, eight classes of GST genes exist: α (GSTA), μ (GSTM), π (GSTP), θ (GSTT), τ (GSTZ), σ (GSTS), o (GSTO) and κ (GSTK) [5]. Glutathione *S*-Transferase P1 (GSTP1) is a major GST, which is ubiquitously expressed in both normal and tumor breast tissue and the GSTP1 gene is located at chromosome 11q13. In GSTP1, an Ile/Val polymorphism has been reported at codon 105, leading to expression of an active but functionally different protein [6, 7]. Our hypothesis was that altered frequencies of GSTP1 genotypes and environmental exposures might be associated with increased susceptibility for the development of breast cancer.

15.2 Experimental

15.2.1 Study Subjects

The study group consisted of 68 breast cancer cases and the control group consisted of 99 healthy women. The breast cancer cases group was comprised of women who had been diagnosed with breast cancer at the Department of Medical Oncology, Mersin University, Turkey. The control group was randomly selected among healthy women at ages similar to the case group. When blood samples were obtained from the individuals and information and permissions were received, a questionnaire was applied to all individuals. The following information was obtained from this questionnaire: age, height, weight, cigarette smoking status, age at menarche, age at menopause, and family history of breast cancer. The body mass index (BMI) was calculated from height and weight measurements using the formula BMI=(kg/m^2).

15.2.2 Genotype Analysis

Venous blood (8 mL) was collected into 15-mL tubes containing 50 mmol/L disodium EDTA, and genomic DNA was extracted by the standard (phenol/chloroform) method. The genotype frequencies for GSTP1 were determined by polymerase chain reaction (PCR)/RFLP-based methods using DNA extracted from peripheral lymphocytes.

15.2.3 Identification of Gstp1 Polymorphisms

GSTP1 exon 5 and exon 6 polymorphisms were determined by using the Polymerase Chain Reaction-Restriction Fragment Length Polymorphisms (PCR-RFLP) method. GSTP1 *ile105va*l (exon 5) genetic polymorphism analysis was performed in a 30-μl reaction mixture containing 25 pmol of each of the following primers: (sense) F 5'-GTA GTT TGC CCA AGG TCA AG-3' and (antisense) R 5'- AGC CAC CTG AGG GGT AAG-3'. Amplification was performed in an automated thermal cycler (Techne Progene, Cambridge, UK). PCR conditions were 1 cycle of 5 min at 94°C, 30 cycles of 1 min at 94°C, 90 s at 59°C and 90 s at 72°C, followed by a final cycle of 7 min at 72°C. The PCR product was digested with *Alw26I* (MBI Fermentas) for 2 h at 37°C. After the 3% agarose gel electrophoresis, the bands at 329 and 107 bp showed wild-type genotype (*Ile105Ile*), bands at 329, 222 and 107 bp showed heterozygous genotype (*Ile105Val*), and the bands at 222 and 107 bp showed homozygous mutant genotype (*Val105Val*) (Fig.15.1).

The GSTP1 exon 5 polymorphism, a 100 bp marker (100 bp DNA ladder; MBI Fermentas) was used as a size standard for each gel line. The gel was monitorized using a visualizing system (Vilber Lourmat, France).

15.2.4 Statistical Analysis

Selected characteristics were compared between cases and controls by using χ^2 test. The analyses of data were performed using the computer software SPSS for Windows version 11.5. Max type I error was accept as 0.05. Binary logistic regression was performed to calculate the odds ratios (ORs), and 95% confidence intervals (CIs) to assess the risk of breast cancer.

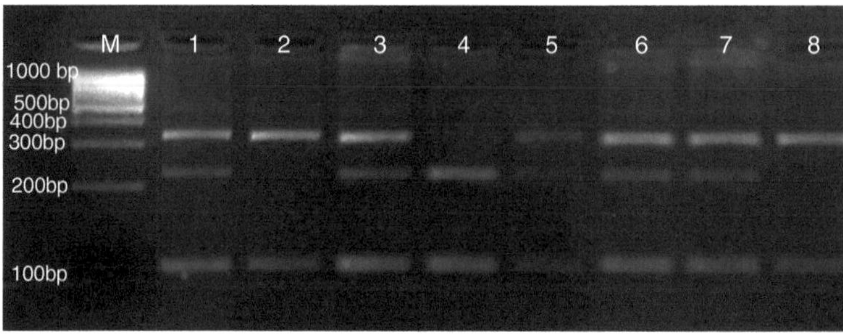

Fig. 15.1 PCR-RFLP patterns of the exon 5 polymorphism. In the wild type sequence (*Ile105Ile*), bands of 222 bp and 107 bp (lane 4) were generated, whereas in the homozygous mutant (*Val105Val*), bands at 329 and 107 bp (lanes 2, 8) were produced. In the heterozygous (*Ile105Val*), all three bands were present (lanes 1,3,5–7)

15.3 Results

Table15.1 depicts the genotype distribution and allele frequencies for GSTP1 in breast cancer patients and the control group. The A allele frequency in the control group was 159 (80.3%) and it was 102 (75%) in the breast cancer group; Polymorphic G allele frequency was 39 (19.7%) in the control group and 34 (25%) in the breast cancer group. For the exon 5 of GSTP1 gene, the distribution of AA, AG, and GG genotypes in the Mersin sample of the Turkish population were 64.5%, 31.5% and 4% in control group whereas the distribution of these genotypes were 57.6%, 35.3% and 7.1% in patients, respectively.

The distribution of major risk factors for breast cancer are shown in Table 15.2. When cases were compared with controls, an increased breast cancer risk was associated with only three of the risk factors examined. Putative risk factors including age≥50 ($P=0.002$ OR: 1.94), body mass index (BMI)≥25 kg/m^2 ($P=0.006$ OR: 1.91) or family history ($P=0.001$ OR:3.32) was found to be correlated with the developing breast cancer risk. However, it was determined that smoking status, age at first pregnancy, age at menarche or menopausal status wasn't associated with breast cancer risk ($P>0.05$). Distribution of GSTP1 genotypes and ORs (%95 CI) for breast cancer according to presumed risk factors among women are shown in Table 15.3.

Table 15.1 Distribution of *GSTP1* alleles and genotypes in cases and controls

			Controls	Cases
Allele Frequencies	A	n (%)	159 (80.3)	102 (75)
	G	n (%)	39 (19.7)	34 (25)
Genotype Frequencies	AA	n (%)	64 (64.5)	39 (57.6)
	AG	n (%)	31 (31.5)	24 (35.3)
	GG	n (%)	4 (4)	5 (7.1)

Table 15.2 Distribution of breast cancer risk factors in cases and controls

Risk factors	Cases	Controls	P-value	OR (95%CI)
Age				
<50 years	32 (47.1%)	54 (54.5%)	0.002	Reference
≥50 years	36 (52.9%)	45 (45.5%)		1.94 (1.28–2.94)
Family history				
No	16 (23.5%)	15 (15.2%)	0.001	3.32 (1.71–6.23)
Yes	52 (76.5%)	84 (84.8%)		Reference
Smoking status				
Yes	19 (27.9%)	33 (33.3%)	0.575	0.87 (0.55–1.39)
No	49 (72.1%)	66 (66.7%)		Reference
Menopausal status				
Premenopausal	22 (32.4%)	55 (55.6%)	0.054	Reference
Postmenopausal	46 (67.6%)	44 (44.4%)		1.49 (0.99–2.26)
BMI				
<25 kg/m^2	17 (25%)	29 (29.2%)	0.006	Reference
≥25 kg/m^2	51 (75%)	70 (70.8%)		1.91 (1.19–3.04)
Age at first pregnancy				
<20	17 (25%)	39 (39.4%)	0.120	Reference
≥20 or no birth	51 (75%)	60 (60.6%)		0.71 (0.46–1.09)
Age at menarche				
<13	10 (14.7%)	17 (17.2%)	0.053	1.50 (0.99–2.26)
≥13	58 (85.3%)	82 (82.8%)		Reference

Table 15.3 Distribution of GSTP1 genotypes and ORs (%95 CI) for breast cancer according to presumed

Risk factors	AA	AG	GG	AG/GG
Age		*P* <0.001		*P*=0.001
<50 years	Reference	3.4 (1.75–6.59)	–	2.9 (1.54–5.62)
≥50 years	Reference	0.4 (0.19–0.84)	2.6 (0.76–8.86)	0.62 (0.32–1.18)
Family history				
No	Reference	1.13 (0.66–1.94)	1.74 (0.62–4.87)	1.2 (0.73–2.01)
Yes	Reference	1.75 (0.61–4.97)	–	2 (0.71–5.59)
Smoking status				
Yes	Reference	0.7 (0.3–1.9)	1.6 (0.2–12.)	0.8 (0.33–2.0)
No	Reference	1.5 (0.9–2.6)	2.2 (0.7–6.7)	1.6 (0.92–2.67)
Menopausal status		*P*<0.001	*P*=0.052	*P*<0.001
Premenopausal	Reference	3.4 (1.59–7.26)	4.33 (0.98–18.99)	3.52 (1.70–7.29)
Postmenopausal	Reference	0.63 (0.33–1.2)	1.25 (0.33–4.67)	0.7 (0.38–1.28)
BMI				
<25 kg/m^2	Reference	1.42 (0.56–3.98)	–	2.13 (0.50–5.07)
≥25 kg/m^2	Reference	1.24 (0.71–2.15)	0.72 (0.2–2.51)	1.16 (0.68–1.86)
Age at first pregnancy				
<20	Reference	1.26 (0.5–3.17)	2.77 (0.79–9.72)	1.58 (0.7–3.59)
≥20	Reference	1.23 (0.7–2.15)	2.6 (0.46–14.6)	1.3 (0.75–2.24)
Age at menarche		*P*=0.058	*P*=0.051	
<13	Reference	3.46 (0.96–12.5)	2.6 (0.32–21.04)	3.2 (0.99–10.59)
≥13	Reference	1.07 (0.64–1.78)	2 (0.66–6.02)	1.16 (0.71–1.88)

Women aged <50 years with the AG genotype were found to have 3.4 fold increased risk of developing breast cancer (OR = 3.4, 95% CI = 1.75–6.59, $P < 0.001$), and women ages <50 years with AG/GG genotypes were found to have almost a 3 fold increased risk of developing breast cancer (OR = 2.9 95% CI = 1.54–5.62, $P = 0.001$). No significant interaction was observed between the GSTP1 genotypes and women aged ≥ 50 years. Premenopausal women with Val allele containing genotypes were found to have almost a 3.5 fold increased risk of breast cancer ($P < 0.001$). GG genotype was associated with a 4.3 fold increased risk of developing breast cancer, but this association was not statistically significant ($P = 0.052$). The association was not apparent among women with postmenopausal breast cancer. Women carrying the AG or AG/GG genotype with a longer duration of menstruation had almost a 3.5-fold increased risk for breast cancer. The ORs were not statistically significant (OR = 3.46, 95% CI = 0.96–12.5, OR = 3.2 95% CI = 0.99–10.59, respectively). Smoking status, age at first pregnancy, BMI, and family history of breast cancer also did not show any effect modification. There was no evidence of interaction between GSTP1 genotypes and these stratifying variables.

15.4 Discussion

Our results suggest that GSTP1 genotype do not play a strong role in susceptibility to breast cancer, in agreement with most previous studies. Of the few studies that have been conducted in Korea [6], in Finland [8], and in North Carolina [9], none have found an overall association between the GSTP1 polymorphism and breast cancer risk. Our results contrast with [10] who found women with the GSTP1 GG genotype to be at an almost two-fold increased risk. [11] in Shanghai, found the GSTP1 GG genotype was significantly associated with greater breast cancer risk (OR 1.50; 95% CI: 1.12–1.99). In our study, the GSTP1 genotypes were significantly associated with a higher risk of premenopausal breast cancer. Our results are in agreement with [11] but contradict Helzlsouer et al. [1998] who reported no association for GSTP1 Val/Val genotype in pre and postmenopausal women. Similar to [9], putative risk factors BMI ≥ 25 kg/m^2 or family history was not found to be correlated with the developing breast cancer. As for the environmental exposures, consistent with two studies [8, 12], smoking status did not significantly modify the effect of GSTP genotypes in breast cancer risk.

This study was conducted in a Mersin sample, and the GSTP Ile105Val polymorphism allele, genotype percentages for the Turkish population were determined. Our findings in Mersin, located in the Eastern Mediterranean region, have important contributions as to whether there is a relationship in the Turkish population between the GSTP gene Ile105Val polymorphism and breast cancer risk. The determination of the percentages of this gene polymorphism for the Mersin sample will not only be a significant contribution for the Turkish population, it will also provide important information for the determination of other illnesses related to this gene polymorphism in the future.

References

1. Kalemi TG, Lambropoulos AF, Gueorguiev M et al (2005) The association of p53 mutations and p53 codon 72, Her 2 codon 655 and MTHFR C677T polymorphisms with breast cancer in Northern Greece. Cancer Lett 222:57–65
2. Mutluhan H, Akbas E, Eras-Erdogan N et al (2008) The influence of HER2 genotypes as molecular markers on breast cancer outcome. DNA Cell Biol 27:575–579
3. Boring CC, Squires TS, Tong T, Montgomery S (1994) Cancer statistics, 1994. CA Cancer J Clin 44:7–26
4. Ambrosone CB, Coles BF, Freudenheim JL, Shields PG (1999) Glutathione-s-transferase (gstml) genetic polymorphisms do not affect human breast cancer risk, regardless of dietary antioxidants. J Nutr 129:565–568
5. Katoh T, Yamano Y, Tsuji M, Watabane M (2008) Genetic polymorphisms of human cytosol glutathione S-transferases and prostate cancer. Pharmogenomics 9:93–104
6. Kim SU, Lee KM, Park SK et al (2004) Genetic polymorphism of glutathione -transferase pl and breast cancer risk. J Biochem Mol Biol 37(5):582–585
7. Vogl FD, Taioli E, Maugard C et al (2004) Glutathione S-transferases M1, T1, and P1 and Breast Cancer: A Pooled Analysis. Cancer Epidem Biomar 13(9):1473–1479
8. Mitrunen K, Jourenkova N, Kataja V et al (2001) Glutathione s-transferase m1, m3, p1, and t1 genetic polymorphisms and susceptibility to breast cancer. Cancer Epidem Biomar 10: 229–236
9. Millikan R, Pittman G, Tse CK et al (2000) Glutathione s-transferases ml, tl, and pl and breast cancer. Cancer Epidem Biomar 9:567–573
10. Egan KM, Cai Q, Shu XO et al (2004) Genetic polymorphisms in GSTM1, GSTP1, and GSTT1 and the risk for breast cancer: Results from the shanghai breast cancer study and meta-analysis. Cancer Epidem Biomar 13:197–204
11. Lee SA, Fowke JH, Lu W et al (2008) Cruciferous vegetables, the GSTP1 Ile105Val genetic polymorphism, and breast cancer risk. Am J Clin Nutr 87:753–760
12. Helzlsouer KJ, Selmin O, Huang HY et al (1998) Association between glutathione s-transferase ml, pl, and tl genetic polymorphisms and development of breast cancer. J Natl Cancer I 90:512–518

Chapter 16
The New Biotechnological Medication "FarGALS" and Its Antimicrobial Properties

L.G. Bajenov, Sh.Z. Kasimov, E.V. Rizaeva, and Z.A. Shanieva

Abstract The purpose of this work was to study the antimicrobial activity of a new medication "FarGALS" and to determine the prospects of its clinical application to treat nosocomial infections. It was established that "FarGALS" possessed pronounced antimicrobial activity against a wide spectrum of pathogenic microorganisms, such as Gram-positive, Gram-negative, nonspore-forming and spore-forming bacteria, as well as *Candida spp.* and *H. pylori.* It has been concluded that the given medication can be used as an antimicrobial agent in the treatment and prevention of various purulent and inflammatory processes, mycosis and other infectious diseases.

Keywords FarGALS • Antimicrobial activity • Pathogenic microorganisms • Antiseptic • Wound healing remedies

16.1 Introduction

The second half of the XXth century, undoubtedly, was an era of antibiotics, and their use contributed to a great success in the fight against serious infections and as a whole to the progress of medicine, "population explosion" and increase in life expectancy. However during this era a substantial growth in resistance of clinically significant bacteria to these medications has been observed. As a consequence, an increase in the number of diseases caused by polyresistant microorganisms has been observed [1]. There is, therefore, a great and urgent need for development and production of new effective medications against pathogenic microorganisms resistant to currently used antibiotics and chemotherapeutic treatment.

L.G. Bajenov (✉), Sh.Z. Kasimov, E.V. Rizaeva, and Z.A. Shanieva
V.Vakhidov Republican Specialised Center of Surgery, Tashkent, Uzbekistan
e-mail: leobaj@tps.uz

S. Mikhalovsky and A. Khajibaev (eds.), *Biodefence*, NATO Science for Peace and Security Series A: Chemistry and Biology, DOI 10.1007/978-94-007-0217-2_16,

16.2 Experimental

The medication "FarGALS" manufactured by FarGALS Ltd, Tashkent, belongs to the group of "antiseptic and wound healing remedies" [2, 3]. It has been registered and licensed by the Pharmacological Committee of the Ministry of Health, Republic of Uzbekistan and has been authorized for clinical application since 2006.

The medication is a sterile water extract from autotrophic bacteria *Ferrooxidans spp.* culture medium. It is a reddish liquid with acidic reaction (pH 3.0) and astringent action. The preparation does not cause irritation of tissues and is intended for external use. However, at present the possibility of its oral administration is being studied.

Antimicrobial activity of the medication was determined by the agar diffusion method [4, 5]. A wide spectrum of pyogenic microflora (Table 16.1) as well as *Candida spp.* and *Helicobacter pylori* were studied as test cultures.

For testing antimicrobial activity of FarGALS the following nutrient media were used: for aerobic bacteria – Müller-Hinton agar, for *Candida spp.* – Saburo agar, for *H. pylori* - blood cardiocerebral agar ("HiMedia", India) [4–6]. Petri dishes with a nutrient medium were inoculated with a microbial suspension of the daily test-cultures in a physiological solution at concentrations of 10^8 microorganisms/mL. The preparations were dried, then holes of 7 mm in diameter were cut out in the agar and 0.01 mL of medication FarGALS was instilled. Each experiment was done in 5 replicates. Dishes were incubated at 37°C for 24–48 h (*H. pylori* – for 96 h). To assess results the diameter of growth inhibition zones of test-cultures was measured around each hole. The cultures were considered to be resistant when inhibition zones measured less than 10 mm, moderately resistant at 11–14 mm, and sensitive at 15 mm and above.

Table 16.1 Antimicrobial activity of the preparation FarGALS

N	Test culture	Number of strains	Zone of growth inhibition, mm (M ± m)
1	*Staphylococcus aureus*	8	20.1 ± 1.5
2	*Streptococcus pneumoniae*	8	21.0 ± 1.2
3	*Haemophilus influenzae*	6	18.6 ± 1.3
4	*Serratia marcescens*	6	13.3 ± 1.1
5	*Escherichia coli*	8	18.1 ± 1.4
6	*Klebsiella pneumoniae*	8	19.5 ± 1.5
7	*Pseudomonas aeruginosa*	8	18.3 ± 1.6
8	*Bacteroides fragilis*	5	18.8 ± 1.3
9	*Clostridium perfringens*	5	17.9 ± 1.4
10	*Bacillus subtilis*	5	21.2 ± 2.0
11	*Candida albicans*	5	16.6 ± 1.4
12	*Candida tropicalis*	5	12.5 ± 1.1
13	*Helicobacter pylori*	8	23.4 ± 2.1

The clinical efficiency of the FarGALS to treat wound infection was studied in patients ($n=12$). Patients with a similar pathology treated by conventional methods formed the control group ($n=12$).

16.3 Results and Discussion

The results of testing the antimicrobial activity of FarGALS are presented in Table 16.1. FarGALS has shown an antimicrobial effect in all tested microorganisms however, the intensity of the effect was different depending on the individual microorganism. The majority of cultures were inhibited by FarGALS with the inhibition zones greater than 15 mm, and the activity of *S. marcescens* and *C. tropicalis* was moderately inhibited (inhibition zone less than 15 mm) (Fig. 16.1). The highest sensitivity to the preparation was noted in *H. pylori*, the pathogen which causes gastritis and ulcerous disease.

The use of FarGALS in the treatment of wound infections caused by polyresistant hospital microorganisms resulted in profound clinical improvement, as the wounds treated with FarGALS showed decreased exudation and increased decontamination rates by 2nd–3rd day of treatment, whereas in the control group the same effects were achieved by the 5th–6th day.

The positive results were obtained in all patients treated by Fargals, but only in 75% patients of the control group, in which chronization of purulent and inflammatory processes were observed in 25% of the patients. The medication was well tolerated by the patients and no side effects were noted.

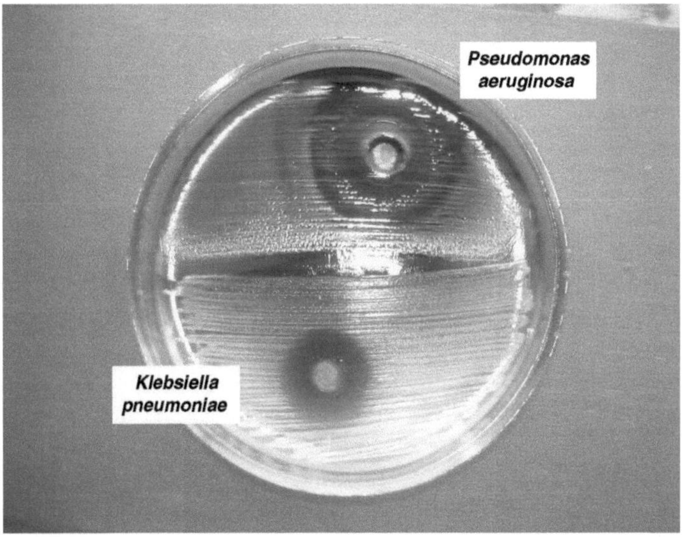

Fig. 16.1 Antimicrobial activity of the medication Fargals in polyresistant strains of pathogens

Preliminary estimates suggest that FarGALS therapy is cost effective when compared with conventional therapy.

16.4 Conclusions

The medication FarGALS has shown both *in vitro* and *in vivo* profound antimicrobial activity against a wide spectrum of pathogenic microorganisms, including Gram-positive, Gram-negative, nonspore-forming and spore-forming bacteria, as well as *Candida spp.* and *H. pylori*. It can be recommended as an antimicrobial agent in the treatment and prevention of various purulent and inflammatory processes, mycosis and other infectious diseases. The high activity of this medication against *H. pylori* suggests that it could be effective in treatment of gastroduodenal diseases associated with this pathogen.

References

1. Global Strategy of the WHO on Suppression of Resistance to Antimicrobial Preparations (2001) World Health Organization. Geneva, Switzerland, 20 pp
2. Babajanova GA et al. (2008) Eurasian Patent 009618
3. Babajanova GA et al. (2002) Uzbek Patent 03242
4. Adarchenko AA, Krasilnikov AP, Nikolaev HE et al (1992) Comparative activity of antibiotics and antiseptics on Enterobacteriaceae spp. Sample Public Health Care of Belarus N6:35–40
5. Afinogenov GE, Elinov NP (1987) Antiseptics in Surgery. Medicine, Leningrad, 144 pp
6. Bajenov LG, Artemova EV, Rizaeva EV (2005) Microbiological Diagnostics of Helicobacteriosis: Methodical Recommendations. Tashkent, Uzbekistan, 18 pp

Chapter 17
Design of Adsorption Cartridges for Personnal Protection from Toxic Gases

G. Grévillot and C. Vallières

Abstract To design an adsorption cartridge, it is necessary to be able to predict the service life as a function of several parameters. This prediction needs a model of the breakthrough curve of the toxic from the activated carbon bed. The most popular equation is the Wheeler-Jonas equation. We study the properties of this equation and show that it satisfies the constant pattern behaviour of travelling adsorption fronts. We compare this equation with other models of chemical engineering, mainly the linear driving force (LDF) approximation. It is shown that the different models lead to a different service life. And thus it is very important to choose the proper model. The LDF model has more physical significance and is recommended in combination with Dubinin-Radushkevitch (DR) isotherm even if no analytical solution exists. A numerical solution of the system equation must be used.

Keywords Adsorption • Activated carbon • Cartridges • Personnal protection

List of Abbreviations

a	specific particle external surface area ($m^2 m^{-3}$)
C	solute concentration in gas phase ($mol\, m^{-3}$)
K	Langmuir constant ($m^3 mol^{-1}$)
k_a	reaction rate constant ($m^3 mol^{-1} s^{-1}$)
k_v	overall adsorption rate parameter (s^{-1})
k_q	intra-particle mass transfer coefficient (s^{-1})
W	adsorbent mass (kg)
N	number of transfer units
Q	volumetric flow rate ($m^3 s^{-1}$)
q	solute concentration in solid phase ($mol\, kg^{-1}$)

G. Grévillot and C. Vallières (✉)
Reactions and Process Engineering Laboratory-CNRS- Nancy University,
1, rue Grandville, 54001 Nancy, France
e-mail: Cecile.Vallieres@ensic.inpl-nancy.fr

S. Mikhalovsky and A. Khajibaev (eds.), *Biodefence*, NATO Science for Peace and Security Series A: Chemistry and Biology, DOI 10.1007/978-94-007-0217-2_17,

q_0 q value in equilibrium with C_0
r_0 particle radius (m)
R separation factor
t time (s)
T throughput parameter
v gas superficial velocity ($m\,s^{-1}$)
X gas phase dimensionless concentration ($=C/C_0$)
Y solid phase dimensionless concentration ($=q/q_0$)
z axial distance (m)
ρ_b bed bulk density ($kg\,m^{-3}$)

17.1 Introduction

Adsorption is a physicochemical phenomenon namely the uptake of gases or vapours on solids. The word "uptake" represents mainly three phenomena: pure adsorption of molecules on a solid surface, vapour condensation in micro pores and chemical reaction of gases with chemicals which are impregnated in the pores of a solid grain. In order to have large amounts of adsorbed gases, large surface areas (or large volumes of pores) per unit volume of adsorbent are required. This is obtained with porous adsorbents, typically, such porous adsorbents are activated carbons with internal surface area in the range 1,000–2,000 m^2/g.

A cartridge contains a given amount of activated carbon. In principle the activated carbon has been chosen to retain the expected toxic gases. Thus the question is: how long can this cartridge protect from toxic gases? To answer this question [1] it is necessary to analyse the behaviour of cartridges from a chemical engineering point of view.

17.2 Breakthrough Curve and Service Time

Consider a cylindrical cartridge of fresh activated carbon grains. Typical dimensions are: 10 cm diameter and 2.5 cm thickness. The feed is air containing a toxic gas. The gas molecules adsorb on the first layers of the carbon bed while the air molecules (oxygen and nitrogen) are not adsorbed. Thus, clean air exits from the cartridge on the mouth side and can be inhaled. At a given time **t**, the bed comprises three zones (Fig. 17.1): a saturated zone near the input and a clean zone near the mouth separated by a so-called "mass transfer zone" (MTZ) or "adsorption front". The front moves at constant velocity if the air flow rate is constant and keeps a constant shape (this point will be discussed later). The cartridge is no longer efficient when the front attains the end of the bed. If the experiment is continued, the front exits the bed. The monitoring of the concentration as a function of time is called "breakthrough curve". The "breakthrough point" B is the point on this curve at which the concentration C_B is too high to have an acceptable inhaled air. It corresponds to the time $\mathbf{t_B}$ which is the

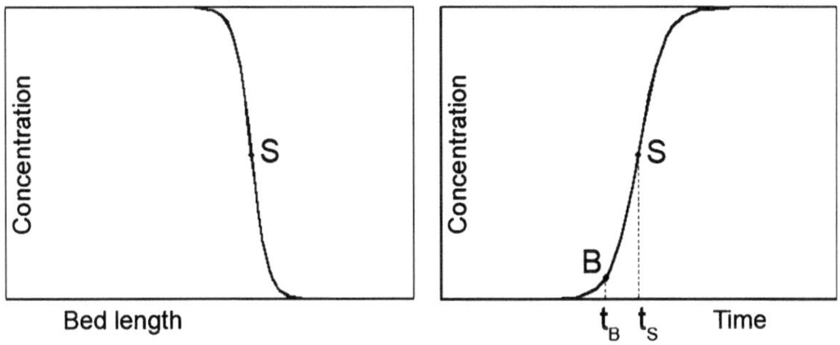

Fig. 17.1 Adsorption front (*left*) and breakthrough curve (*right*)

"service time" of the cartridge. The breakthrough point is generally defined as a percentage of the feed air concentration of the toxic gas (1–10%). The sole objective being to foresee the service time of a cartridge, we need a cartridge model accurately representing the adsorption front or, equivalently, the breakthrough curve.

17.3 Position and Shape of the Breakthrough Curve

The position and shape of the breakthrough front are determined by two almost independent phenomena.

The position in the time scale is given by the adsorption equilibrium isotherm, which is a relationship between the concentration of the toxic gas in air and in the adsorbent. This relationship depends only on the temperature and is unique for each couple adsorbate-adsorbent (we consider here a single toxic gas in dry air). If we imagine a vertical breakthrough front, the front would exit at a time t_S (stoechiometric time) given only by the isotherm. Because the front is always dispersed, the isotherm determines the position of the barycentric point S of the front. Point S exits at $\mathbf{t_S}$. The stoechiometric time can be easily calculated knowing the isotherm, toxic concentration, carbon mass and flow rate. It is given by a mass balance between the starting time and the breakthrough time and considering a vertical front (Eq.17.1):

$$t_S = \frac{W_e W}{C_0 Q} \tag{17.1}$$

where: $\mathbf{C_0}$ is the inlet concentration, **Q** is the volumetric flow rate, **W** is the weight of charcoal and $\mathbf{W_e}$ is the adsorption capacity corresponding to $\mathbf{C_0}$. The isotherm must be measured or estimated with a model. The Dubinin-Radushkevich model is often used to predict adsorption isotherms [2].

The shape of the front is given by the spreading of the front around the point S. The spreading depends mainly on toxic mass transfer kinetics between gas and solid phases. Thus numerous parameters can be considered: air flow rate, size of the toxic molecule, pore sizes of the carbon, carbon grain diameter. With large pores and small grains, the mass transfer from gas to carbon is very fast: the spreading would be very weak leading to an almost vertical breakthrough curve. On the contrary, the front can be spread to a greater extent. A second source of spreading is the so-called "axial dispersion". It is a phenomenon related to flow through porous media, occurring even if the bed is made of glass beads. It includes molecular diffusion in the gas phase. So we see that the modelling of the spreading of the front is generally more difficult than to predict the time of point B.

17.4 Constant Pattern Behaviour

A question arises: how does the front shape change when travelling through the bed? This is an important question because the shape and thus the breakthrough point would change with the bed length.

It has been shown that the spreading of the front tends to a limit after a certain travel in the bed. The front is thus named "constant pattern front". This is due to the usual curvature of the isotherm. The non-linearity of the isotherm leads to compressive effects on the front: if the spreading phenomenon is absent, the front would be vertical (shock type, analogous to shock wave in supersonic flows). This shows that there is competition between compressive forces due to the curvature of the isotherm and dispersive forces leading to spreading. The dynamic equilibrium between these forces leads to a constant pattern front. The constant pattern is usually attained after several millimeters of bed travel. Constant pattern behaviour is characterised by duration Δt between stoechiometric and breakthrough times which is independent of the bed length (Eq.17.2):

$$\Delta t = t_S - t_B \tag{17.2}$$

or:

$$t_B = \frac{W_e W}{C_0 Q} - \Delta t \tag{17.3}$$

The constant pattern concept is associated with the non-linear theory of chromatography but seems to be not known from researchers working on protection cartridges. Experimental evidence for cartridges has been demonstrated for a long time, but not recognized as constant pattern behaviour. A large amount of experimental work was completed by Wood and co-workers at Los Alamos Laboratory. For example, Wood and Moyer [3] performed 48 experiments on the adsorption of acetone at different bed carbon masses and different flow rates. They showed a linear relationship between 1% breakthrough time and total charcoal weight on the one hand and bed residence time on the other hand. All the 48 results are collected in Fig. 17.2. Figure 17.2 shows that $\mathbf{t_B}$ is a linear function of the ratio W/Q as predicted by Eq. 17.3, with a value of **Δt** independent of carbon mass **W**. The constant pattern behaviour is thus proved for the part of the fronts near 1% breakthrough concentration.

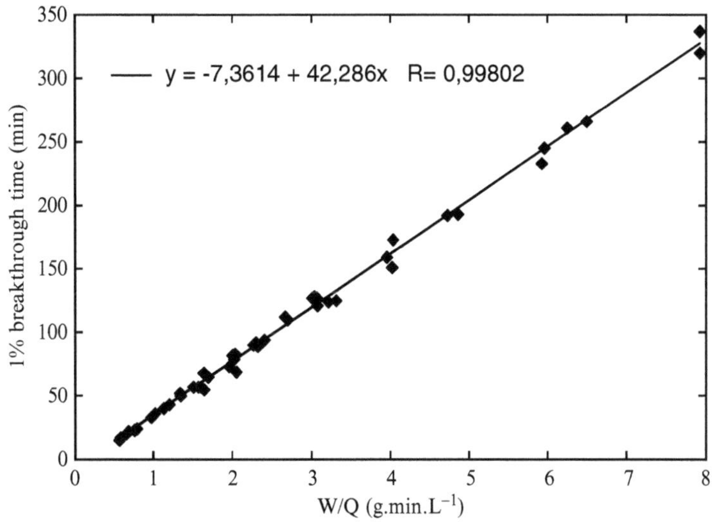

Fig. 17.2 1% Breakthrough time as a function of W/Q for 48 experiments

Very recently, experiments using new techniques have been performed by Lodewyckx et al. [4]. X-ray microtomography coupled with image analysis allows visualising dynamic adsorption of organic vapour and water vapour on activated carbon. Figure 17.3 in [4] shows profiles inside the bed at different times. It is remarkable that the fronts seem to be of constant pattern shape.

17.5 Model for Breakthrough Curve: The Wheeler Equation

The most popular and almost uniquely used equation for representing breakthrough curves is the Wheeler [5] or Wheeler –Jonas equation (Eq.17.4):

$$t_B = \frac{W_e W}{C_0 Q} - \frac{W_e \rho_b}{k_v C_0} \ln\left(\frac{C_0 - C_B}{C_B}\right) \tag{17.4}$$

where: ρ_b is the bulk density of the bed, C_B the concentration at time t_B and k_v an overall adsorption rate coefficient [6]

This equation can be rearranged using Eq.17.1 to give:

$$t_B = t_S - \Delta t \tag{17.5}$$

With:

$$\Delta t = \frac{W_e \rho_b}{k_v C_0} \ln\left(\frac{C_0 - C_B}{C_B}\right) \tag{17.6}$$

Equation 17.5 shows that the Wheeler equation has the form of a constant pattern front because Δt is independent of the bed length. In addition, Eq.17.5 shows that the front is symmetrical relatively to $\mathbf{t}_S$. Notice that constant pattern and symmetry are independent: a front could be symmetrical but not of constant pattern shape and the inverse is true.

The Wheeler equation seems to be very simple with only one adjustable parameter $\mathbf{k}_v$. However it has been discovered that it is difficult to correlate $\mathbf{k}_v$ to operating parameters, mainly the flow rate **Q**. In addition, research conducted in other fields of adsorption such as volatile organic compounds adsorption for air purification, have shown that the breakthrough front is usually not symmetrical. In this case, it is useless to try to correlate $\mathbf{k}_v$.

17.6 Comparison of Several Breakthrough Curve Equations

In a review paper, LeVan [7] studied constant pattern models for gas adsorption. The model is based on the differential mass balance for the solute:

$$\rho_B \frac{\partial q}{\partial t} + \varepsilon \frac{\partial C}{\partial t} + v \frac{\partial C}{\partial z} = D_{ax} \frac{\partial^2 C}{\partial z^2} \tag{17.7}$$

In case of no axial dispersion, the right-hand side is zero. The adsorption equilibrium is represented by Langmuir equation:

$$q = \frac{q_m KC}{1 + KC} \tag{17.8}$$

For adsorption rate, LeVan considered four models: axial dispersion (this is not really a "rate" model but rather a flow model), external mass transfer, linear driving force approximation (LDF) and reaction kinetics. The purpose of this development was to restore these very compact equations with the variables of Wheeler equation for comparison.

17.6.1 Reaction Kinetics Model

We shall firstly consider the last model [Equation 46 in [7]] in the original paper), which seems to be that of Wheeler. The rate equation for the reaction kinetic mechanism is:

$$\frac{\partial q}{\partial t} = k_a \left[(q_m - q)C - \frac{1}{K} q \right] \tag{17.9}$$

where $\mathbf{k_a}$ is a forward reaction rate constant. The rate equation is combined with the Eqs. 17.7 and 17.8 and constant pattern is assumed. This approach leads to the following Eq. 17.10 for the adsorption front:

$$\frac{1}{1-R}\ln\left[\frac{1-X}{X}\right] = N - NT \tag{17.10}$$

where **X** is a dimensionless concentration, **T** a time-space relation called "throughput parameter", **N** a space variable and **R** a parameter related to the Langmuir constant. For that purpose, we clarify the right hand side member **N-NT** of these equations. For the reaction kinetics model, we have:

$$N = k_a \frac{(1+KC_0)}{K}\frac{q_0\rho_b z}{C_0 v} \tag{17.11}$$

$$T = \frac{C_0}{q_0}\frac{vt}{\rho_b z} \tag{17.12}$$

$$R = \frac{1}{1+KC_0} \tag{17.13}$$

Equations 17.11–17.13 lead to:

$$t = \frac{q_0\rho_b z}{C_0 v} - (N - NT)\frac{K}{k_a(1+KC_0)} \tag{17.14}$$

By combining with (17.1) and clarifying R and X we obtain:

$$t = \frac{q_0\rho_b z}{C_0 v} - \frac{1}{k_a C_0}\ln\left(\frac{C_0 - C}{C}\right) \tag{17.15}$$

Writing the equation at z=Z, we obtain a breakthrough front equation. Introducing the bed carbon mass **W** and noting that $\mathbf{q_0}$ is $\mathbf{W_e}$ in the Wheeler's notation, we finally have:

$$t = \frac{W_e W}{C_0 Q} - \frac{1}{k_a C_0}\ln\left(\frac{C_0 - C}{C}\right) \tag{17.16}$$

In Eq. 17.16, a value of **t** corresponds to a concentration **C**. If we choose a concentration value $\mathbf{C_B}$, for example as 10% of $\mathbf{C_0}$, the corresponding time would be $\mathbf{t_B}$. Thus Eq. 17.16 is exactly the Wheeler equation, with the definitions of $\mathbf{k_a}$ and $\mathbf{k_v}$ related by:

$$k_a = \frac{k_v}{W_e\rho_b} \tag{17.17}$$

Both units of **k** are coherent. Also note that the hypothesis of Langmuir isotherm is not necessary, because its parameter **K** is absent from Eq.17.16. This equation gives a perfectly symmetric front around the stoichiometric point.

17.6.2 Linear Driving Force Model

The time variation of local amount adsorbed is represented by the so-called LDF model in place of Eq.17.9:

$$\frac{\partial q}{\partial t} = k_q a\left(q^* - q\right) \tag{17.18}$$

where **q*** is the solute concentration in the particle that would exist in equilibrium with the gas phase concentration at the exterior of the particle. The intra-particle mass transfer coefficient $\mathbf{k_q}$ is given by:

$$k_q a = \frac{15 D_e}{r_0^2} \tag{17.19}$$

where $\mathbf{D_e}$ is an effective intra-particle diffusion coefficient. The constant pattern equation for this model is given by LeVan as:

$$\frac{1}{1-R}\ln\left[\frac{1-X}{X^R}\right] + 1 = N - NT \tag{17.20}$$

with:

$$N = k_q a \frac{q_0 \rho_b z}{C_0 v} \tag{17. 21}$$

As previously, we obtain:

$$t = \frac{W_e W}{C_0 Q} - \frac{1}{k_q a}\left(1 + \frac{1 + KC_0}{KC_0}\ln\left[\frac{1-X}{X^R}\right]\right) \tag{17.22}$$

This equation is different from the Wheeler equation. The first term on the right-hand side is identical and is the stoichiometric time $\mathbf{t_s}$, but the second term includes the Langmuir coefficient **K** explicitly and in **R**. Thus no link with the Wheeler equation can be found. In addition this equation is valid solely with the Langmuir isotherm. This is a serious limitation because it has been recognized that Dubinin-Radushkevich (DR) approach is very useful. No analytical solution exists for the particular case of DR equation. A solution to this problem is to solve the system of equations by numerical methods.

17.6.3 Comparison of Models

The two other models of LeVan do not give the Wheeler equation and will not be discussed here.

Figure 17.3 compares the calculated breakthrough fronts of the four models using a value of $R = 0.5$. The horizontal axis is a time scale, the zero value being the

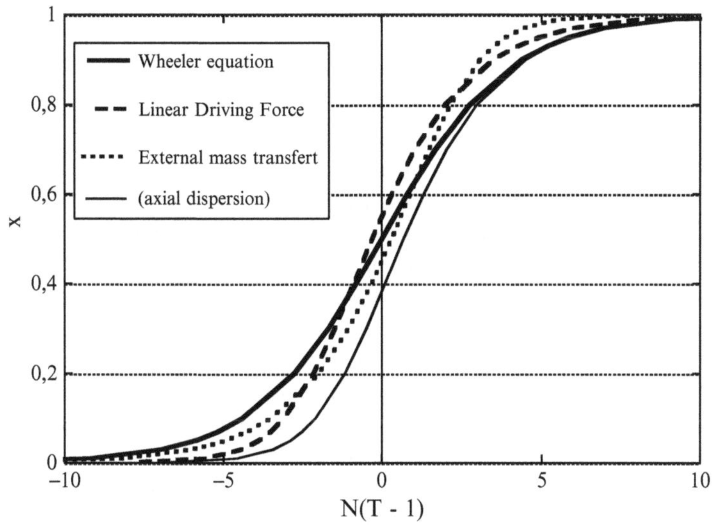

Fig. 17.3 Breakthrough curves calculated using different models

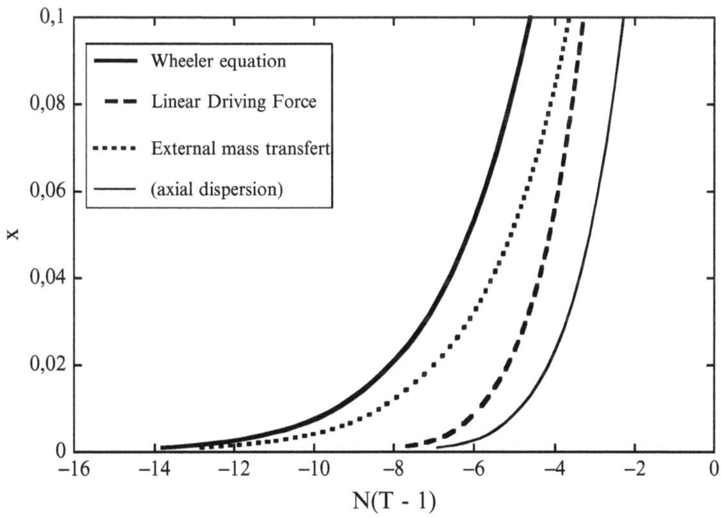

Fig. 17.4 Breakthrough curves at low breakthrough concentrations

stoechiometric time $\mathbf{t_S}$. The Wheeler front is symmetrical and as a consequence, X = 0.5 at $\mathbf{t_S}$. The other fronts are not symmetrical.

Figure 17.4 enlarges the breakthrough parts at X < 0.1 that is below 10% of the feed. If we choose a given percentage of the feed, we can see that the models foresee different service times. Thus the model choice is of primary importance for calculating service time of cartridges.

17.7 Conclusions

The major disadvantage of the Wheeler equation is that the rate coefficient $\mathbf{k_v}$ has no physical significance. In fact it is recognized that the adsorption reaction itself is very fast, almost instantaneous at time scale of the cartridge life time, and the overall kinetics is controlled by mass transfer between the gas and solid phase. Thus it is useless to find correlations of $\mathbf{k_v}$ with operating parameters. Of course such correlations can be established using several adjustable coefficients. This has been done and, taking into account the very large number of experiments which have been performed, the correlations seem to work rather well.

The linear driving force model has much more physical significance. It has been derived from a two-dimensional model of intra-particle diffusion, solution of which is a series development. The particle size appears explicitly. The effective diffusion coefficient is related to the particle porosity and to the size of the adsorbate molecule. Thus it makes sense to search for correlation of $\mathbf{D_e}$ with these properties. However such relations are complex and it is rather difficult to predict $\mathbf{D_e}$ for a given carbon and a given molecule.

In conclusion, it is recommended for future work to use the LDF model. Because Langmuir isotherm has severe limitations, the use of the DR equation is also recommended. But in this case analytical solutions no longer exist and numerical calculations of the system of equations must be performed.

References

1. Wood GO (1994) Estimating service lives of organic vapour cartridges. AIHA J 55(13):11–15
2. Wood GO (1992) Activated carbon adsorption capacities for vapors. Carbon 30:593–599
3. Wood GO, Moyer E (1989) A review of the Wheeler equation and comparison of its application to organic vapor respirator cartridge breakthrough data. AIHA J 50(8):400–407
4. Lodewyckx P, Blacher S, Léonard A (2006) Use of x-ray microtomography to visualise dynamic adsorption of organic vapour and water vapour on activated carbon. Adsorption 12:19–26
5. Lodewyckx P, Wood GO, Ryu SK (2004) The Wheeler–Jonas equation: a versatile tool for the prediction of carbon bed breakthrough times. Carbon 42:1351–1355
6. Wu J, Claesson O, Fangmark I, Hammarstrom LG (2005) A systematic investigation of the overall rate coefficient in the Wheeler–Jonas equation for adsorption on dry activated carbons. Carbon 43:481–490
7. LeVan MD (1989) Asymptotic fixed bed behavior: proportionate and constant patterns. In: "Adsorption: Science and Technology", vol 158, **NATO-ASI Series**. Kluwer, Amsterdam, pp 149–168

Chapter 18
Using Silver Nanoparticles as an Antimicrobial Agent

R.R. Khaydarov, R.A. Khaydarov, S. Evgrafova, and Y. Estrin

Abstract Antimicrobial and antifungal properties of silver nanoparticles, silver ions, acrylate paint and cotton fabric impregnated with Ag nanoparticles were assessed against *Escherichia coli* (Gram-negative bacterium); *Staphylococcus aureus* and *Bacillus subtilis* (Gram-positive bacteria); *Aspergillus niger, Aureobasidium pullulans* and *Penicillium phoeniceum* (cosmopolitan saprotrophic fungi). The silver ions used in the bacterial susceptibility tests were released from pure silver electrodes using a 12 V battery-operated direct current generator. The water-based silver colloidal solution was obtained by electroreduction of silver ions in water. Nanosilver was less effective against *E. coli, S. aureus, B. subtilis* and *P. phoeniceum* compared to silver ions. However silver nanoparticles have prolonged bactericidal effect as a result of continuous release of Ag ions in sufficient concentration and thus nanoparticles can be more suitable in some bactericidal applications. The synthesized silver nanoparticles added to water paints or cotton fabrics have demonstrated a pronounced antibacterial and antifungal effect.

Keywords Silver • Nanoparticles • Bacteria • Eukaryotes

R.R. Khaydarov (✉) and R.A. Khaydarov
Institute of Nuclear Physics, Tashkent, Uzbekistan
e-mail: renat2@gmail.com

S. Evgrafova
V.N. Sukachev Institute of Forestry SB RAS, Krasnoyarsk, Russia

Y. Estrin
Department of Materials Engineering, ARC Centre of Excellence for Design in Light Metals, Monash University and CSIRO Division of Materials Science and Engineering, Clayton, VIC, Australia

S. Mikhalovsky and A. Khajibaev (eds.), *Biodefence*, NATO Science for Peace and Security Series A: Chemistry and Biology, DOI 10.1007/978-94-007-0217-2_18,

18.1 Introduction

Silver has been well known for its antimicrobial properties since ancient times. In ancient Greece, Rome, and Macedonia, silver was used to control infections and spoilage. Since 20th century silver and its compounds have been used extensively in many bactericidal applications including wound healing, water treatment, as flower preservatives, etc. [1]. Due to their unique size-dependent optical, electrical and magnetic properties, silver nanoparticles up to 100 nm in size were extensively investigated and have found applications in catalysis [2], optics [3], electronics [4] and other areas of science and technology [5]. At present most of silver nanoparticles applications are associated with their use as antibacterial/antifungal agents [6]. This makes according to a recent market research report produced by Bourne Research group in 2006, nanosilver "one of the fastest growing product categories in the nanotechnology industry". For instance, as ordinary cotton fabrics provide an excellent environment for microorganisms to grow, owing to their ability to retain moisture [7], there is an interest growing in preparation of bactericidal cotton fibres containing silver nanoparticles for the textile industry [8, 9]. Impregnating silver nanoparticles into commercially available paints is also a promising trend. Nanosilver-based wall paint would prevent the formation of mould inside buildings and the growth of algae on outside walls [10].

However the mechanism of the antimicrobial effect of silver nanoparticles is not well understood. It has been recently reported that "Nanosilver represents a special physicochemical system which confers its antimicrobial activities via $Ag+$" [11]. According to Morones et al., the bactericidal effect of silver nanoparticles on microorganisms is connected not merely with the release of silver ions in solution [12]. Silver nanoparticles can also be attached to the surface of the cell membrane and drastically disturb its proper function [12]. They could also penetrate inside the bacteria and cause further damage by interacting with sulfur and phosphorus-containing compounds such as DNA.

The purpose of our study was (a) to quantitatively estimate antimicrobial effect of silver nanoparticles comparing it with that of silver ions; and (b) to study the efficacy of nanosilver as an antimicrobial agent against a range of microbes on the surface of paints and 100% cotton fabrics.

18.2 Experimental

18.2.1 *Preparation of Silver Ions and Nanoparticles*

The silver ions used in the bacterial susceptibility tests were released from pure silver electrodes using a 12 V battery-operated direct current generator. The apparatus used for silver ion generation was described previously in [13]. The water-based silver colloidal solution was obtained by a three-stage process based on the

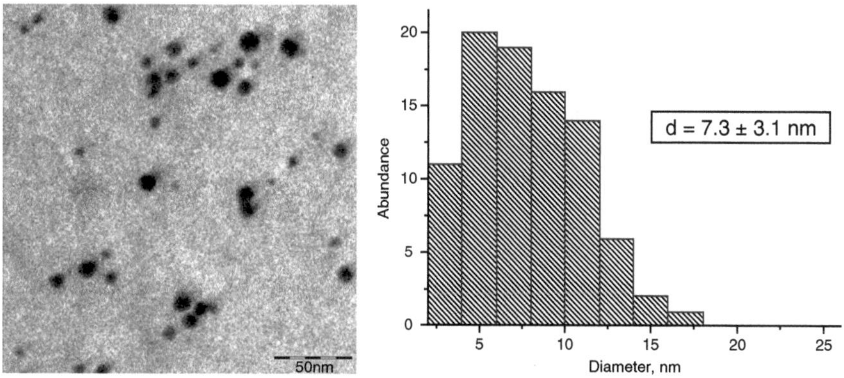

Fig. 18.1 TEM image (the scale bar is 50 nm) and histogram of silver nanoparticles prepared by the electrochemical method (adapted with permission from [14]

electroreduction of silver ions in water [14]. The nanosilver particles were spherical with a mean diameter of 7 ± 3 nm (Fig. 18.1).

The concentration of silver nanoparticles and ions in solutions was determined by neutron activation analysis [15]. Samples were irradiated in the nuclear reactor at the Institute of Nuclear Physics, Tashkent, Uzbekistan. The product of nuclear reaction $^{109}Ag(n,\gamma)^{110m}Ag$ has the half-life $T_{1/2} = 253$ days. The silver concentration was determined by measuring the intensity of gamma radiation with the energy of 0.657 MeV and 0.884 MeV emitted by ^{110m}Ag. A Ge(Li) detector with a resolution of about 1.9 keV at 1.33 MeV and a 6,144-channel analyzer were used for recording gamma-ray quanta.

The morphology of silver nanopartilces on the cotton surface and paint samples was observed by field emission scanning electron microscopy (FE-SEM; JSM-6700F, JEOL, Japan). The size and shape of the nanoparticles in solution were determined with transmission electron microscopy (TEM) (LEO-912-OMEGA, Carl Zeiss, Germany).

18.2.2 Assay for Antimicrobial Activity

Antibacterial and fungicidal properties of silver particles were assessed using the *Escherichia coli* (Gram-negative bacterium); *Staphylococcus aureus* and *Bacillus subtilis* (Gram-positive bacteria); *Aspergillus niger, Aureobasidium pullulans* and *Penicillium phoeniceum* (cosmopolitan saprotrophic fungi). The minimum inhibitory concentrations (MIC) of solutions for various microbes were determined using the macrodilution broth susceptibility test. Nutrient broth used in the macrodilution method contained 50.00 $g L^{-1}$ of peptic digest of animal tissue; 1.5 $g L^{-1}$ of beef extract; 5.00 $g L^{-1}$ of sodium chloride and 5 $g L^{-1}$ glucose, pH was 7.4 ± 0.2. A standardized suspension with approximately 10^6 CFU mL^{-1} was obtained by inoculating the culture in nutrient broth (Hi-Media) and incubating the tubes at 37 °C for 3 h.

(CFU = colony forming units). A serial dilution of the Ag ions dispersion and the silver nanoparticles dispersion was prepared within a desired range. Ten mL of the standardized culture suspension was then inoculated and tubes were incubated at 37 °C for 24 h. MIC was defined as the lowest concentration of the inhibiting agent that completely inhibited bacterial growth; the unit for MIC was chosen as mg (Ag) per L. MIC was examined visually, by checking the turbidity of the tubes.

18.2.3 Antimicrobial Finishing of Cotton and Paint Samples

Common household acrylic paint widely used for repairing and decorating purposes has been used in our studies. Ag-nanoparticle-embedded acrylic paint was obtained by diluting the initial paint sample with a colloidal solution of required nanosilver concentration in the range of 2–50 ppm. For the antibacterial tests a 22 × 22 mm pasteboard was covered with Ag-nanoparticle-embedded acrylic paint.

The bleached woven cotton fabric of 98 $g\,m^{-2}$ density was cut into equal-sized square pieces of 15 mm × 15 mm. The samples were immersed in a colloidal solution bath for 1 min, then squeezed thoroughly and dried at 60°C for 5 min.

The antibacterial and fungicidal properties of Ag nanoparticles were evaluated as follows. Cotton fabric and an acrylic paint samples treated with different compositions of Ag nanoparticles were immersed in a thin layer of beef-extract agar. One mL aliquots of suspension with approximately 10^5 $CFU\,mL^{-1}$ density of the microorganisms were withdrawn and distributed uniformly on agar surface and incubated at 28 °C. Antimicrobial activity was evaluated according to the presence or absence of microbial growth just above the sample after 24 h incubation for bacteria and 72 h incubation for fungi. All microbiological tests were performed in triplicate.

18.3 Results and Discussion

18.3.1 MIC Assays

To compare the bactericidal efficacy of silver nanoparticles and silver ions, the minimum inhibitory concentration (MIC) assays were conducted for gram-negative bacterium *E. coli*, gram-positive bacteria *S. aureus* and *B. subtilis* and fungus *P. phoeniceum.* The data on MICs are summarized in Table 18.1. The results demonstrated that the antimicrobial activity of silver ions was superior to that of silver nanoparticles against all microbes tested.

Despite the pronounced antimicrobial effect, silver ions have only limited usefulness as an antimicrobial agent in applications such as medicine, clothing, and household products. This is due to their rapid binding to or inactivating by components of the medium. This limitation can be overcome by using as an antimicrobial agent, silver nanoparticles, which continuously release Ag ions in sufficient concentration [16].

Table 18.1 Minimum inhibitory concentrations (*MIC*) of silver nanoparticles and silver ions

	Electrically generated	Silver nanoparticles
	Silver ions	(Average particle size 7 nm)
Microbe	MIC (mg(Ag) L^{-1})	MIC (mg(Ag) L^{-1})
E. coli	1.0	5
S. aureus	0.6	3
P. phoeniceum	0.5	2
B. subtilis	2.4	29

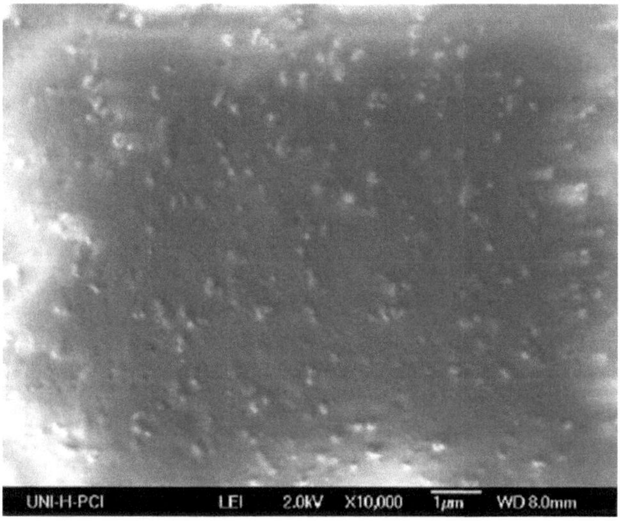

Fig. 18.2 Water paint sample with immobilized silver nanoparticles

18.3.2 Silver Modified Water Paint

Water paints were impregnated with nanosized silver colloids. Most of initial silver nanoparticles agglomerated into up to 200 – nm clusters as a result of attractive interaction forces between the particles (Fig. 18.2).

Antibacterial and antifungal effects of nanosilver-based water paint are summarized in Table 18.2

Figure 18.3 shows photographs of growth of *A. pullulans, P. phoeniceum* and *S. aureus* cultures on pasteboard samples modified by silver nanoparticles.

Increase of the nanosilver concentration in water paint up to 5–6 $\mu g\,cm^{-2}$ suppressed *B. subtilis* and *E. coli* growth. On the other hand larger concentrations of nanosilver can potentially lead to undesirable color change of the water paint with time.

Table 18.2 Antimicrobial effect of samples of water paint impregnated with nanosilver

	Modified Paint	
	№1	№2
Microbe	(Unmodified)	(Modified with 0.8 $\mu g\,cm^{-2}$ nanosilver)
Aspergillus niger	+	–
Penicillium phoeniceum	+	–
Aureobasidium pullulans	+	–
Staphylococcus aureus	+	–
Bacillus subtilis	+	+
Escherichia coli	+	+
Control (samples on beef-extract agar)	+	–

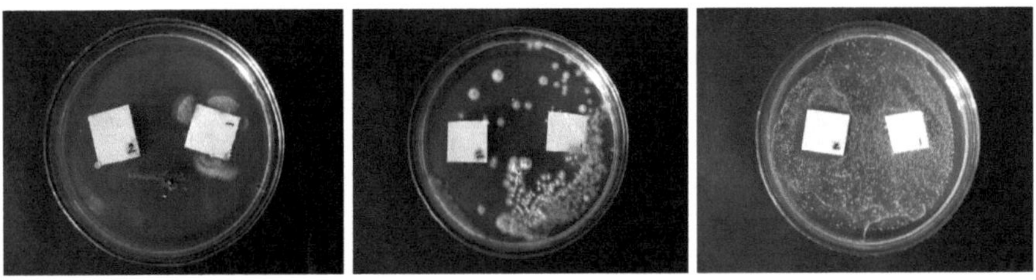

Fig. 18.3 Growth of *A. pullulans* (*left*), *P. phoeniceum* (*middle*) and *S. aureus* (*right*) cultures on pasteboard samples modified by silver nanoparticles.(Note: the white spots correspond to microbial colonies). The sample №1 is a control sample, unmodified paint; the sample №2 is modified with silver nanoparticles of 0.8 $\mu g\,cm^{-2}$ paint

The color change of the exterior side of the wall of the house (Tashkent, Uzbekistan) painted with the nanosilver-modified (0.8 $\mu g\,cm^{-2}$) paint was monitored. The neutron activation analysis tests conducted over the period of six months (March-October, 2008) showed no significant loss of silver nanoparticles in the wall paint. Thus addition of silver nanoparticles could be suggested for using in the paint industry. Microbes can come into contact with walls in a number of ways: via deposition of dust and fine aerosols, human skin contact, and by splashes from liquids. The nanosilver-based wall paint would prevent the formation of mould inside buildings and the growth of algae on exterior walls.

18.3.3 Modified Cotton Fabrics

Cotton fabrics were impregnated with nanosized silver colloids synthesized by the electrochemical technique. The particles had good dispersibility on the surface of

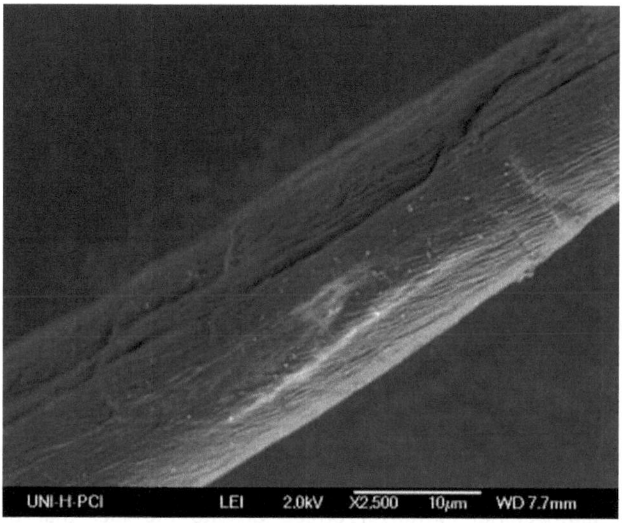

Fig. 18.4 Cotton sample with immobilized silver nanoparticles

Table 18.3 Laundering durability of silver nanoparticles on modified cotton fabric samples

	Ag concentration ($\mu g\,cm^{-2}$)
Before washing	5.0
After 2 cycles	3.5
After 5 cycles	1.8
After 10 cycles	1.0

modified cotton spread. Agglomeration of silver nanoparticles into larger clusters was also observed (Fig.18.4).

Cotton fabrics with immobilized silver nanoparticles (mean size of 15 nm) inhibited growth of *A. niger, P. phoeniceum* and *S. aureus* cultures, at nanoparticles concentration 5 $\mu g\,cm^{-2}$, 3 $\mu g\,cm^{-2}$ and 1 $\mu g\,cm^{-2}$, respectively [17]. In the present study aqueous dispersion of 7 ± 3 nm silver nanoparticles was used during the finishing process. It allowed reducing size of silver nanoparticles on the surface of cotton fabric from the micron-size down to ~100 nm (Fig. 18.4) compared to our previous work [17].

Antifungal/antibacterial effect of cotton fabric surface for *A. niger, P. phoeniceum* and *S. aureus* has been confirmed even at as low nanosilver concentration as 1 $\mu g\,cm^{-2}$. The same experiments conducted for *E. coli, B. subtilis* and *A. pullulans* cultures also demonstrated a pronounced antimicrobial effect at concentrations of nanosilver of 7 $\mu g\,cm^{-2}$, 5 $\mu g\,cm^{-2}$ and 3 $\mu g\,cm^{-2}$, respectively.

The laundering durability of the bacteriostasis of the silver-treated cotton fabric was also studied. The concentration of silver particles on fabrics surface before washing and after two, five, and ten washings was estimated (Table 18.3).

The results showed that silver particles are sufficiently bound to the cotton fabric, which can retain good bacteriostatic properties even after 10 cycles of washing.

Thus nanosilver-based textile materials have great promise in various areas, for example in hospitals to prevent wounds from contamination with microorganisms, in particular fungi and bacteria such as *S. aureus.*

18.4 Conclusions

Silver nanoparticles synthesized by a cost-effective three-stage electrochemical technique have demonstrated great promise as antimicrobial agents. Nanosilver was less effective against *E. coli, S. aureus, B. subtilis* and *P. phoeniceum* compared to silver ions. However silver nanoparticles have prolonged bactericidal effect as a result of continuous release of Ag ions in sufficient concentration and thus nanoparticles can be more suitable in some bactericidal applications. The synthesized silver nanoparticles added to water paints or cotton fabrics have demonstrated a pronounced antibacterial/antifungal effect, despite the fact that they tend to agglomerate into clusters up to 200 nm.

References

1. Klasen HJ (2000) Historical review of the use of silver in the treatment of burns. I Early uses Burns 26:117–130
2. Lewis LN (1993) Chemical catalysis by colloids and clusters. Chem Rev 93:2693–2730
3. Murphy CJ, Sau TK, Gole AM et al (2005) Anisotropic metal nanoparticles: Synthesis, assembly, and optical applications. J Phys Chem B 109:13857–13870
4. Li Y, Wu X, Ong BS (2005) Facile synthesis of silver nanoparticles useful for fabrication of high-conductivity elements for printed electronics. J Am Chem Soc 127:3266–3267
5. Niemeyer CM (2001) Nanoparticles, proteins, and nucleic acids: Biotechnology meets materials science. Angew Chem Intl Ed 40(22):4128–4158
6. Buzea C, Pacheco II, Robbie K (2007) Nanomaterials and nanoparticles: Sources and toxicity. Biointerphases 2(4):MR17–MR71
7. Chen C-Y, Chiang C-L (2008) Preparation of cotton fibers with antibacterial silver nanoparticles. Mater Lett 62(21–22):3607–3609
8. Lee HJ, Jeong SH (2004) Bacteriostasis of nanosized colloidal silver on polyester nonwovens. Text Res J 74:442–447
9. Lee HJ, Jeong SH (2005) Bacteriostasis and skin innoxiousness of nanosize silver colloids on textile fabrics. Text Res J 75:551–556
10. Egorova EM, Revina AA, Rumyantsev BV et al (2002) Stable silver nanoparticles in aqueous dispersions obtained from micellar solutions. RUSS J APPL CHEM+ 75(10):1585–1590
11. Lok C-N, Ho C-M, Chen R et al (2007) J Biol Inorg Chem 12:527–534
12. Morones JR, Elechiguerra JL, Camacho A et al (2005) The bactericidal effect of silver nanoparticles. Nanotechnology 16:2346–2353
13. Khaydarov RA, Khaydarov RR, Olsen RL, Rogers SE (2004) Water disinfection using electrolytically generated silver, copper and gold ions. J Water Supply Res T 53:567–572
14. Khaydarov RA, Khaydarov RR, Gapurova O et al (2009) Electrochemical method of synthesis of silver nanoparticles. J Nanopart Res 11(5):1193–1200

15. de Soete D, Gijbels R, J Hoste J (1972) Neutron activation analysis. Wiley-Interscience, London, UK
16. Kim JS, Kuk E, Yu KN et al (2007) Antimicrobial effects of silver nanoparticles. Nanomed: Nanotech, Biol, and Med 3(1):95–101
17. Khaydarov RA, Khaydarov RR, Estrin Y et al (2009) Silver nanoparticles: Environmental and human health impacts. In: Linkov I, Steevens J (eds) Nanomaterials: Risk and benefits. Springer, Netherlands, pp 287–297

Chapter 19
Immobilization and Controlled Release of Bioactive Substances from Stimuli-Responsive Hydrogels

S.E. Kudaibergenov, G.S. Tatykhanova, and Zh.E. Ibraeva

Abstract Drugs and proteins were immobilized within the spatial structure of thermo- and pH sensitive hydrogels. The release of drugs and proteins in response to environmental changes were studied. The temperature of swelling-shrinking behavior change of hydrogels decreased in the following order: NIPA-APSA (35°C) > NIPA-AA (34.4°C) > NIPA-AA/Richlocaine (33.8°C) > PNIPA (32.7°C). Oscillating "on-off" release mechanism of drug and proteins from the PNIPA and NIPA-AA hydrogels were observed in the course of cyclic shrinking and swelling of hydrogels in water and phosphate buffer at 25°C and 40°C.

Keywords Stimuli-responsive hydrogels • Drug delivery

19.1 Introduction

Delivering biologically active substances in a strictly defined dose to target tissues of the body is one of most important challenges of modern medicine and biotechnology [1,2]. Presently, about 25% of drugs are produced as drug delivery systems. Due to their excellent swelling in water, softness, elasticity and biological compatibility polymer hydrogels are widely applied for designing of drug delivery systems. Stimuli responsive hydrogels capable of transporting and releasing drugs at target sites within the body, have attracted considerable attention [3–5]. The morphology, size and shape of stimuli-responsive polymers, such as homo- and copolymers of acrylamide (AA) and N-isopropylacrylamide (NIPA), change under the action of external stimuli [6]. The wounded and diseased body organs usually

S.E. Kudaibergenov (✉), G.S. Tatykhanova, and Zh.E. Ibraeva
Institute of Polymer Materials and Technology, Panfilov str. 52/104, Almaty 050004, Kazakhstan
and
Laboratory of Engineering Profile, K.I. Satpaev Kazakh National Technical University, Satpaev str. 22, Almaty 050013, Kazakhstan
e-mail: skudai@mail.ru; ipmt-kau@usa.net

S. Mikhalovsky and A. Khajibaev (eds.), *Biodefence*, NATO Science for Peace and Security Series A: Chemistry and Biology, DOI 10.1007/978-94-007-0217-2_19,

have higher temperature and pH compared to healthy organs. Stimuli-responsive hydrogels therefore, could deliver the drug to a wounded tissue and release it in this location by changing its structure under the external stimuli. Both linear and cross-linked PNIPA undergo a sharp conformational and volume transition at 32–34°C (close to the normal body temperature). Copolymerization of NIPA with other monomers provides the possibility to control the transition temperature, adapting it for special needs. Thus materials that release drugs at certain temperatures could be obtained. The immobilization of biologically active substances, such as drugs, proteins, DNA, enzymes and living cells within stimuli-responsive hydrogels is of great interest for medicine, pharmaceutics, biotechnology, bio- and genetic engineering. Polymer-protein systems can also be used as biosensors, for instance, to determine the concentration of sugar in blood or toxic substances in the environment.

19.2 Experimental

An anesthetic drug, Richlocaine, developed jointly by scientists from Kazakhstan and Russia, and commercially available biologically active substances bovine serum albumin, lysozyme, and catalase were used. Hydrogels of acrylamide and acrylic acid copolymer (AA-AAc), poly(N-isopropylacrylamide) (PNIPA), N-isopropylacrylamide and acrylic acid copolymer (NIPA-AAc), N-isopropylacrylamide and 2-(acrylamido)-2-propanesulfonic acid copolymer (NIPA-APSA) were synthesized. Diffusion parameters of bioactive substances into hydrogel matrices were calculated using Eq. (19.1):

$$M_t / M_\infty = kt^n \tag{19.1}$$

where M_t is the mass of hydrogel at time t, M_∞ is the mass of hydrogel at equilibrium-swollen state, k is the characteristic swelling constant, and n is the swelling exponent that describes the diffusion mechanism of bioactive agents.

19.3 Results and Discussion

Figure 19.1 shows the temperature-dependent volume-phase transitions of NIPA-based hydrogels. It is suggested that formation of a complex between bioactive molecules and functional groups of hydrogels is responsible for immobilization of the former. The lower critical solution temperature (LCST) of PNIPA can be tuned to the required value by introducing hydrophobic or hydrophilic fragments.

The temperature of the swelling-shrinking behavior change of hydrogels decreased in the following order: NIPA-APSA (35°C) > NIPA-AA (34.4°C) > NIPA-AA/Richlocaine (33.8°C) > PNIPA (32.7°C) [4]. The swelling dynamics of

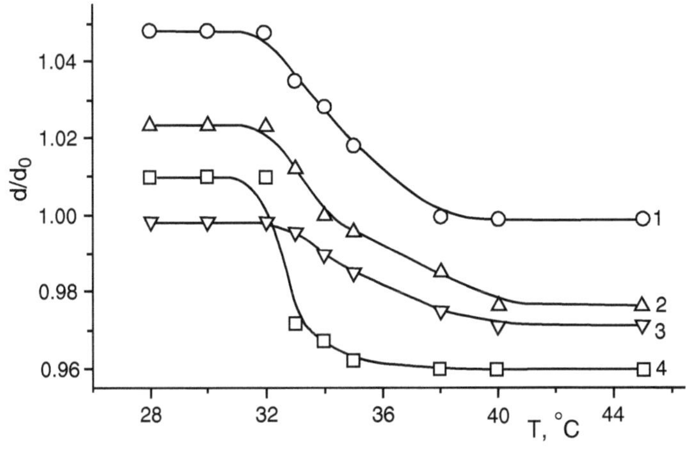

Fig. 19.1 Temperature dependence of the diameter d of NIPA-AA (1), NIPA-AA-Richlocaine (2), NIPA-APSA (3) and PNIPA (4)

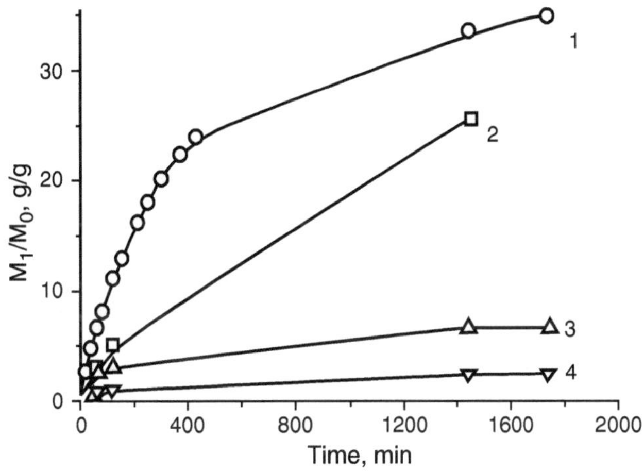

Fig. 19.2 Swelling of NIPA-AA (1,2) and PNIPA (3,4) in $1\cdot10^{-3}$ mol L^{-1} aqueous solution of richlocaine (1), 0.05% lysozyme in phosphate buffer, pH = 7.4 (2), 0.1% bovine serum albumin, BSA in aqueous solution (3) and phosphate buffer, pH = 7.4 (4)

PNIPA, NIPA-APSA and NIPA-AA in aqueous solution of richlocaine, BSA and lysozyme are shown in Fig. 19.2.

Dynamic swelling parameters of bioactive substances into hydrogel matrices are summarized in Table 19.1. The values of $n > 0.5$ indicate that the loading mechanism of bioactive substances deviates from Fickian diffusion. For NIPA-APSA and NIPA-AA/Richlocaine systems the diffusion mechanism is relaxation-controlled because their n values are close to 1. Temperature-dependent release of richlocaine from the NIPA-AA hydrogels is shown in Figs. 19.3 and 19.4.

Table 19.1 The values of *n* and *k* for NIPA-based hydrogels with encapsulated bioactive substances

	In watcr		In phosphate buffer	
Hydrogel/Bioactive substances	n	$k \cdot 10^2$	n	$k \cdot 10^2$
NIPA-APSA (1:1 mol/mol)	1.01	1.4	–	–
NIPA-APSA (1:1 mol/mol)/ Richlocaine	0.93	9.1	–	–
NIPA-APSA (3:1 mol/mol)	0.82	8.9	–	–
NIPA-APSA (3:1)/ Richlocaine	0.84	2.5	–	–
NIPA-AA (3:1 mol/mol)	0.90	2.7	–	–
NIPA-AA (3:1 mol/mol)/Richlocaine	1.03	2.1	–	–
PNIPA/BSA	0.42	18	0.63	10.0
NIPA-AA (3:1 mol/mol)/BSA	0.68	5.3	0.74	4.5
PNIPA/Lysozyme	0.71	9.9	–	–
NIPA-AA (3:1 mol/mol)/Lysozyme	–	–	0.53	19.2

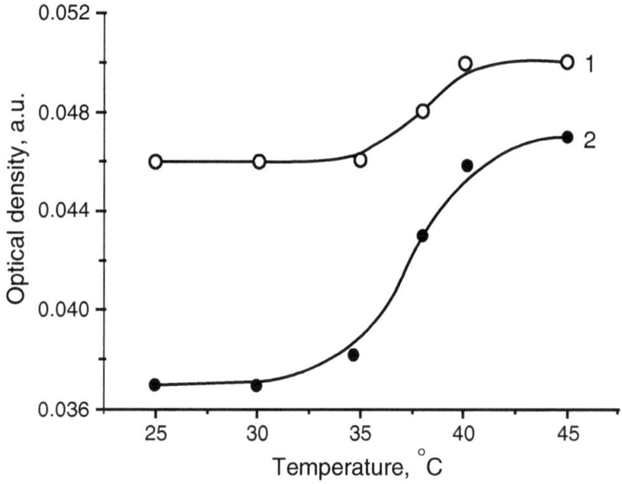

Fig. 19.3 Temperature-dependent release of richlocaine from NIPA-AA (3:1 mol/mol) hydrogel matrix at pH=5.5 (1) and in phosphate buffer at pH=7.4 (2). $C_{Richlocaine} = 1 \cdot 10^{-3}$ mol·L^{-1}

As seen from Fig. 19.3, a sharp increase of optical density of richlocaine coincides with volume transition of NIPA-AA (see also Fig. 19.1). The percentage of released richlocaine was 44.5% and 7.0% at 40°C and 35°C, respectively. The *n* value equal to 0.52 at 40 °C reflects the Fickian diffusion while the $n = 0.26$ at 35°C is characteristic of anomalous diffusion of richlocaine [7]. The rate of drug release from NIPA-AA was minimal at pH 5. It gradually increased with increasing pH and leveled off at pH 8 (Fig. 19.5).

The pH dependence of drug release reflects strong electrostatic interactions between COO^- groups of NIPA-AA and NH^+ groups of richlocaine at pH 5. In these conditions the carboxylic groups of AA are partly ionized while the richlocaine molecules are in a salt form. In strong acidic conditions the ionization of carboxylic

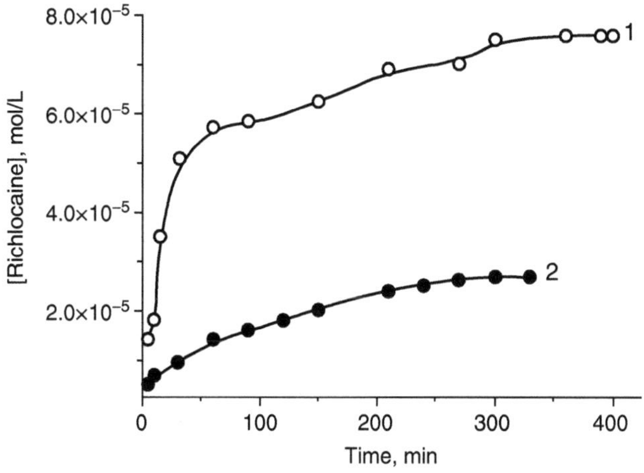

Fig. 19.4 Kinetics of richlocaine release from NIPA-AA (3:1 mol/mol) hydrogel at 40 °C (1) and 35 °C (2). Phosphate buffer, pH = 7.4, 0.15 M NaCl

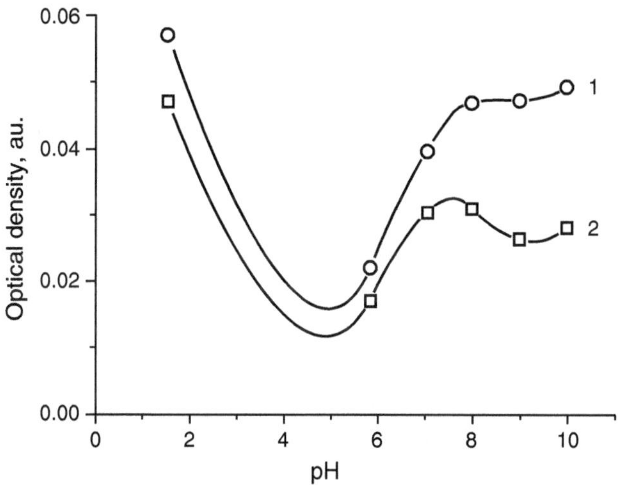

Fig. 19.5 pH-dependent release of richlocaine from NIPA-AA hydrogel. $C_{Richlocaine} = 3 \cdot 10^{-3}$ (1) и $1 \cdot 10^{-3}$ (2) mol L^{-1}

groups is fully suppressed and the electrostatic interactions between COOH and NH^+ groups are weak. This leads to richlocaine release from the hydrogel. In basic conditions the carboxylic groups are fully ionized whilst the richlocaine molecules are in deprotonated form. This leads to destruction of ionic bonds between NIPA-AA and richlocaine and consequently to the drug release into the medium. The optical density of proteins sharply increases in the range of 35–45 °C in aqueous solutions (Fig. 19.6).

The protein release has discontinuous character and occurs between 22 °C and 32 °C in phosphate buffer. The latter is probably due to charge effects of proteins.

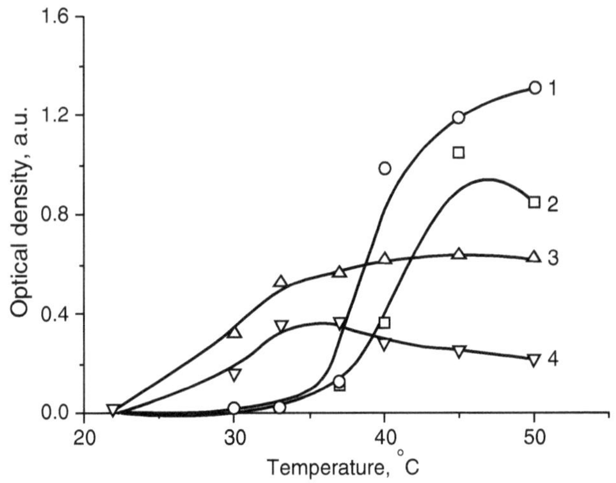

Fig. 19.6 Temperature-dependent release of lysozyme (1,4) and BSA (2,3) from PNIPA in water (1,2) and phosphate buffer (3,4). $C_{BSA} = 0.1\%$; $C_{Lysozyme} = 0.05\%$

The kinetics of the oscillating swelling-shrinking of hydrogels in response to the temperature change is shown in Figs. 19.7 and 19.8. The hydrogels are swollen at 25 °C and shrink at 40 °C. The drug and protein release profiles exhibit a trend similar to swelling-shrinking behavior of hydrogels [8,9]. The initial release of bioactive substances is due to their squeezing out during the first temperature pulse. Release of richlocaine, BSA and lysozyme at temperatures below LCST is governed by diffusion. At temperatures above LCST the hydrogel surface shrinks instantaneously and forms an impermeable "skin" layer restricting the release of immobilized bioactive molecules. The second and third temperature pulses lead to a decrease of the release rate due to decreasing concentration of bioactive substances in hydrogel volume.

Kinetics of catalase sorption by hydrogels is diffusion limited. The equilibrium swelling degree of dry samples in the course of catalase sorption and the activity of the immobilized enzyme changed in the following order: AA-AAc > NIPA-AAc > PNIPA [10]. This can be explained by the fact that binding of catalase by the hydrogel matrix proceeds via electrostatic interaction with participation of carboxylic groups of the hydrogel network and amine groups of the enzyme. Maximal swelling and binding degree of catalase by hydrogels corresponds to neutral region. The relative activity of catalase encapsulated into AA-AAc and NIPA-AAc networks after 74 days decreased twofold while the activity of catalase in solution decreased by 46 times (Table 19.2). The activity of immobilized and free catalase in the temperature range from 25 to 70°C decreased threefold and 10 fold, respectively. These results reveal that the hydrogel-immobilized catalase preserved its catalytic activity for a longer time and at a higher temperatures than the native enzyme.

Regulation of enzymatic activity of catalase in the temperature range from 25 tot 40°C is demonstrated in Fig. 19.9.

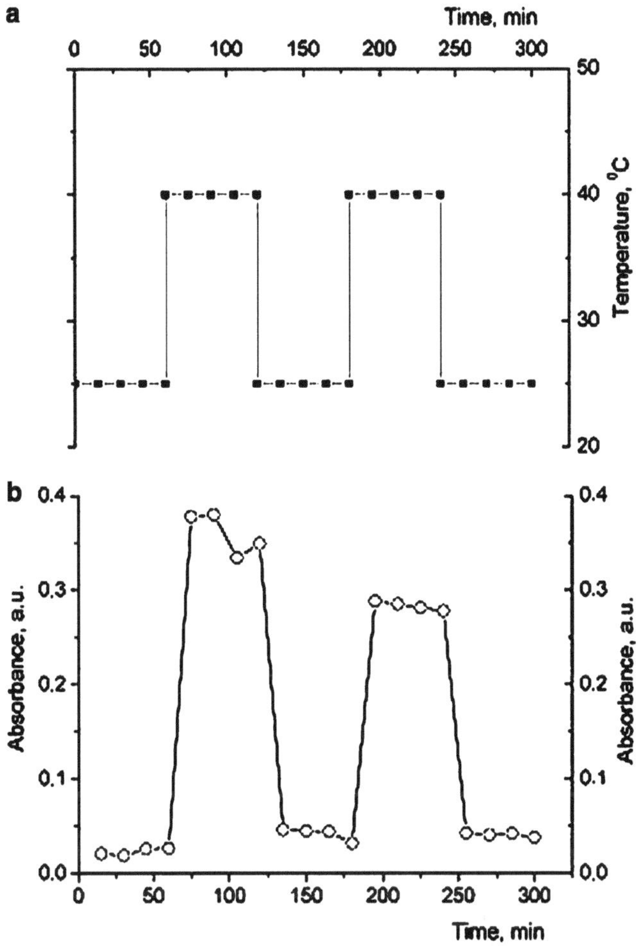

Fig. 19.7 Oscillating change of temperature (**a**) and time-dependent pulsatile release of BSA (**b**) PNIPAM hydrogel in phosphate buffer, pH = 7.4 (1) and water (2) at 25°C and 40°C

19.4 Conclusions

Richlocaine, bovine serum albumin, lysozyme and catalase were immobilized within the thermo- and pH-sensitive hydrogel matrix – PNIPA, NIPA-APSA and NIPA-AA. The values of *n* and *k* characterizing the sorption mechanism of bioactive substances by hydrogels were calculated. Oscillating "on-off" release mechanism of richlocaine and proteins from PNIPA and NIPA-AA hydrogels were observed in the course of cyclic shrinking and swelling of hydrogels in water and phosphate buffer at 25 and 40°C.

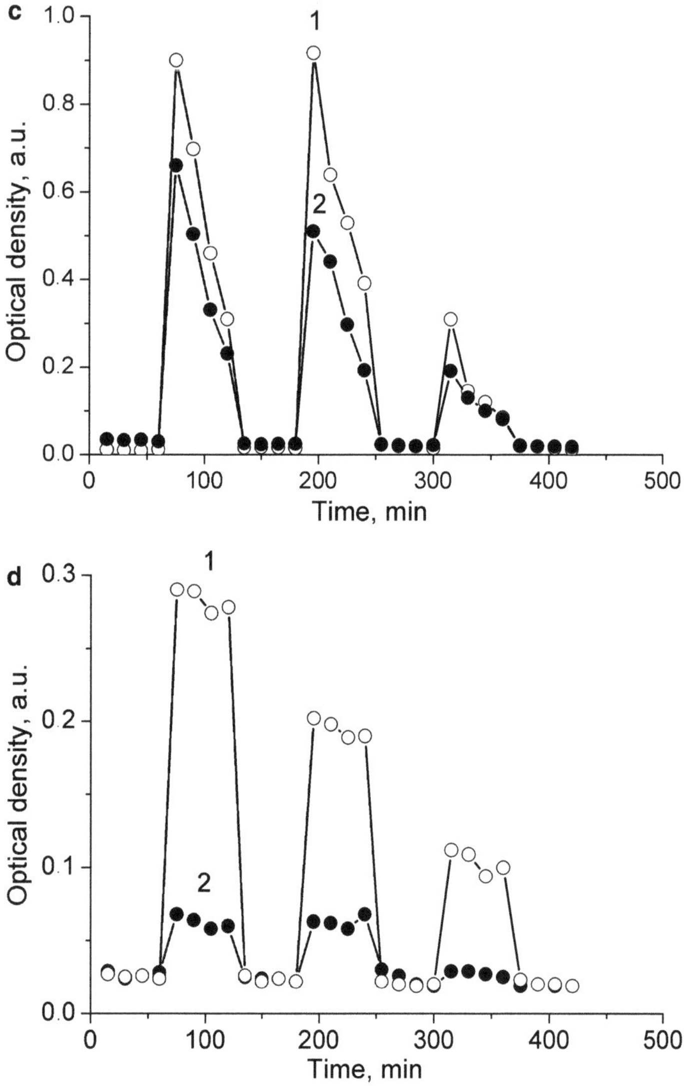

Fig. 19.8 Time-dependent pulsatile release of richlocaine (**c**) and lysozyme (**d**) from PNIPAM hydrogel into phosphate buffer (1) and water (2) at 25 and 40°C

Table 19.2 Enzymatic activity of catalase immobilized within AA-AAc and NIPA-AAc hydrogels

Catalase immobilized within hydrogel	Days					
	1	16	40	50	55	74
	Enzymatic activity of catalase stored at +4°C (%)					
AA-AAc	99.1	86.9	60.2	54.6	51.0	41.2
NIPA-AAc	100	98.4	72.2	63.0	58.0	51.3
Free catalase	100	58.0	25.0	7.2	5.2	2.14

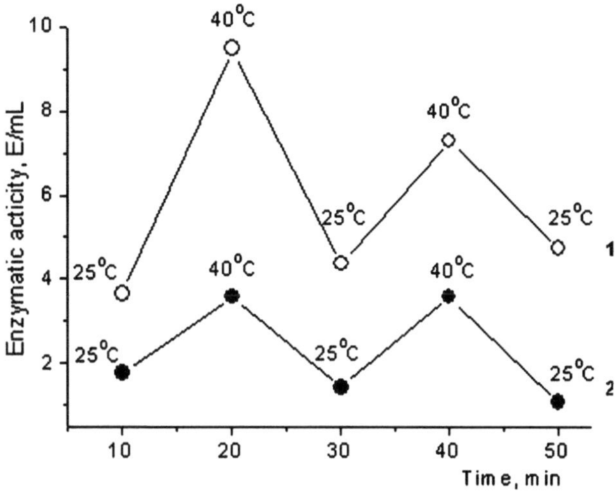

Fig. 19.9 Time-dependent change of enzymatic activity of catalase immobilized within PNIPA gel by sorption (1) and in aqueous solution (2) at temperature interval 25–40°C

References

1. Peppas NA et al (2006) Hydrogels in biology and medicine: from molecular principles to bionanotechnology. Adv Mater 18:1345–1360
2. Peppas NA et al (2000) Hydrogels in pharmaceutical formulations. Eur J Pharm Biopharm 50:27–46
3. Hoffman A, Stayton PS (2004) Bioconjugates of smart polymers and proteins: Synthesis and application. Macromol Symp 207:139–151
4. Lee KY, Yuk SH (2007) Polymeric protein delivery systems. Prog Polym Sci 32:669–697
5. Rzaev ZM, Dinçer S, Pişkin E (2007) Functional copolymers of N-isopropylacrylamide for bioengineering applications. Prog Polym Sci 32:534–595
6. Galaev IYu, Mattiasson B (2000) 'Smart' polymers and what they could do in biotechnology and medicine. Trends Biotechnol 17:335–340
7. Kim B, Flamme KL, Peppas NA (2003) Dynamic swelling behavior of pH-sensitive anionic hydrogels for protein delivery. J Appl Polym Sci 89:1606–1613
8. Kudaibergenov SE, Dolya NA, Tatykhanova GS et al (2007) Semi-interpenetrating polymer networks of polyelectrolytes. Eurasian Chemical Technological Journal 9:177–192
9. Tatykhanova GS, Kudaibergenov SE. (2008) Controlled release of local anesthetic drug richlocaine from the pH- and thermosensitive hydrogels-copolymers of N-isopropylacrilamide and acrylic acid. New smart materials via metal mediated macromolecular engineering: from complex to nanostructures. Antalya, Turkey, 1–12 September 2008.
10. Tatykhanova GS, Bektenova GA, Kudaibergenov SE (2008) Sorption immobilization of catalase within the matrix of pH and thermosensitive polymeric hydrogels. Chemistry Journal of Kazakhstan 21:271–276

Part IV
Medical Treatment

Chapter 20
Critical Care Organization During Mass Hospitalization

A.N. Kosenkov, A.K. Zhigunov, A.D. Aslanov, and T.A. Oytov

Abstract This paper represents the experiment of organization of work of the Nalchik Republican Clinical Hospital on October 13th, 2005 (on the date of an attempt of assault upon the city). During 5 h, 66 people had been hospitalized with different injuries. Owing to organizational arrangements diagnostic research was effectively carried out and there was not any surgery delay. On the whole 98 surgical interferences to 64 wounded patients were performed. Four injured victims died (6.1%), including three (5%) victims dying in the first few hours after being admitted due to the massive destruction of the internal organs and a state of shock, and one person died of sepsis following multiple operations as a result of injury to the abdomen and perineum. The remaining 62 (93.9%) patients were discharged at different times after successful treatment.

Keywords Emergency medical aid • Mass hospitalization • Trauma • Military municipal surgery

20.1 Introduction

At present trauma is one of the three main causes of mortality along with cardio-vascular and oncological diseases in the population of the Russian Federation. Amongst different variants of combined injuries, vascular-osseous injuries occupy a considerable place and are followed up by a high frequency of post operative complications (39–46%), amputations (up to 25%) and lethality (12–21%) [1–5].

A.N. Kosenkov (✉)
I.M. Sechenov First Moscow State Medical University (MSMU), Moscow, Russia
e-mail: Alenkos@rambler.ru

A.K. Zhigunov, A.D. Aslanov, and T.A. Oytov
K.M. Berbekov Kabardino-Balkarian State University, Nalchik, Russia

S. Mikhalovsky and A. Khajibaev (eds.), *Biodefence*, NATO Science for Peace and Security Series A: Chemistry and Biology, DOI 10.1007/978-94-007-0217-2_20,

The president of the American Association of Trauma Surgeons, A. Meyer in his report "Death and Disability from Injury: A Global Challenge" published in 1998 predicted that by the year 2020 the main causes of mortality will become accidents, wars and violence [6]. Unfortunately, judging by events of the last decade, this prognosis is turning into reality. The increase in number of technogenic and anthropogenic disasters accompanied by major human casualties and losses, nowadays often disturb the normal working rhythm of hospitals. Although the lethality in specialised Chest and Abdominal Cavity Trauma Units does not exceed 10–20%, the majority of hospital losses are due to these types of injuries [7]. That is why the organization of emergency surgical care in multi-specialty hospitals is so important, as these hospitals are the first points of response to deal with consequences and effects of emergency situations.

20.2 Organization of Medical Aid in case of Mass Hospitalization

It is important to emphasize that until recently, neither Russian nor foreign civil surgeons were familiar with the organization of emergency surgical care in civil clinical institutions, in the case of mass hospitalization. The principles of organization of surgical aid initially developed for protection of military staff against warfare were adapted in the last decade to protect civilians. This has significantly advanced the emergency medical care, however the specific conditions of megalopolises have additional requirements for surgical aid organization in case of mass hospitalization [8, 9]. Therefore a concept of the military-municipal surgery was proposed by B.V. Petrovsky [10]. Usually, to deal with warfare injuries patients are taken through definite stages of the military medical care: (1) first aid; (2) pre-medical aid; (3) first medical aid; (4) qualified aid; and (5) specialized aid. However, going through all the stages may result in loss of precious time, whereas in urban areas patients can be admitted directly to multi-specialty hospitals, where immediate specialized treatment can be provided. This decreases lethality from blood loss and shock, and allows for saving the life of patients with serious injuries who otherwise would not stand a chance of survival in field conditions.

One of the big differences in organizing this type of aid from the system of field surgery, is that the deployment and functioning of the mass hospitalization emergency system is unexpected and interferes with normal hospital work routines [11]. More than 20 years ago J.E. Waeckerle wrote: "Catastrophe at first is scary and shocking, later confuses and creates confusion in all areas, where to start from and what to do" [12].

At present, the improvement in treatment results of the injured with multiple trauma during mass hospitalization depends in the first place on the organization of aid.

Specialized aid is divided into surgical and general aid.

Main types of specialized surgical medical aid are:

- For trauma of head, neck and spine - neurosurgical, ophthalmological, ENT (ear, nose and throat), and dental
- Traumatological
- Thoracic
- Abdominal and urological
- Burns
- Pediatric
- Gynecological
- Vascular surgery
- Nephrological

Main types of specialized general aid are:

- Toxicological
- Radiological
- Help for general patients
- Psycho-neurological
- Help for patients with infectious diseases
- Pediatric

Causes of trauma during mass admissions are:

- Anthropogenic
- Natural
- War activities

In all cases the trauma is caused by a high impact agent. The state of shock which frequently develops in patients with trauma is mainly due to the dimensions and localisation of damaged tissue on the one hand, and the time interval from the moment when trauma was induced. The degree of shock is largely responsible for the development of multi-organ failure and prognosis of the outcome for the patient. It is therefore of utmost importance to admit patients to a specialized hospital as soon as possible. According to Y. Volynskiy-Basmanov, the lethality in a large group of patients receiving specialized treatment within 1 h is up to 30%, within 3 h up to 60%, and 9 h - 90% [13].

20.3 Organization of Medical Aid in the Aftermath of a Terrorist Attack in Nalchik, Russia

In this paper we analyze the work carried out in the Nalchik Republican Clinical Hospital, in the aftermath of an armed attempt to take over the city of Nalchik on 13 October 2005.

During the 5 h period there were 66 injured people admitted to the hospital who were brought either by medical or civil transport, including 40 military servicemen (60.6%), 23 civilians (34.8%) and three patients (4.5%) were from the armed terrorist group who

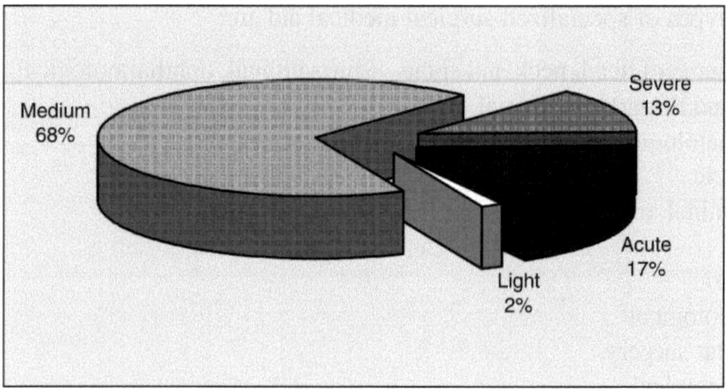

Fig. 20.1 Severity of injuries

also received medical aid. The medium age of the injured was 33.8±2.6 years varying from 19 to 79 years, the majority were males – 63 (95.5%), and three females (4.5%). Only one of these women had a non-penetrating injury of the abdominovesical pouch, whereas the other two were admitted to the ICU with poisoning.

According to their severity, the injuries were classified as shown in Fig. 20.1: the majority of patients had injuries of medium severity. The severity of injury was defined mainly in accordance with its localization, dimensions, type, and blood loss. Individual features such as sex, age, associated illnesses, etc. were also taken into account. It is important to point out that 19 (28.8%) patients had severe and very severe injuries.

The structure of trauma injuries is given in Table 20.1. There were on average 1.5 injuries per injured person. The most common localization of injuries was in the lower limbs - 59.4%, of which shin – 47.4%, upper limbs and head – 25.0% each. The injuries with high lethality included injuries of the chest and abdominal cavities, and also pelvis, which were accompanied by a deep shock condition.

To ensure the smooth running of patient care institutions during the mass hospitalization in the Nalchik Republican Clinical Hospital, short training courses were given to all medical staff. During previous cases of mass hospitalization which had occurred on several occassions due to technogenic and natural disasters, the hospital personnel were aware of all responsibilities and procedures required and followed them to handle the situation effectively. According to these principles the work was also organized on 13 October 2005.

Organization of advance instructions was given according to the following principles:

- Once in 3 months.
- Distribution of functions of every person working in the hospital.
- In advance areas where extra beds could be placed in the existing sections of the hospital.

Timely information and effective communication are the most important principles in handling emergency situations. The Head Doctor was the first person to receive

Table 20.1 Characterization of injuries during the mass hospitalization

Localization of damage	Quantity	Percent
The upper limbs, including	16	25.0
Shoulder	9	56.3
Forearm	6	37.5
Hand	1	6.2
The lower limbs, including	38	59.4
Pelvis	3	7.9
Hip	13	34.2
Knee joint	1	2.6
Lower leg	18	47.4
Ankle joint	1	2.6
Foot	2	5.3
The main limb vessels	5	7.8
Head, including	16	25.0
Facial part	4	25.0
Eye	3	18.8
Neck	3	4.7
Thorax, including	11	17.2
Lungs	5	45.5
Oesophagus	1	9.1
Diaphragm	2	18.2
Abdominal cavity, including	9	14.1
Stomach	1	11.1
Small intestine	3	33.3
Large intestine	3	33.3
Spleen	1	11.1
Pelvic organs	5	7.8
Damages to pelvic bones	3	4.7

Percentage is according to number of admitted injured with trauma (n=66). In every subgroup percentage is given depending on number injured in the group

information about the situation. He then informed his deputy and the deputy gave the information to all the heads of departments and services in turn, who were responsible for informing their subordinates. The mass hospitalization situation is treated as an emergency with 24/7 readiness and all the personnel are required by hospital rules to report immediately to the hospital.

The Head Doctor took full responsibility and the command to deal with the emergency situation of mass hospitalization of injured victims. In this kind of situation the strict principle of centralization was put into effect.

The functions of the Head Doctor of the hospital were:

- Administration, Change of planned procedures: Surgical, Diagnostic, Hospitalization, Consultations, Visits, Increase donor service for doctors and medical personnel, Use of emergency reserves.

The functions of the Deputy Head Doctor of the hospital were:

- Organization of patient admittance in emergency situations
- Opening of new operating theatres
- Regulation of surgical procedures
- Organisation of consultations about severely injured patients

Medical assessment of the injured victims was headed by an experienced surgeon, Head of the Surgical Department of Emergency Surgery. Doctors of all specialties were involved with medical assessment. Every injured patient was personally supervised by an assigned doctor starting from the time when the patient was admitted to the operating theatre.

Each Head of Department had the following duties:

- To inform all personnel to immediately arrive at the hospital
- To organize the treatment and surgical procedures during mass admissions
- To allocate the space for the injured
- To discharge or transfer patients to the general wards.

Within 1 h from the beginning of admissions 28 surgical brigades were formed comprised of trauma surgeons, general surgeons, vascular surgeons and neurosurgeons, all of them being the most experienced specialists. In case additional help was required, the doctors of non-surgical specialties and those undergoing academic career development from non-surgical departments were available on call.

All non-emergency clinical tests and manipulations were put on hold to allow all the personnel to perform emergency procedures. In case of ambiguous situations, the Council of Physicians comprised of the Director of the Hospital and other clinical department personnel were consulted to resolve the situation.

At each incident 14 operating theatres were functional. Two halls which were transformed into temporary operating theatres were ready as reserve in case of increase in hospitalizations.

The average duration of surgical procedures was 67.3±4.3 min (15–350 min). The patients had blood loss of 1,500 mL before operation and 2,700 mL during operations. To cover this amount of donor blood use and its components, the amount in the blood bank was increased with the help of doctors and other medical personnel from other departments.

To increase the number of beds available, the planned non-emergency hospitalization to surgical departments was put on hold and patients who recovered and patients waiting for non-urgent planned operations were either discharged or transferred to non-surgical departments.

As a result of all these changes undertaken, all the surgical procedures were performed on time, totaling 98 in 66 injured patients. Four injured victims died (6.1%), including three (5%) victims dying in the first few hours after being admitted due to the massive destruction of the internal organs and a state of shock, and one person died of sepsis following multiple operations as a result of injury of the abdomen and perineum. The remaining 62 (93.9%) patients were discharged at different times after successful treatment.

20.4 Conclusions

The analysis of the emergency medical aid provided during mass hospitalization in the Nalchik Republican Clinical Hospital can be summarized as follows: The term "military field surgery" coined by the famous Russian surgeon NI Pirogov in the nineteenth century [14] equally applies to situations which involve both injured people and doctors during mass trauma accidents in big cities and can be described as "military municipal surgery".

Rapid first aid and transportation of the injured to specialized hospitals in big cities help to reduce blood loss, state of shock and create better chances for saving the lives of the majority of the injured victims.

Patients with massive injuries are usually admitted to hospitals, whereas patients with the same injuries in other situations out of the city would have little chance of survival.

To give adequate aid to the injured with severe traumas in big cities, it is important to have all specialty surgical hospitals available for immediate and proper medical aid.

Correctly organized work of medical care providers in case of mass admittance of injured victims will avoid unnecessary delays in diagnostics and treatment, which in turn is very important in reducing the lethality and rate of complications.

References

1. Ankin LN (2004) Polytrauma (organizational, tactical and methodological problems) (in Russian). Moscow, p 174
2. Sokolov VA (2006) Multiple traumas: practical guidance for traumatology doctors (in Russian). Moscow, p 510
3. Bondarenko AV (2005) The organization of the specialized help for polytrauma treatment in a large city. Bull Traumatol Orthop (in Russian) 4:81–84
4. Yucel N, Lefering R, Maegele M et al (2006) Trauma associated severe hemorrhage (TASH)-Score: probability of mass transfusion as surrogate for life threatening hemorrhage after multiple trauma. J Trauma 60(6):1228–1236
5. Waydhas C, Seekamp A, Sturm JA (2006) The trauma surgeon's role in intensive care. Chirurg 77(8):682–686
6. Meyer AA (1998) Death and disability from injury: a global challenge. J Trauma 44(1):1–12
7. Abakumov MM (2005) Rendering of the surgical help at mass receipt of victims in hospitals of a mega-city. Khirurgiia (Moscow) (in Russian) N1:8–12
8. Hrupkin VI (2000) The organization of the urgent specialized surgical help to the population in extreme situations. In: Medicine of accidents, the urgent and extreme medicine (in Russian), Moscow, pp 162–165
9. Nechaev EA, Brusov PG, Eruhin IA (1993) The qualified and specialized surgical help in modern system medical maintenance. Mil Med J 1:17–21
10. Petrovsky BV (1998) Selected lectures on military surgery (Military field surgery and Military municipal surgery). Meditsina, Moscow, (in Russian)
11. Mirzoian AE, Shved SI (2001) Modern representations about principles of the organization and volume of the surgical help at mass accidents (Review of literature). In: The genius of orthopedy (in Russian), Kurgan, Kazakhstan 2:61–68

12. Waeckerle JE (1983) The skywalk collapse: a personal response. Editorial. Ann Emerg Med 12:651
13. Volynskiy-Basmanov Yu (2004) Rescue operations after an explosion. World and security №3, p 12, (in Russian)
14. Burdenko NN (1941) Foundations of military field surgery, Vol. I. Moscow

Chapter 21
Enterosgel: A Novel Organosilicon Enterosorbent with a Wide Range of Medical Applications

Volodymyr G. Nikolaev

Abstract Enterosgel® is a polymethylsiloxane based hydrogel produced by polycondensation of methylsilicic acid with the loss of water and formation of siloxane bonds (≡Si-O-Si≡). Upon organosilica gel drying, a solid mesoporous adsorbent (xerogel) with specific surface area of up to 300 $m^2 g^{-1}$ is formed. The xerogel content in the medicinal preparation Enterosgel is about 7%. The sorption process by Enterosgel follows two mechanisms – molecular adsorption and co-sedimentation in the gel. Compared with activated carbons most commonly used as oral sorbents (enterosorbents), Enterosgel possesses lower capacity towards compounds with molecular weight below 1,500 Da, but it is a much more potent adsorbent than activated carbons in its binding ability towards high molecular weight compounds such as proteins and bacterial endotoxins. In many experimental and clinical studies which evaluated oral use of Enterosgel for treatment of wound infection, abdominal sepsis, ischemic hypoxia, acute intestinal infections, viral hepatitis, complications of chemo- and radiotherapy of cancer, it has been demonstrated that enterosorption led to normalization of intestinal microflora, suppression of lipid peroxidation and oxidative modification of plasma proteins, restoration of detoxifying and synthetic liver functions, improvement of renal functions, as well as decreased manifestations of systemic toxicity. These useful sorptive properties along with positive clinical results allow the consideration of Enterosgel as an effective enterosorbent and open a wide potential for its use in combined treatment of diseases requiring long-term oral chemotherapy, such as tuberculosis, AIDS, rheumatoid arthritis and viral hepatitis C.

Keywords Oral sorption (enterosorption) • Polymethylsiloxane • Hydrogel • Chemotherapy

---

V.G. Nikolaev (✉)
R.E. Kavetsky Institute of Experimental Pathology, Oncology and Radiobiology, NAS of Ukraine, 45, Vasylkivska street, Kiev 03022, Ukraine
e-mail: aos@onconet.kiev.ua

S. Mikhalovsky and A. Khajibaev (eds.), *Biodefence*, NATO Science for Peace and Security Series A: Chemistry and Biology, DOI 10.1007/978-94-007-0217-2_21,

21.1 Introduction

The term "enterosorption" has been proposed to define a method of sorption therapy based on daily oral administration of "enterosorbents", i.e. significant (20–50 g) doses of highly activated synthetic carbons [1]. These carbons are produced as microbeads of 0.25–0.40 mm diameter and with specific surface area of 1,200–2,000 $m^2 g^{-1}$ and bulk density of 0.28–0.32 $g cm^{-3}$. They are obtained by pyrolysis of different porous polymeric resins. It is necessary to note that practically all initial results that attracted clinicians to the new therapy, were obtained with this high quality sorption material. The initial studies allowed us to formulate the main mechanisms of curative action of enterosorption [2, 3]. The proposed term has been accepted in the scientific literature, and is used along with a more English term of 'oral adsorption'. Soon a multitude of medicinal preparations and dietary supplements were named enterosorbents, despite the fact that they often have only two properties in common with their namesake – they were administered at large doses up to several dozen of grams per day and were used for similar medical indications. Apart from different types of activated carbon, ion exchange and neutral resins, silicon-containing adsorptive materials, dietary fibers and various combinations of above mentioned materials were called enterosorbents. An important common feature of enterosorbents, is the absence of classic pharmacokinetics that is caused by their localization exclusively in the gastro-intestinal tract, and also an ability to elevate significantly the volume of indigestible food residue, which allows them to perform the functions of dietary fibers [4, 5] (Belyakov 1991, Nikolaev 2005).

The subject of the present review is properties of silicon-organic enterosorbent Enterosgel currently manufactured as a medicinal preparation by the Ukrainian enterprise "Creoma-Pharma Ltd".

21.2 Structure and Adsorptive Properties of Enterosgel

Enterosgel belongs to a class of silicon-containing enterosorbents, the same class as different types of clays and zeolites, and amorphous silicon dioxide (Aerosil®). It is interesting to note that silicon-containing materials rather than activated carbon should be considered the first enterosorbents, because the tradition of eating natural clays for improvement of well-being, jugulation of diarrhea, and, possibly, for treatment of deficiency in microelements, goes back to bygone times, and as a phenomenon known as geophagia it is observed particularly in primates [6, 7].

Methylchlorosilane serves as the initial stock for synthesis of Enterosgel. Enterosgel, i.e. polymethylsiloxane, is a hydrogel of methylsilicic acid obtained in the process of its polycondensation (Fig. 21.1), when molecules of methylsilicic acid lose water and form silanol (≡Si-O-Si≡) bonds.

This hydrogel has structure of a globular porous substance that may be described in terms of traditional structure-sorption parameters such as size of a globule, specific surface area, size and volume of pores, and pore size distribution.

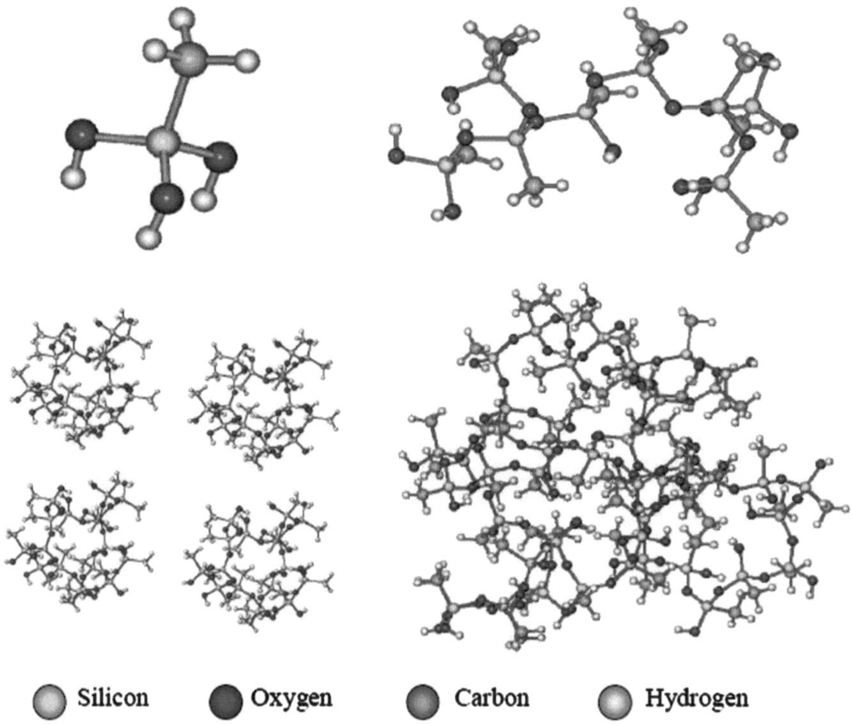

Fig. 21.1 Formation of spatial structure of a hydrogel of methylsilicic acid

Stable hydrogen bonds of the type≡Si-O•••HO-Si≡play an important role in formation of the hydrogel structure [8, 9]. The preparation of a methylsilicic acid hydrogel is an intermediate stage of polymethylsiloxane synthesis, the final solid product of which is a xerogel of methylsilicic acid obtained from hydrogel by its desolvatation (dehydration) at 120°C according to Eq. (21.1):

$$(CH_3SiO_{1,5} \cdot nH_2O)_m \rightarrow (CH_3SiO_{1,5})_m + nmH_2O \tag{21.1}$$

This xerogel has well developed porosity mainly in the mesopore range, which is partially regulated during synthesis, with specific surface area up to 300 $m^2 g^{-1}$ and total pore volume up to 1 cm^3g^{-1} (Fig. 21.2). However, the hydrogel rather than xerogel has attracted most interest as an enterosorbent.

In terms of surface chemistry methylsilicic acid hydrogel, or polymethylsiloxane is a polyfunctional adsorbent which contains both hydrophobic CH_3–groups and hydrophilic OH–groups. It is considered that the porous structure of the hydrogel is created by adjoining nano-granules with the size of approximately 50 nm, and with the interstitial space filled with water. These granules form larger agglomerates, which are organoleptically felt; that is why during production Enterosgel undergoes careful cavitation treatment to shift particle size distribution towards a range of 10–20 μm and to improve the taste of the preparation. Polymethylsiloxane hydrogel

Fig. 21.2 Scanning electron microscopy image of a methylsilicic acid xerogel

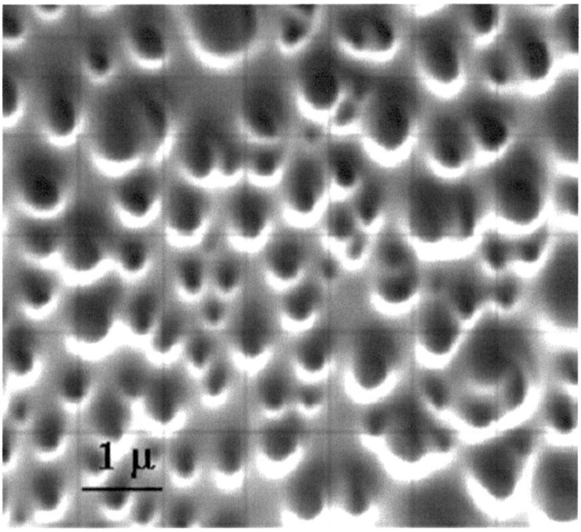

Table 21.1 Adsorption of low and high molecular weight solutes, in mg g^{-1} of silicon matrix, on dispersed xerogel and on native Enterosgel

Adsorbate adsorbent	Methylene blue, 373.9 Da	Human serum albumin, 67,000 Da
Xerogel	11.4	25.0
Enterosgel paste	17.0	714.0

contains nearly 6–7% of the solid matrix, the rest being water. This hydrogel has unusual sorption properties different from those of the xerogel (Table 21.1).

Enterosgel and the dispersed xerogel have near the similar adsorption capacity for methylene blue, but a completely different picture is observed in the case of adsorption of human serum albumin, a large molecular weight solute. The adsorption capacity ratio of Enterosgel to xerogel for HSA is 28.5:1. This result indicates existence of two mechanisms of adsorption by Enterosgel, (1) physical adsorption of low and medium molecular weight solutes, and (2) co-precipitation in the gel of compounds of high molecular weight, such as blood plasma proteins, enzymes, and bacterial toxins.

Being mixed with water, Enterosgel forms a milky white dispersion that separates into two layers, producing a stable suspension in the lower layer, and the upper layer is water. The preparation can be precipitated as a more solid layer by centrifugation. If the dispersion contains protein, then the upper aqueous protein solution does not undergo any chemical or conformational alterations. At the same time the protein co-precipitated with Enterosgel cannot be qualitatively detected with the use of common methods, such as biuret reaction, Lowry, Bradford method, or immunoenzymatic method [10]. In the same study using an example of casein-trypsin couple, it has been shown that co-precipitation with Enterosgel drastically decreases availability of the substrate as well as activity of respective enzymes.

Table 21.2 Ratio of adsorptive capacity (A, mg g^{-1}) of enterosorbents Enterosgel (*ESG*)/ Carboline (*CARBO*) adjusted to their daily doses

Solute	Molecular weight, Da	A_{ESG}/A_{CARBO}
Paracetamol	251	0.0025
Uric acid	168	0.0056
Methyl orange	327	0.0095
Methylene blue	374	0.0465
Rifampicin	823	0.0565
Salicylic acid	138	0.061
Vitamin B_{12}	1,355	0.263
Veronal	184	0.538
Serum albumin	67,000	25.0
Lipopolysaccharide, LPS	From 10,000 (monomer) to >500,000	1.79
Trypsin	23,3000	50
IgG	150,000	100

A daily dose of carbon enterosorbent Carboline is 6 g, Enterosgel – 45 g

The sorption capacity of Enterosgel adjusted to a daily dose of the native preparation demonstrates a sharp difference from a common activated carbon enterosorbent Carboline® (Table 21.2).

As follows from Table 21.2, sorption capacity of a conventional carbon enterosorbent for adsorbed compounds, including medicinal preparations with molecular weight <1.5 kDa, is significantly higher than that of Enterosgel both in absolute values (mg/g) and adjusted to an average daily dose. For high molecular weight solutes the ratio A_{ESG}/A_{CARBO} is higher than unity. The higher binding capacity of Enterosgel could be possibly explained by co-precipitation of these compounds with the gel. Meanwhile, low capacity of enterosorbent for solutes with molecular weight <1,500 Da is very important in practice, because molecular weight of the majority of medicinal preparations administered orally, are low molecular substances with molecular weight in this range. In principle, this fact allows the use of Enterosgel alongside the main drug therapy without the risk of depleting the prescribed drug by adsorption with the gel.

For evaluation of efficiency of medical sorbents, the issue of their deliganding properties, i.e. an ability to withdraw toxic protein bound compounds (ligands) is of great importance. If a sorbent possesses strong deliganding capability as, for example, some types of modern carbon hemosorbents do [11, 12], then after contact with such an adsorbent, the ratio of molar concentrations of ligand - protein carrier (M_L/M_P) decreases, i.e. the transport protein transforms into a more purified state than it was initially (Table 21.3).

Contrary to carbon enterosorbents, Enterosgel does not possess an ability for selective removal of albumin-bound ligands regardless of their affinity with the protein carrier – weak (L-tryptophane), medium (sodium caprylate, deoxycholic acid), or strong (indole-3-carboxylic acid and unconjugated bilirubin). It means that if protein-bound toxins are removed by Enterosgel, this occurs simultaneously with adsorption of the carrier protein.

Table 21.3 Comparative efficacy (M_L/M_P) of organosilicon and carbon enterosorbents for removal of protein bound ligands

Ligand M_L/M_P	L-Tryptophan 104 Da	Sodium caprylate 166 Da	Deoxycholic acid 392 Da	Indole-3-carboxylic acid 161 Da	Unconjugated bilirubin 584 Da
Initial	82.9	13.3	9.36	1.0	10.0
After contact with Enterosgel	81.5	13.6	8.8	1.0	10.8
After contact with Carboline	54.8	2.9	3.33	0.68	2.34

Experimental conditions: 3% human serum albumin, phosphate buffer solution, pH 7.2, containing ligands with different degrees of affinity to the protein

In contact with donor blood plasma at 1:5 w/w ratio, Enterosgel reduces concentration of total protein on average by 18%, albumin by 15%, α_1-, α-$_2$, β- and γ-globulins by 34, 16, 25 and 12%, respectively. In parallel, total cholesterol decreases by 48%, approximately by an equal degree for high and low density cholesterols; concentration of phospholipids falls by 53% and triglycerides by 29%. This data is important for assessing the potential effect of Enterosgel as an extracting agent in extracorporeal detoxification. Enterosgel mixed with bovine bile, reduces the total cholesterol by 12%, triglycerides by 19%, phospholipids by 10%, and total bile acids by 18%, indicating a moderate decholesterolisation effect of the preparation.

21.3 Toxicology of Enterosgel

In experiments assessing acute toxicity of Enterosgel carried out on rats (5 dose levels, from 50 to 10,000 mg kg^{-1} per day), mice and guinea pigs (500 and 5,000 mg kg^{-1} per day) it has been shown that Enterosgel paste is a low-toxic preparation (class IV toxicity). It has also been shown that the preparation expresses neither topical-induced irritation nor general sensitizing action towards mucosa and skin.

The study of sub-chronic toxicity of Enterosgel has been performed on male rats that for 3 months received daily doses of the preparation at 200, 400, 650, and 1,300 mg kg^{-1}. No significant differences between animals in control and experimental groups were found by comparing their general behavior, orexia, body weight and weight of separate organs, morphological and biochemical blood composition, parameters of pro-oxidant and antioxidant homeostasis, with exception of total cholesterol level in animals that received the doses of 400 and 650 mg kg^{-1} body weight (2.12 ± 0.05 and 2.02 ± 0.07 mmol L^{-1} vs 2.55 ± 0.1 mmol L^{-1} in control group).

Morphological studies performed by light and electron microscopy did not reveal any signs of toxicity of Enterosgel administered to animals at sub-chronic regimen.

In detailed studies of pregnant rats and their fetuses, no signs of embryotoxicity or teratogenic action of Enterosgel have been found, and this fact is very important due to traditional use of enterosorption for treatment of gestosis of first and second half of pregnancy. It is interesting to note that analysis of fetuses of experimental animals that received Enterosgel, for anomaly of bone system by Dawson's method showed a decrease in the number of cases with delayed ossification of cranium and breast bone compared to the control.

Safety of Enterosgel preparation in terms of mutagenic action has been shown in the tests for induction of chromosome aberrations in bone marrow cells, in cultured human peripheral blood lymphocytes, and in the Ames test for induction of reversible gene mutations in *Salmonella typhimurium.*

In experiments on BALB/c mice Enterosgel administered at the dose of 116 mg per animal for 2 weeks have not demonstrated immunotoxic properties according to key indices of humoral and cellular immunity. At the same time its positive influence on activity of peritoneal macrophages of experimental animals has been registered.

In experiments on rats with 2-week administration of Enterosgel at the dose of 1,500 $mg\,kg^{-1}$ body weight, the possibility of silicon accumulation in the tissues of spleen, kidneys, lungs, stomach, small and large intestines, and cardiac muscle, was examined. No aberrations in silicon content were found in tissues and organs of experimental animals compared to control group that did not receive the preparation. No accumulation of silicon was found in organs and tissues of animals with injuries of gastro-intestinal tract mucosa caused by experimental induction of peptic gastric ulcer and ulcerative colitis, except for some elevation of silicon concentration in the gastric wall. There was no accumulation of silicon in spleen, lungs, kidneys liver, and muscles of rats after 2-week and 4-week application of Enterosgel-containing preparation over the large fascial skin wound [10].

The conclusion derived from the data described above is that Enterosgel does not possess any noticeable toxicity, and its use in experiments on rats has not led to silicon deposition in internal organs and tissues.

21.4 Enterosgel for Treatment of Diseases of the Gastro-Intestinal Tract

LG Nikolaeva used enterosorbents Enterosgel, activated carbon KAU and lignin sorbent Polyphepan for treatment of patients with Flexner dysentery and salmonellosis [13]. Oral adsorbent therapy accelerated the regression of symptoms of acute intestinal infection, decreased the expression of endogenous intoxication, and reduced by 2–3 days the period of contamination by enteric pathogens in the patients. In Table 21.4, the data characterizing the effect of Enterosgel administration (1–1.5 $g\,kg^{-1}$ body weight per day) on treatment of rotaviral infection (intestinal influenza) in 50 newborns, are presented [14].

This result is of special importance if one takes into account the wide spread rotaviral infection of newborns in third world countries.

L.A. Valenskaya *et al* showed that in children suffering from dysentery, Enterosgel administration improves digestion of maltose, studied by the method of

Table 21.4 Clinical and laboratory indices of efficacy of Enterosgel in treatment of rotaviral infection in newborns (adapted from [14])

Clinical or laboratory index	Treatment with Enterosgel, days	Control group, days
Clinically manifested intoxication	3.2±0.3[a]	7.9±0.1
Respiratory disturbance	4.4±0.4[a]	8.3±0.7
Hyperbilirubinemia	3.2±0.3[a]	7.3±1.2
Disturbed thermoregulation	1.7±0.3[a]	5.4±0.4
Tympanitis	2.0±0.2[a]	5.8±1.5
Posseting of milk	1.8±0.5[a]	6.7±0.8
Diarrhea	2.1±0.8[a]	7.3±1.2
Duration of dysbiocenosis	10.7±2.8[a]	24.5±2.3
Duration of stay in hospital	12.3±2.7[a]	33.2±3.1
Duration of excretion of rotaviruses with stool	2.3±1.0[a]	13.4±2.3
Rate of complications (%):	12.3±2.8[a]	42.5±4.7
a) Necrotic colitis	11.2±2.4[a]	28.3±3.4
b) Toxicosis with exicosis	7.3±0.7[a]	18.7±4.8
Rate of development of nosocomial infections, (%)	16.8±2.1[a]	52.7±4.8

[a]Significant compared with control

carbohydrate load test [15]. O.A. Putilina *et al.* reported positive experience of Enterosgel use for treatment of dysentery and salmonellosis in adults and children, also noting a significant reduction of the period of intestinal malfunction [16].

According to Yu.A. Sukhov *et al*, administration of Enterosgel to patients with acute intestinal infections led to significant decrease of the plasma concentration of pro-inflammatory cytokines TNF-α and IL-2 [17]. In the work of M.A. Andreichin *et al*, Enterosgel was administered to patients with acute intestinal infection (AII) caused by opportunistic flora and shigella Sonne [18]. It was shown that enterosorption promoted regression of pathogenic symptoms, decrease of integral indices of endogenous intoxication as well as normalization of such indices of intestinal mucosa injury as the level of I-FABP protein in blood plasma, and content of lyzozyme in faeces. Furthermore, a number of positive consequences of using Enterosgel were observed in reconvalescent patients during the study of their intestinal microbiocenosis. In general, it has been shown that enterosorption significantly increases the number of reconvalescents with minimal grade I dysbiosis along with simultaneous decrease of the number of cases of grades III and IV dysbiosis. The same researchers found that 10-day administration of Enterosgel to 20 clinically healthy individuals resulted in positive alterations of intestinal microflora via increase of titers of bifidobacteria and lactobacilli, and decrease of present opportunistic microorganisms. A similar result was obtained during the study of Enterosgel in rats: 90-day administration of the enterosorbent led to improvement of the state of microflora of experimental animals with disappearance of bacteria non-characteristic of intestinal ecotopes, and predominance of lactobacilli in the small intestine [10]. These experimental and clinical results undoubtedly open

Table 21.5 Dynamics, in days, of the main clinical manifestations in patients with chronic diseases of digestive system organs

Index	Control group, $n=15$	Main group, $n=24$
Normalization of number of stools	20.5±1.5	6.0±1.4
Formation of fecal masses	21.4±2.5	15.4±2.5
Disappearance of pain syndrome	19.4±1.6	10.6±1.9
Disappearance of meteorism	18.5±1.0	10.5±1.8

prospects for use of Enterosgel in prophylaxis of dysbiosis and treatment of its widespread sub-clinical forms. Introduction of Enterosgel in the conventional therapy of intestinal dysbacteriosis leads to marked positive alterations in microbiocenosis indices in 98% patients [19]. Positive influence of Enterosgel on enteric microflora has also been observed upon administration of this preparation to patients with viral hepatitis [19], and children with severe burns [20].

Of significant interest is an attempt to use Enterosgel for therapy of chronic hard-to-treat diseases of gastro-intestinal tract such as malabsorption syndrome, gluten enteropathy, exacerbation of chronic enteritis, post-resection syndrome and the syndrome of irritated large bowel.

As follows from Table 21.5, administration of Enterosgel significantly accelerates remission of patients compared with the control group.

Prophylactic and therapeutic administration of Enterosgel to rats with experimental peptic ulcer and ulcerative colitis, significantly decreased the number and surface area of lesions on gastro-intestinal tract (GIT) mucosa and reduced the severity of the syndrome of endogenous intoxication that accompanied these injuries [21, 22]. The first evidence of clinical use of Enterosgel in combined therapy of peptic gastric ulcer and duodenum was reported by S.M. Tkach, who had noted that enterosorption significantly reduced the number of side effects of treatment, and the rate of *Helicobacter* eradication increased from 83.3 to 93.3% [23].

Some preliminary data concerning Enterosgel use in the treatment of nonspecific ulcerative colitis in clinic have also been published. Local disbalance of the immune system of the gastro-intestinal tract plays a significant role in pathogenesis of this autoimmune disease, and there is a potential for therapeutic treatment of ulcerative colitis by enterosorption. This statement is supported in particular by results reported by O.I. Osadchaya *et al*, who studied the influence of Enterosgel on humoral immunity, indices of lipid peroxidation, and level of endogenous intoxication [24]. Positive influence of Enterosgel administration was detected in such indices as content of diene conjugates, Schiff bases, circulating immune complexes (CIC), percentage of patients with positive test to serum cryoglobulins, plasma concentration of cryoglobulins and plasma concentration of IL-10. These changes were moderate and did not lead to significant normalization of the altered indices. A tendency for improvement compared to the control group was revealed in many other parameters, such as content of C-reactive protein and ceruloplasmin, degree of oxidative damage of blood plasma proteins, concentration of sodium nitrite, binding ability of blood plasma proteins, ethanol test, ratio of content of immunoglobulins of different classes, concentration of serum albumin, content of compounds with medium molecular weight ("medium molecules"), and pro-inflammatory cytokines TNF-α, IL-1β and IL-6. Being moderate in absolute value, all these shifts nevertheless are of unidirectional character and could be interpreted as a result of positive alteration of nonspecific ulcerative colitis, due to the use of Enterosgel.

21.5 Hepatic and Renal Insufficiency

In the study of N.A. Gorchakova *et al*, Enterosgel was used for the treatment of fulminant hepatitis in rats caused by administration of tetrachloromethane [25]. It was noted that enterosorption hampered lipid peroxidation in liver tissue of experimental animals, elevated activity of enzymes of the antioxidant pool and decreased activity of serum transaminases, which indicates better preservation of hepatocyte membranes. O.R. Grek *et al*, used multiple administrations of CCl_4 in combination with drinking of 5% ethanol for modeling of chronic hepatitis in rats. They demonstrated a stable positive effect of Enterosgel administration on activity of serum transaminases and alkaline phosphatase, as well as the rate of hepatic metabolism of xenobiotics [26].

A number of authors reported positive influence of Enterosgel on the course of acute viral hepatitis A and B in children and adults [27–33]. Patients who received enterosorbents had faster relief of cholemic syndrome and hyperenzymemia, attenuation of skin itching, and improvement of biochemical indices compared to patients from control group. M.A. Andreichin *et al*, administered Enterosgel to patients with chronic hepatitis C, who also received interferon inducers as basic therapy. It was shown that along with positive subjective effects, enterosorption leads to a decrease in the activity of serum alanine-aminotransferase (ALAT) and decrease in concentration of serum thrombomodulin that serves as an indicator of the degree of endothelial malfunction occurring as a consequence of viral dependent injury of vascular endothelium [18].

V.V. Gebesh and I.G. Semenchenko compared the results of surgical treatment of patients with mechanical jaundice in groups that received or did not receive Enterosgel, and concluded that enterosorption led to significant improvement in the state of patients prepared for surgery and during post-surgical period [32]. Such an improvement was seen not only in indices of cholemia and enzymemia, but also in nitrogen-excreting renal function, electrolytic balance, serum concentration of albumin, and leukocyte formula. The average reduction of patients' stay in hospital was 3.5 days, and mortality in the group treated with Enterosgel decreased from 25 to 15% compared to the control group.

In the work of I.M. Skalich and N.I. Zhigarenko (1998), Enterosgel was used as a part of combined therapy for liver pathology of alcohol etiology [34], while O.I. Osadchaya *et al*, showed that in patients of this category, transport function of albumin due to Enterosgel administration increased from 35 ± 7 to 57 ± 7 mg of an organic dye (Congo red) per 1 g of protein versus 36 ± 4 and 39 ± 5 mg g^{-1} in the control group and 90 ± 10 mg g^{-1} in healthy donors [24].

Table 21.6 Functional indices in rats with glycerol model of renal insufficiency

	3 days		45 days		
Index	Main group, $n=16$	Control, $n=14$	Main group, $n=14$	Control, $n=8$	Intact animals, $n=8$
Survival, %	100	100	87	63	100
GFR, ml min^{-1}	0.10±0.01	0.08±0.01	0.15±0.02*	0.08±0.02	0.16±0.02
Protein loss with urine, mg/100 g	0.18±0.003	0.21±0.03	0.28±0.03*	0.46±0.04	0.16±0.02
Blood creatinine, μmole L^{-1}	197.0±0.2[a]	286.0±20.	157.0±16.8*	272.8±18.6	62.9±4.3

*Significant difference from untreated control ($P<0.05$)

Use of Enterosgel for treatment of renal pathologies is of particular interest. A 2-week administration of Enterosgel had positive influence on the indices of kidney function and survival of rats with a glycerol model of renal insufficiency (Table 21.6) [35].

The use of different enterosorbents including Enterosgel for treatment of chronic renal insufficiency of II and III stages was studied in detail by N.A. Kolesnik, who showed that an optimized dose of Enterosgel of 90 g daily administered for 3 months, was able to decrease azotemia levels in 35% of patients, and to prevent its elevation in 25–30% of patients [36]. This is in agreement with results on the use of carbon enterosorbents obtained a decade earlier [1, 37]. M.F. Valentis suggested to administer Enterosgel to patients with chronic renal insufficiency for 6 months or longer, and noticed an improvement of their state as early as 4–5 days after start of treatment, particularly decrease of azotemia grade and metabolic acidosis, which allowed patients to increase their daily protein consumption [38]. These experimental and clinical results are especially interesting, because unlike activated carbon, Enterosgel has low adsorptive capacity towards low molecular uremic metabolites such as urea, creatinine, and uric acid. It is also incapable of breaking down the protein-bound uremic toxins as opposed to synthetic activated carbon enterosorbent SCN used in the former USSR, and more recently activated carbon AST-120, administered as oral sorbent to pre-dialysis patients with chronic renal insufficiency [39, 40].

21.6 Diabetes Mellitus and Dyslipidemia

In experiments on rats with streptozotocin induced diabetes, Enterosgel preparation was shown to have normalizing influence on the indices of lipid profile, parameters of pro-oxidant-antioxidant homeostasis in liver tissue, and its histological structure [41]. Decrease in concentrations of glycosylated hemoglobin, total cholesterol, triglycerides, lipoproteins of low and high density, urea and lipid hydroperoxides along with simultaneous decrease in activity of reduced glutathione, catalase, superoxide dismutase, cytochrome oxidase, and succinate dehydrogenase were significant compared to the control group. Certain positive shifts in lipidogram were also observed in rats with a simple model of alimentary cholesterolosis, as well as some decrease of activity of blood plasma ALAT and alkaline phosphatase, compared with animals from the control group [42]. It is interesting to note that, as in case with renal insufficiency, the effect of Enterosgel could not be explained by direct sorption of certain metabolites, because capacity of this sorbent towards triglycerides, cholesterol, urea, etc., is evidently insufficient. However, the experimental results were in good agreement with clinical data for Enterosgel use in patients with diabetes and dyslipidemia. For example, M.N. Dolzhenko *et al*, showed that in patients with insulin-dependent diabetes complicated with ischemic heart disease, administration of Enterosgel resulted in the decrease of low density lipoproteins by 20% on average, along with simultaneous increase of high density lipoproteins by 39% In addition to significant (compared to the control group) decrease of transaminase activity, and decrease of serum concentration of C-reactive protein – the most important marker of systemic inflammatory reaction [43, 44]. In diabetic patients with clear symptoms of non-alcoholic steatohepatosis, who received Enterosgel, total cholesterol of blood plasma decreased from 8.05 ± 1.15 to 6.45 ± 1.18 but remained unchanged in the control group. In patients with diabetes complicated with acute coronary syndrome, administration of Enterosgel resulted in improvement of biochemical indices and had a positive effect on systolic and diastolic function of the left ventricle, and led to the decrease of ventricular extrasystolia [43, 44]. In the study of E.A. Dotsenko and T.F. Zhiznevskaya, Enterosgel was administered for 1 month in a single dose of 15 g at night or 15 g twice a day to 48 patients with hypercholesterolemia (>6.5 $\mathrm{mmol\,L^{-1}}$), hypertriglyceridemia (>4 $\mathrm{mmol\,L^{-1}}$), or with a level of high density cholesterol below 0.7 $\mathrm{mmol\,L^{-1}}$ [45]. The scheme with double administration of the preparation per day was found to be more effective and led to a decrease of total cholesterol by 9%, triglycerides by 47% and index of atherogenicity by 8%. In parallel, in the control group (40 patients), concentration of triglycerides increased on average by 3%.

21.7 Treatment of Endogenous Intoxications in Surgical Clinic

Prophylactic administration of Enterosgel to rats 4 days before acute blood loss at the level of 20–25% of the circulating blood volume was found to be effective for mitigation of biochemical manifestations of oxidative stress caused by hemic hypoxia [10]. In comprehensive experimental work of A.V. Nedelyaeva, Enterosgel was studied along with other enterosorbents in experiments with a model of severe burns in rats and mice [46]. It was shown that enterosorption had a positive influence on protein-synthesizing liver function and concentrations of serum albumin in wounded animals. Activity of serum transaminases and the content of products of lipid peroxidation decreased, while concentration of ceruloplasmin, a protein with antioxidant properties, increased. Administration of Enterosgel led to a decrease of the level of serum peptides of medium molecular weight and total plasma toxicity, as well as preserved glycogen content in hepatocytes. Combination of a fibrous carbon sorbent, Enterosgel, and polyvinylpyrrolidone was found to be the most effective for treatment of burned animals, and reduced their mortality from 35 to 16% [46]. In experimental work of I.V. Naida et al, (1993), administration of Enterosgel to rats with a deep burn of 15–20% of total body surface, in the dose of 1 $g kg^{-1}$ of body weight promoted reactivation of cytochrome P-450-dependent reactions, decreased activity of serum transaminases, and improved dynamics of wound healing in burned animals [47].

O.I. Osadchaya and A.M.Boyarskaya recently studied the effect of Enterosgel on the plasma concentration of pro-inflammatory cytokine TNF-α. Its level is significantly increased in severely burned patients, however, in patients treated with Enterosgel, concentration of TNF-α was significantly lower by day 19–21 compared to the control group (184.2 ± 14.4 versus 256.0 ± 15.7, and 24.2 ± 6.0 $pg mL^{-1}$ in healthy individuals). In addition, simultaneous elevation of interleukin IL-4 concentration was seen in these patients to 107.0 ± 9.0 versus 94.4 ± 9.8 in the control group, and 32.7 ± 7.5 $pg mL^{-1}$ in healthy individuals [48].

Taking into account the fact that carbonyl groups in blood plasma proteins are generated upon interaction of oxygen with histidine, arginine, lysine, and proline, their concentration could be used as an indicator of oxidative stress. The data presented in Table 21.7 provide evidence of the systemic action of Enterosgel directed at mitigation of oxidative stress.

V.N. Losytska *et al.* found that in patients with severe burns treated with Enterosgel, total binding of congo red by blood plasma on the 19th day after trauma increased to 80 ± 15 versus 50 ± 12 $\mu g mg^{-1}$ of protein in the control group with the healthly standard being 100 $\mu g mg^{-1}$ [49]. B.S. Sheiman *et al*, reported a significant decrease in concentration of "middle molecules" by the 10th day, and diene conjugates by the 20th day after the trauma in patients with large burns was treated with Enterosgel [50, 51]. They also observed a tendency for more rapid normalization of phagocytic activity of neutrophils in these patients compared to the control group. In patients with severe burns treated with Enterosgel some deceleration of the reaction of rosette formation occurred upon the use of autologous serum or its fractions in toxemic and in septico-toxemic stages of burn disease. This observation may indicate a mitigation of autoimmune processes influenced by enterosorption [50, 51]. O.I. Osadchaya *et al*, revealed an increase of functional activity of B-lymphocytes in reactions of spontaneous blast-transformation induced by autologous serum in

Table 21.7 Influence of Enterosgel administration on the content of products of protein oxidative modification in blood plasma of patients with severe burns. Carbonyl groups were determined using 2,4-dinitrophenylhydrazine

	Content of carbonyl groups ($\mu mol L^{-1}$) on different days after burn trauma			
Patient group	3–4 days	9–11 days	19–21 days	Healthy individuals
Control	6.80±0.36*	11.34±0.2*	9.85±0.78*	4.13±0.35
Main	6.75±0.65**	5.49±0.34**	4.44±0.23**	

* Significant compared with the indices of healthy individuals (P<0.05);
** Significant compared with the indices of control group (P<0.05)

burned patients who underwent treatment with Enterosgel [52]. I.V. Naida *et al,* reported a favorable influence of Enterosgel on some factors of cell immunity in elderly patients with severe burn disease [47], whereas A.M. Boyarskaya *et al,* explained the positive result of Enterosgel use in therapy of intestinal dysbacteriosis in burn disease, not only by local action of the enterosorbent, but also with elevation of non-specific immune resistance to the organism caused by it [20]. V.A. Mastchenko also reported a positive influence of Enterosgel on enteric microbiocenosis in children with severe and extremely severe burn trauma [53]. N.V. Pasechko and L.P. Polivanova, who treated pigs with partial-thickness and deep burns (20% of body surface) with Enterosgel, detected a significant improvement of morphofunctional state of intestines including mucosa and structure of myocytes of the intestinal wall, compared to the controls [54]. Summarizing the experience of Enterosgel use in 400 patients of the Novosibirsk Burns Center, A.A. Shmarin noted that 2-week-long use of enterosorption in the therapy of injured individuals starting on day 3–4 after the trauma, decreased the number and intensity of pyretic reactions in patients, improved appetite and decreased the number of GIT complications [47, 55]. As a rule, in these patients leukocytosis was lower, deficiency of body weight less pronounced, superficial drying and scab sequestration occurred more rapidly, and edging epithelization of burn wound began earlier. The period of treatment of superficial and partial-thickness burns was reduced by 3–5 days, whilst in deep burns the period of wound preparation for autografting was reduced by 2–3 days.

V.V. Nikonov *et al,* proposed use of massive doses of Enterosgel combined with Fortrans laxative and various eubiotics as the means for prophylaxis of endotoxemia, oxidative stress and bacterial translocation during preparation for surgery associated with the risk of massive blood loss, and in critical state patients with multi-organ insufficiency, severe burns, sepsis, and polytrauma [56]. This scheme may be used for therapy of different pathologies such as chronic hepatitis, allergy and exacerbation of bronchial asthma.

V.V. Luzin proposed to use Enterosgel slurry in nasogastric drainage of intestine in patients with acute enteric insufficiency and expressed paresis of small intestine [57]. T.I. Chernysh, who administered Enterosgel through nasogastric pathfinder in patients with diffuse peritonitis, showed that such manipulation significantly reduced the period of enteric paresis by more than 40 h [58]. A.G. Lebedev *et al,* performed intestinal lavage with Enterosgel slurry through a pathfinder with double opening placed during surgery, or enterostoma, and this was found to be beneficial for symptom relief of postsurgical paresis in patients with intestinal commissure and necrotic pancreatitis [59]. Some authors suggested that administration of Enterosgel proved to be useful at different localizations of purulent inflammatory process [60].

21.8 Oncological Diseases

T.A. Ageev *et al,* studied efficiency of the scheme "cyclophosphane-vincristine-prednisolone" for the therapy of transplanted lymphosarcoma, and found that administration of Enterosgel to animals decreased liver cell damage and concentration of «middle molecules» in blood serum to 0.433 ± 0.043 a.u. vs 0.704 ± 0.037 a.u. in the control group, without interfering with chemotherapy [61].

In the opinion of some researchers, Enterosgel is a useful means of application in oncological surgery, which reduces the number of postsurgical complications and relieves the course of postsurgical period in patients with mechanical jaundice, improves indices of enteric microbiocenosis, decreases concentration of «medium molecules» and intensity of local proteolysis [62–64]. According to their data, use of Enterosgel in patients undergoing intense courses of polychemotherapy, reduced intensity of nausea and vomiting, decreased the value of hematological indexes of intoxication, and improved the structural and functional state of the erythrocyte membrane. The number of patients with expressed ($<2 \times 10^9$ L^{-1}) leukopenia was reduced on average from 33% to 18%, whilst in patients undergoing chemotherapy due to tumors of the digestive system, these differences were 21.2% vs 54.6% in the control. L.V Guta considered administration of Enterosgel during polychemotherapy of ovarian cancer of III – IV stages useful, noting better tolerability of treatment and decrease of «middle molecules» concentration in the plasma of these patients [65]. M.I. Loseva *et al*, used Enterosgel for therapy of patients with acute lymphoblastic and myeloid leukosis, and registered more rapid remission of the patients along with a number of positive biochemical and clinical effects [66].

21.9 Allergy and Skin Diseases

O.Yu. Pobereznik *et al*, used oral administration of Enterosgel in combination with its cutaneous application for treatment of 70 patients with eczema and allergic dermatitis, while 70 patients with the same diagnosis were assigned to the control group. The authors noted that in the group of patients treated with sorption therapy, cutaneous rash disappeared 4 days earlier than in the control group, and their stay in clinic was 15.7 ± 1.5 days versus 19.5 ± 1.8 days for patients not treated with Enterosgel [67].

A.A. Baranov *et al*, reported a notable acceleration of jugulation of obstructive syndrome and usefulness of Enterosgel for liquidation of signs of endogenous intoxication and decrease of IgE plasma content in children with bronchial asthma, periodermitis, recurrent urticaria and Quincke's edema [68]. N.V. Banadina noted milder expression of lactase insufficiency and endotoxemia in children with bronchial asthma treated with this enterosorbent [69]. V.V. Batov confirmed significant acceleration of eczema syndrome regression in patients receiving Enterosgel and their robust remission occurred 8.0 ± 3.5 days earlier than in control group (25.0±4.1 days) [70].

21.10 Enterosgel in Other Medical Applications

A.I. Pal'tsev (1999), recommended to use Enterosgel for treatment of gestosis in the first and second half of pregnancy [71], and Yu.K. Gusak *et al* [72], and L.N. Ilyenko *et al* [73, 74] successfully applied a combination of oral and intravaginal administration of this sorbent for treatment of nonspecific colpitis and vaginitis.

Favorable influence of Enterosgel on the course of postsurgical period upon surgery of organs of small pelvis was reported by a number of authors, who also recommended introducing this sorbent in therapy of placental dysfunction [73–75]

Despite its low capacity towards compounds of low and middle molecular weight, Enterosgel has attracted the attention of specialists in professional pathology, who propose to include it into the therapy of chronic professional intoxications with aromatic hydrocarbons, benzene, cyclohexane, aldehydes, heavy metals, and organophosphate pesticides [76–79]. Such recommendations are based on the positive influence of Enterosgel on the state of pro-oxidant-antioxidant homeostasis and detoxifying function of liver and kidneys, as well as its ability to mitigate systemic manifestations of endogenous intoxication syndrome and to correct intestinal dysbiosis.

Summarizing their 5-year experience of Enterosgel use in a psychiatric clinic, T.N. Pushkareva and A.P. Chuprikov proposed a few schemes for use of the preparation in treatment of different forms of schizophrenia, and noted that enterosorption did not affect concentration of psychotropic drugs in urine [80].

A.M. Mosunov and A.V. Pozdnyakov used Enterosgel for acceleration of regression of hepato-depressive syndrome in patients with severe diffuse liver pathology, and reported shortened terms of disability of these patients from 29.4 ± 3.8 to 18.3 ± 2.4 days [81]. A.B. Kaydulov and I.V. Vasilenko observed fast reduction of toxic and abstinent events as well as improved functional state of the liver and decreased requirement for transfusion therapy in patients with alcoholic intoxication and in patients with abstinence syndrome of moderate severity, treated with Enterosgel [82].

Some publications described successful use of Enterosgel for treatment of systemic osteoporosis in post-menopausal women [83], reactive arthritis associated with chlamydia or/and yersiniosis infections [84], and severe forms of acute pneumonia in children [85, 86].

21.11 Prospects of the Use of Enterosgel for Treatment of Chronic Pathologies

Enterosgel and other enterosorbents, particularly activated carbons, have an extremely wide range of clinical applications.

The magnitude of this range has certain explanations. Firstly, Enterosgel, as any other enterosorbent, is not a pharmacological preparation in the conventional sense. It is rather related to the same category of biomaterials as, for example, membranes for plasmapheresis that are also used for numerous indications. Secondly, there are a number of typical responses of the organism associated with Enterosgel use, which are repeated in the laboratory and in the clinic in the treatment of various pathological states. These responses include normalization of intestinal microbiocenosis, suppression of lipid peroxidation processes and activation of antioxidant defense, improved indices of lipidogram, decreased plasma concentration of "middle molecules", decreased plasma content of circulating immune complexes and pro-inflammatory cytokines, and positive immune modulation of many parameters of cellular and humoral immunity. One should also add improvement of detoxifying and synthetic functions of the liver and restoration of properties of hepatocyte membranes, improved renal functions, and elevation of regenerative-reparative potential of a number of organs and tissues in general. Many of these phenomena are long term characteristics and poorly correspond to the properties of Enterosgel shown *in vitro*, and this fact once again points out the complexity and depth of mechanisms of therapeutic action of enterosorption.

By its therapeutic action, Enterosgel is a typical enterosorbent with proven therapeutic efficacy. Among the most important patterns of Enterosgel use linked to the spectrum of its adsorptive properties, is a possibility to prescribe it in parallel with administration of practically any oral pharmacological preparation. This pattern is based on a low (compared with activated carbon sorbents) sorption ability of Enterosgel towards compounds with molecular weight below 1,500 Da, to which the large majority of medicinal compounds administered orally belong.

In Table 21.8 comparative data on sorption of some antituberculosis and antiretroviral preparations by Enterosgel and a modern activated carbon enterosorbent Carboline, are presented.

As it follows from Table 21.8, Enterosgel has low capacity towards medicinal preparations studied as opposed to activated carbon. It does not mean that carbon sorbents should not be used for elimination of toxic effects of prolonged drug therapy – for this purpose one could separate drug administration from sorbent administration by 1-2 hours, and introduce meal consumption between them, however, in such cases Enterosgel is surely more suitable.

The results described above suggest a large potential for use of Enterosgel in minimization of iatrogenic intoxications and other side effects of prolonged pharmacotherapy in combined treatment of such diseases as tuberculosis, HIV-infection and AIDS, rheumatoid arthritis, unspecific ulcerative colitis, Crohn's disease, some forms of syphilis and leprosy, and upon complications of decholesterolisation therapy. In all mentioned cases, the other important element of Enterosgel use is its ability to interfere with pathogenesis of these diseases based on the listed useful effects.

These properties of Enterosgel are of great interest for treatment of HIV-infected patients. In Table 21.9 the preliminary results of Enterosgel use for treatment of diarrheic syndrome in HIV-infected patients treated with highly active antiretroviral therapy are presented [87].

As follows from Table 21.9, Enterosgel accelerates the reduction of clinical symptoms in HIV-infected patients with diarrheic syndrome. At present diarrheic

Table 21.8 Adsorptive capacity of Enterosgel and carbon enterosorbent Carboline towards some antituberculosis and antiretroviral preparations

A

Preparation	Molecular weight, Da	Enterosgel, mg g^{-1}	Carboline, mg g^{-1}
Isoniazide	137.1	0.02±0.01	9.11±0.41
Pyrazinamide	123.1	0.15±0.02	9.94±0.48
Rifampicine	823.0	1.50±0.18	19.77±0.72
Stavudine	224.2	0.00±0.00	25.14±0.01
Lamivudine	229.3	0.96±0.01	140.78±0.00

Table 21.9 Influence of Enterosgel on the rate of disappearance of clinical symptoms in HIV-infected patients with diarrheic syndrome (adapted from [87])

Group	Normalization of performance status	Disappearance of abdominal distension	Pain relief	Double decrease of number of stools	Normalization of stools
Main	3.67 ± 1.12	4.28 ± 1.93	4.56 ± 2.66	3.47 ± 1.25	6.03 ± 1.71
Control	5.35 ± 2.21	5.36 ± 2.31	4.94 ± 2.49	5.15 ± 2.18	8.00 ± 3.32
Statistical significance	$p<0.005$	$p<0.2$	$p>0.5$	$p<0.005$	$p<0.02$

syndrome in HIV-infected patients is considered to be linked with development of malabsorption syndrome and general nutrition malfunction, and with decreased efficacy of antiretroviral preparations towards HIV, persistent immunocompetent cells in the intestine, which make an important impact on disease progression [88, 89].

Apart from mitigation of various types of toxicity that are characteristic of antiretroviral preparations, and jugulation of diarrheic syndrome, Enterosgel may be useful for treatment of HIV-infected patients as a means of supportive treatment of concomitant diseases such as tuberculosis, viral hepatitis, acute pneumonia, and malignant neoplasm.

21.12 Conclusions

Enterosgel is an organosilicon material possessing unusual sorptive properties. It has low capacity towards compounds with molecular weight below 1,500 Da, but it is a much more potent adsorbent than activated carbons in its binding ability towards high molecular weight compounds such as proteins and bacterial endotoxins. Numerous experimental and clinical studies have shown a wide range for its medical applications. Enterosgel administration as an oral sorbent led to normalization of intestinal microflora, suppression of lipid peroxidation and oxidative modification of plasma proteins, restoration of detoxifying and synthetic liver functions, improvement of renal functions, as well as decreased manifestations of systemic toxicity.

Due to an unusual relationship between its sorptive properties and the molecular weight of substances adsorbed, Enterosgel practically does not bind medicinal compounds administered orally, because in the majority of cases they have molecular weight below 1,500 Da. This characteristic of Enterosgel opens many prospective avenues for its use in combined treatment of chronic diseases associated with prolonged use of toxic pharmacologic preparations.

References

1. Nikolaev V, Strelko V, Korovin Yu et al (1982) Theoretical basis and practical use of enterosorption method. In: Sorption methods of detoxication and immunocorrection in medicine, Kharkiv, Ukraine (In Russian), pp 112–114

2. Nikolaev V (1984) Method of hemocarboperfusion in experiment and clinic. Naukova Dumka, Kyiv (In Russian), 359 pp
3. Nikolaev V (1990) Peroral application of synthetic activated charcoal in USSR. Biomat Art Cells Art Org 4:555–568
4. Belyakov N, Martinyuk V, Fridman M (1991) Peculiarities of use of enterosorption in presurgical period in patients with large intestine. In: Belyakov N (Ed) Enterosorption, Center of sorption technologies publ., St-Petersburg (In Russian)
5. Nikolaev V, Mikhalovsky S, Gurina N (2005) Modern enterosorbents and mechanisms of their action. Efferentnaya Therapiya 4:3–17 (In Russian)
6. Wilson M (2003) Clay: Mineralogical and related characteristics of geophagic materials. J Chem Ecol 7:1525–1547
7. Dominy NJ, Davoust E, Minekus M (2004) Adaptive function of soil consumption: an in vitro study modeling the human stomach and small intestine. J Exp Biol 207(2):319–324
8. Slinyakova I, Denisova T (1988) Organosilicon adsorbents. Synthesis, properties, and applications. Naukova Dumka, Kiyv (In Russian)
9. Shevchenko Yu, Dushanin B, Yashina N (1996) New silicon compounds – porous organosilicon matrices for technology and medicine. In: Silicon for Chemical Industry. Sandefjord, Norway
10. Nikolaev V, Olestchuk O, Klishch I et al (2009) Administration of preparation «Enterosgel» for prophylaxis of oxidative stress at acute blood loss. Visnyk Naukovykh Doslidzhen' 1:69–71 (In Ukrainian)
11. Sarnatskaya V, Lindup W, Walther P et al (2002) Albumin, bilirubin and activated carbon: New edges of an old triangle. Art Cells Blood Subs and Immob Biotech 2:113–127
12. Sarnatskaya V, Yushko L, Nikolaev A et al (2007) New approaches to the removal of protein-bound toxins from blood plasma of uremic patients. Artif Cells Blood Substit Immobil Biotechnol 3:287–308
13. Nikolaeva LG (1993) Microbiological aspects of use of enterosorbents in acute enteric infections. Likarska Sprava 8:81–83 (In Russian)
14. Dzyublik I, Shun'ko E, Barbova A (1997) Use of Enterosgel for treatment of rotavirus infections in newborns. In: Biosorption methods and preparations in prophylactic and therapeutic practice, First Conference, Kyiv (In Ukrainian), pp 17–18
15. Valenskaya L, Alexeenko L, Nikityuk S (1997) Enterosgel in therapy of acute dysentheriae in children. In: Biosorption methods and preparations in prophylactic and therapeutic practice, First Conference, Kiyv (In Russian), pp 45–46
16. Putilina O, Safronova T, Piskareva I (2000) Comparative characteristic of efficacy of enterosorbents of different groups in Salmonella infection. In: Comparative characteristic of efficacy of enterosorbents of different groups in Salmonella infection. In: Clinical use of Enterosgel preparation in patients with pathology of organs of digestive system, (In Russian), pp 121–122
17. Sukhov Yu, Gebesh V, Golub A (2007) Influence of enterosorption on the level of proinflammatory cytokines upon intestinal infection and measles. Klin Immunologiya 6:76–78 (In Russian)
18. Andreichin M, Koncha V, Klyimyuk S (2010) Influence of Enterosgel preparation on cytolysis of hepatocutes and endothelial disfunction in patients with chronic hepatitis C. In press (In Ukrainian)
19. Moroz L, Paliy I (2006) Study of influence of detoxicant Enterosgel on clinical and laboratory indexes in acute viral hepatitis. In: Medico-biological aspects of enterosorbent "Enterosgel" Use for therapy of different diseases, Kyiv (In Russian), pp 71–76
20. Boyarskaya G, Osadchaya O, Zhernov A, Kovalenko O (2006) Use of enterosorbent Enterosgel in combined therapy of enteric disbacteriosis in children with burn disease. In: Medico-biological aspects of enterosorbent "Enterosgel" Use for therapy of different diseases, Kyiv (In Russian), pp 83–90
21. Yastremskaya S, Klishch I, Nikolaev V et al (2010) Evaluation of efficacy of administration of Enterosgel preparation in medicinal form – paste for oral use in animals with peptic gastric ulcer. Comparative characteristic of efficacy of enterosorbents of different groups in Salmonella infection. In: Clinical use of Enterosgel preparation in patients with pathology of organs of digestive system(in Ukrainian)

22. Yastremskaya S, Klishch I, Nikolaev V et al (2010) Efficacy of use of Enterosgel enterosorbent in experimental ulcerative colitis. In press (In Russian)
23. Tkach S (2006) Efficacy of enterosorbent Enterosgel in combined antihelicobacter therapy of peptic ulcer. Zhurnal Praktychnogo Likarya 5–6:55–58 (In Russian)
24. Osadchaya O, Boyarskaya G, Sheiman B et al (2008) Informativity of numerical methods of evaluation of endogenous intoxication in patients with severe burns with the use of enterosorption. Klinichna Imunologiya, Alergologiya, Infectologiya 1:77–79 (In Russian)
25. Gorchakova N, Chekman I, Surok V et al (2005) Study of pharmacological activity and safety of Enterosgel preparation. Mystetstvo Likuvannya 4:5–10 (In Russian)
26. Grek O, Kolpakov M, Bashkirov Yu et al (2000) Use of Enterosgel for correction of disturbance of liver function in experimental chronic toxic hepatitis. In: Clinical use of Enterosgel preparation in patients with pathology of organs of digestive system, Moscow (In Russian), pp 63–66
27. Vozianova Zh, Korchinskiy N, Pashnovaya E et al (1990) Enterosorption in combined therapy of patients with viral hepatitis. Vrachebnoe Delo 4:117–120 (In Russian)
28. Garnitskaya L (1994) Use of Enterosgel in combined therapy of patients with viral hepatitis B on the background of mechanical jaundice. Vrachebnoe Delo 5–6:138–140 (In Russian)
29. Nikityuk S, Alexeenko L, Volynska L (1997) Correction of immunological disbalance in children with viral hepatitis A using Enterosgel. In: Biosorption methods and preparations in prophylactic and therapeutic practice, First Conference, Kyiv (In Ukrainian), p 59
30. Olkhovnikova E, Gavrilova N, Golovanova L (1999) Enterosgel preparation in treatment of viral hepatitis in children. In: Proceedings of the Conference«Enterosgel and Enterosorption Technology in Medicine», Novosibirsk – Moscow (In Russian), pp. 44–45
31. Myasnikov V (2002) Report on the results of clinical trials of Enterosgel preparation in therapy of patients with viral hepatitis, part IV. Kreoma Publ, Kyiv (In Russian), pp 22–23
32. Gebesh V, Semenchenko I (2000) Use of Enterosgel in therapy of patients with mechanical jaundice. In: Clinical use of Enterosgel preparation in patients with pathology of organs of digestive system, Moscow, (In Russian), pp 66–68
33. Moroz L, Paliy I, Tkachenko T (2006) Use of Enterosgel preparation in combined therapy of patients with acute viral hepatitis. In: Medico-biological aspects of enterosorbent "Enterosgel" use for therapy of different diseases, Kyiv (In Russian), pp 65–70
34. Skalich I, Zhigarenko N (1998) Efficacy of enterosorbents and antioxidants in therapy of chronic diseases of liver of alcoholic etiology. Vrachebnoe Delo 5:93–95 (In Russian)
35. Fira L, Nikolaev V, Klishch I et al (2010) Study of efficacy of Enterosgel preparation in the treatment of experimental renal insufficiency. In press (In Russian)
36. Kolesnik M (1995) Efferent methods in combined therapy of patients with glomerulonephritis. Thesis for degree of Dr Med Sci, Kyiv (In Ukrainian)
37. Shostka G, Riabov S, Lukichev B et al (1984) Oral sorbents in the treatment of chronic renal failure. Ter Arkh 7:58–63 (In Russian)
38. Valentis M (1999) Use of Enterosgel preparation in combined therapy of patients with chronic renal insufficiency. In: Proceedings of the Conference « Enterosgel and Enterosorption Technology in Medicine», Novosibirsk – Moscow (In Russian), p 18
39. Sanaka T, Sugino N, Teraoka S et al (1988) Therapeutic effects of oral sorbent in undialyzed uremia. Am J Kidney Dis 2:97–103
40. Nakagawa N, Hasebe N, Sumitomo K et al (2006) An oral adsorbent, AST-120, suppresses oxidative stress in uremic rats. Am J Nephrol 5:455–461
41. Tchernyashova V, Olestchuk O, Nikolaev V et al (2008) Study of efficacy of use of Enterosgel in a model of experimental streptozotocine diabetes. Visnyk Farmakologii i Farmatsii 3:33–37 (In Ukrainian)
42. Pokotylo O, Yastremskaya S, Nikolaev V et al (2010) Influence of enterosorbent Enterosgel on indexes of lipid exchange in experimental hypercholesterolemia. In press (In Russian)
43. Dolzhenko M, Shershneva O, Perepel'chenko N, Potashev S (2006) Optimization of therapy of coronary syndrome with the fall of ST segment in patients with diabetes mellitus of type II by method of enterosorption. News of Medicine and Pharmacy № 1-2:8–9

44. Dolzhenko M, Shipulin V, Sokolova L (2005) Role of enterosorption in hypolipidemic therapy of patients with nonalcoholic steatohepatitis with concominant IHD and diabetes mellitus type II. Mystetstvo Likuvannya 9:65–66 (In Russian)
45. Dotsenko E, Zhiznevskaya T (1999) Influence of Enterosgel preparation on the state of lipid-transporting system in patients with hyperlipidemia. In: Proceedings of the conference «Enterosgel and Enterosorption technology in Medicine», Novosibirsk – Moscow (In Russian), pp 22–23
46. Nedelyaeva A (2001) Comparative physiological analysis of different sorbents in the model oh thermal injury. In: Collection of Reports on the use of Enterosgel preparation in medicine, part I, Moscow (In Russian), pp 28–37
47. Naida I, Zapadnyuk V, Povstyanoy N et al (1993) Age-related peculiarities of natural mechanisms of detoxication and curative action of Enterosgel in burn disease. Klinichna Khirurgiya 9-10:53–56, In Russian
48. Osadchaya O, Boyarskaya G (2009) Effect of enterosorption on humoral immunity of patients with nonspecific ulcerative colitis. Consilium Medicum (In Ukrainian) 5(3):20–21
49. Losytska V, Naida I, Tsiganov V (1997) Toxin-binding ability of blood serum proteins in burned patients with the use of Enterosgel. In: Biosorption methods and preparations in prophylactic and therapeutic practice, First Conference, Kyiv (In Ukrainian), pp 121–122
50. Sheiman B, Osadchaya O, Boyarskaya G et al (2007) Use of enterosorption for prophylaxis of autoimmune processes in patients with severe burns. Klinichna Imunologiya, Alergologiya, Infectologiya 3:104–106 (In Russian)
51. Sheiman B, Osadchaya O, Boyarskaya G et al (2007) Influence of enterosorption on functional activity of factors of antimicrobial resistance in patients with severe burns. Klinichna Imunologiya, Alergologiya, Infectologiya 4:61–63 (In Russian)
52. Osadchaya O, Boyarskaya G, Zheriev A, Sheiman B (2006) Study of efficacy of use of Enterosgel preparation in patients upon endogenous intoxication. In: Medico-biological aspects of enterosorbent "Enterosgel" use for therapy of different diseases, Kyiv (In Russian), pp 91–96
53. Maschenko V (1997) Influence of enterosorption on microbiocenosis in children with severe and extremely severe burn trauma. In: Biosorption methods and preparations in prophylactic and therapeutic practice, First Conference, Kyiv (In Ukrainian), pp 120–121
54. Pasechko N, Polivanova L (1997) Influence of enterosorbents on structural components of intestine upon severe thermal burns of skin. In: Biosorption methods and preparations in prophylactic and therapeutic practice, First Conference, Kyiv (In Ukrainian), pp 108-111
55. Osadchaya O (2008) Role of enterosorption in treatment of metabolic intoxication in patients with severe burns. Liki Ukraini 7:56–58, In Russian
56. Nikonov V, Nud'ga A, Kovaleva E (2007) "Fortrans-enterin-eubiotin" therapeutic complex for detoxication of human organism. In: Medico-biological aspects of enterosorbent "Enterosgel" use for therapy of different diseases, Kyiv (In Ukrainian), pp 22–26
57. Luzin V (2001) Surgical aspects of syndrome of enteric insufficiency. In: Collection of Reports on the use of Enterosgel preparation in medicine, part II, Moscow (In Russian), pp 5-9
58. Chernysh T (2001) Enterosorption with Enterosgel for treatment of advanced peritonitis. In: Collection of Reports on the use of enterosgel preparation in medicine, part II, Moscow, (In Russian), pp 10–13
59. Lebedev A, Lyaschenko Yu, Petukhov A (2001) Use of Enterosgel in patients with intestinal obstruction. In: Collection of Reports on the use of Enterosgel preparation in medicine, part II, Moscow (In Russian), pp 23–25
60. Smiyan I, Pavlishin G, Listchenko N (1997) Enterosgel in combined therapy of newborns with purulent-septic pathologies. In: Biosorption Methods and preparations in prophylactic and therapeutic practice, First Conference, Kyiv (In Ukrainian), pp 46–47
61. Ageev T, Kaledin V, Nikolin V (2001) Effects of Enterosgel during chemotherapy of experimental lymphosarcoma. In: Collection of Reports on the use of Enterosgel preparation in medicine, part III, Moscow (In Russian), pp 22–23

62. Kaban O, Gunina L, Shevchenko Yu et al (2001) Efficacy and perspective of use of preparations on the basis of hydrogel and xerogel of methylsilicic acid in patients with malignant neoplasm of digestive tract. Klinichna Khirurgiya 1:34–37 (In Russian)
63. Kaban O, Gunina L, Znamenskiy V et al (1997) Influence of Enterosgel on endogenous intoxication and expression of dysbacteriosis during combined therapy of patients with cancer of digestive tract. Kreoma Publ, Kiyv (In Russian), pp 31–33
64. Gunina L, Litvinenko A (1997) Detoxicating effect of Enterosgel upon polychemotherapy of patients with advanced tumors of peritoneal cavity. Kreoma Publ, Kiyv (In Russian), pp 33–35
65. Guta L, Temchenko O, Sopel' V, Matsela N (1997) Use of silicon-organic sorbents for endogenous intoxication syndrome correction. In: Biosorption methods and preparations in prophylactic and therapeutic practice, First Conference, Kiyv (In Russian), p 35
66. Loseva M, Pospelov T, Mishenin A et al (1999) Efficacy of Enterosgel use in remission therapy in patients with acute leukosis. In: Proceedings of the Conference «Enterosgel and Enterosorption Technology in Medicine», Novosibirsk – Moscow (In Russian), pp 14-15
67. Poberezhnik O, Osolodchenko T, Kutneevich Ya, et al. (1997) Use of immobilized medicinal preparations in combined therapy of patients with eczema. In: Biosorption methods and preparations in prophylactic and therapeutic practice, First Conference, Kyiv (In Ukrainian), pp 59-60
68. Baranov A, Geppe N, Karpushkina A (1997) Efficacy of Enterosgel in therapy of bronchial asthma and atopic dermatitis in children. In: Biosorption methods and preparations in prophylactic and therapeutic practice, First Conference, Kyiv (In Ukrainian), pp. 50-52
69. Banadina N (1997) Influence of various types of sorption therapy on functional state of small intestine of children suffering from bronchial asthma. In: Biosorption methods and preparations in prophylactic and therapeutic practice, First Conference., Kyiv (In Ukrainian), pp 56-57
70. Batov V (2000) Place of Enterosgel preparation in combined therapy of neurodermitis. In: Clinical use of Enterosgel preparation in patients with pathology of organs of digestive system, Moscow (In Russian), pp 74–75
71. Paltsev A (1999) Enterosgel in clinic of innate pathologies...In: Proceedings of the Conference «Enterosgel and Enterosorption Technology in Medicine», Novosibirsk – Moscow (In Russian), pp 53–57
72. Gusak Yu, Gusak N, Pchelintsev V, Tarasova L (1999) Enterosgel in treatment of inflammatory pathologies in gynecology and obstetrics. In: Proceedings of the Conference «Enterosgel and Enterosorption Technology in Medicine», Novosibirsk – Moscow (In Russian), pp 41–43
73. Ilyenko L, Petrovich E (a) (2002) Use of Enterosgel in combined therapy of inflammatory pathologies of uterus and uterine adnexa. In: Collection of Reports on the Use of Enterosgel Preparation in Medicine, part V, Moscow (In Russian), pp 15–25
74. Ilyenko L, Petrovich E (в) (2002) Evaluation of efficacy of use of sorbent Enterosgel in combined therapy of recurrent forms of vaginal candidosis. In: Collection of Reports on the Use of Enterosgel Preparation in Medicine, part V, Moscow (In Russian), pp 26–34
75. Gusak Yu, Morosov V, Chikin V et al (2002) Use of Enterosgel preparation in postsurgical period in obstetric. In: Collection of Reports on the Use of Enterosgel Preparation in Medicine, part V, Moscow (In Russian), pp 46–49
76. Sukharevskaya T, Nikiforova N (1999) Use of Enterosgel preparation in optimization of etiotropic therapy of chronic professional intoxications. In: Proceedings of the Conference «Enterosgel and Enterosorption Technology in Medicine», Novosibirsk – Moscow (In Russian), pp 30–33
77. Shpagina L, Gerasimenko O, Bobrov S (1999) Comparative evaluation of efficacy of use of enterosorbents in therapy of chronic professional intoxications. In: Proceedings of the Conference «Enterosgel and Enterosorption Technology in Medicine», Novosibirsk – Moscow (In Russian), pp 37–39
78. Shpagina L, Gerasimenko O, Tretyakov S et al (1999) Use of different enterosorbents for therapy of chronic professional intoxications. In: Proceedings of the Conference «Enterosgel and Enterosorption Technology in Medicine», Novosibirsk – Moscow (In Russian), p 57
79. Poteryaeva A (2001) Use of Enterosgel in clinic for treatment of occupational diseases. Methodical Recommendations, Moscow, (In Russian)

80. Pushkareva T, Chuprikov A (1997) Use of enterosorption in combined therapy of schizophrenia. In: Biosorption methods and preparations in prophylactic and therapeutic practice, First Conference, Kyiv (In Ukrainian), pp. 77–78
81. Mosunov A, Pozdnyakov A (1999) Clinical study of the efficacy of Enterosgel preparation in diffuse liver pathology accompanied by hepato-depressive syndrome. In: Proceedings of the Conference«Enterosgel and Enterosorption technology in Medicine», Novosibirsk – Moscow (In Russian), pp 15–18
82. Kaydulov A, Vasylenko I (1997) Use of Enterosgel for treatment and mitigation of alcoholic intoxication. In: Biosorption methods and preparations in prophylactic and therapeutic practice, First Conference, Kyiv (In Ukrainian), pp 74–76
83. Povoroznyuk V, Nikonenko P, Bayandina E et al (1997) Use of enterosorbent«Enterosgel»in combined therapy of osteoporosis. In: Biosorption methods and preparations in prophylactic and therapeutic practice, First Conference, Kyiv (In Ukrainian), pp 43–46
84. Babinina L, Viznyak N, Matyukha L (1997) Enterosorbents in combined therapy of reactive arthritis. In: Biosorption methods and preparations in prophylactic and therapeutic practice, First Conference, Kyiv (In Ukrainian), pp 78–79
85. Pasyaka N (1997) State of LPO processes and AOS in children with severe form of acute pneumonia treated with Enterosgel. In: Biosorption methods and preparations in prophylactic and therapeutic practice, First Conference, Kyiv (In Ukrainian), p 58
86. Pasyaka N (1997) Use of Enterosgel for correction of endocytosis in children of early age suffering from severe form of acute pneumonia. In: Biosorption methods and preparations in prophylactic and therapeutic practice, First Conference, Kyiv (In Ukrainian), p 57
87. Yurchenko O, Fedorenko S, Nikolaev V et al (2010) Use of enterosorbent Enterosgel in combined therapy of HIV-infected patients. In press (In Russian)
88. Guadalupe M, Reay E, Sankaran S et al (2003) Severe CD4+ T-cell depletion in gut lymphoid tissue during primary human immunodeficiency virus type 1 infection and substantial delay in restoration following highly active antiretroviral therapy. J Virol 21:11708–11717
89. Guadalupe M, Sankaran S, George MD et al (2006) Viral suppression and immune restoration in the gastrointestinal mucosa of human immunodeficiency virus type 1-infected patients initiating therapy during primary or chronic infection. J Virol 16:8236–8247

Chapter 22
Rehabilitation Methods for Exposure to Heavy Metals Under Environmental Conditions

A.R. Gutnikova, B.A. Saidkhanov, I.V. Kosnikova, I.M. Baybekov, K.O. Makhmudov, D.D. Ashurova, A.KH. Islamov, and M.I. Asrarov

Abstract Heavy metals, anthropogenic toxicants, can penetrate into the human organism in tiny amounts through food and water and then accumulate, promoting development of chronic poisonings and the reduction of human adaptability to the environment. Modeling of heavy metal anthropogenic pollution makes it possible to study the mechanism and nature of heavy metals pathological effect on humans and animals. The knowledge of heavy metals cytotoxic properties and mechanisms of their interaction with living species opens new prospects in the search for a prevention and therapeutic treatment of chronic diseases associated with the effect of xenobiotics. In this paper, pathological disorders in liver due to heavy metals effects and their treatment have been investigated.

Keywords Anthropogenic toxicants • Exposure to heavy metals • Pathological disorders in liver • Rehabilitation

22.1 Introduction

Heavy metals (HM) form a special group of anthropogenic toxicants in many respects, responsible for unfavorable ecological situations and morbidity rise in industrial regions. They can penetrate into the human organism in tiny amounts through food and water and then accumulate, these toxicants promote development of chronic poisonings and the reduction of human adaptability to the environment [1–3]. Not only the health of workers of metallurgical and mining enterprises is

A.R. Gutnikova (✉), B.A. Saidkhanov, I.V. Kosnikova, I.M. Baybekov, K.O. Makhmudov, D.D. Ashurova, and A.KH. Islamov
V.Vakhidov Republican Specialised Center of Surgery, Tashkent, Uzbekistan
e-mail: gutnikova@mail.ru

M.I. Asrarov
Institute of Physiology and Biochemistry, Academy of Sciences, Tashkent, Uzbekistan

S. Mikhalovsky and A. Khajibaev (eds.), *Biodefence*, NATO Science for Peace and Security Series A: Chemistry and Biology, DOI 10.1007/978-94-007-0217-2_22,

affected by heavy metal release into the environment, but also the inhabitants of industrial centers and neighboring regions are subjected to this chemical impact. However, evaluation of the adverse effects of pollution on the human organism is difficult to measure. In reality a human being is exposed to the effect of a mixture of HM species of variable composition rather than a single substance. The nature and composition of pollutants is region specific, and they may have synergetic and antagonistic properties. Modeling of heavy metal anthropogenic pollution makes it possible to study the mechanism and nature of HM pathological effect on humans and animals. The knowledge of HM cytotoxic properties and mechanisms of their interaction with living species, opens new prospects in the search for a prevention and therapeutic treatment of chronic diseases associated with the effect of xenobiotics.

In industrial areas of Tashkent region in Uzbekistan the main HM toxicants are copper, manganese, molybdenum, chromium and their combinations. They enter into the human organism with inhaled air, drinking water and vegetables, which are the main part of the local population's food, and cause an increase in liver diseases. The main type of treatment of such diseases is applying different methods of detoxification of the organism and some methods increase resistance towards these toxic effects. Only a combination of several approaches can ensure fast reduction of the level of toxic substances in biological media and restoration of homeostasis.

In this paper, pathological disorders in liver due to HM effect and their treatment have been investigated.

22.2 Experimental

The investigations were conducted using 190 Vistar rats with a body mass of 140–150 g, housed in a vivarium and fed with standard food rations. The animals were divided into three groups. The first group of somatically healthy animals was used as a control. The second group were rats suffering from sub-chronic poisoning caused by a toxic mixture containing heavy metal salts of copper, manganese, molybdenum and chromium ($CuSO_4$, $KMnO_4$, $(NH_4)_2MoO_4$, $K_2Cr_2O_7$ in doses of 60, 11.2, 10 and 1.19 $mg\,kg^{-1}$ of body mass, respectively). The mixture was injected intraperitoneally for 4 weeks. The metal ratio was similar to the average ratio in soils in the Almalyk mining and metallurgical region of Uzbekistan. Having a pathological process induced by intake of HM mixture, the third group of animals was subjected to a combined treatment course for 3 weeks with sorbent materials and antioxidant therapy. Citric pectin with the molecular mass of 70,000 Da, 50% degree of esterification, and carboxyl group content of 0.6% was used as the sorbent. Daily the animals were given sorbent orally in the dosage of 0.5 g per 100 g of the body mass 1 h before feeding. Hepamal™ was used as an antioxidant agent. Hepamal is an oil extract of immortelle and costmary flowers and sweetbrier fruits. It was introduced orally 2 h after feeding once a day in the dosage of 1 mL per 100 g of the body mass. On completion of the therapy course the animals were weighed and then anesthesized and decapitated. The blood and liver tissue were taken for further assessment.

22.3 Results and Discussion

A 4-week injection of HM mixture caused sub-chronic poisoning in rats with the symptoms of displacement of a number of indices of lipid, protein, carbohydrate, nitrogen and pigment metabolism and homeostasis. The animals' appearance and behavior changed, and 31% body mass loss occurred, and the lethality reached 21%. Anemia was registered in all animals' clinical blood tests. Hemolysis, aggregation of erythrocytes and appearance of pathological forms of red cells were confirmed by photo-optical analysis of blood smears. Redistribution in the erythrocyte pool was noticeable. The number of discocytes was reduced, and the total amount of pathologically changed cells increased by 24%. General and irreversible transformation indices increased by 37% and sevenfold, respectively. On the contrary, reversible transformation index was reduced by 11%. These data confirm that the structural integrity of cellular membranes was damaged (Fig. 22.1a).

The pathological state was verified by a number of metabolic changes: the level of "middle molecules" (MM) increased by 1.5 times, total bilirubin fraction increased by 75%, to a great extent owing to the increase of direct fraction, and the activity of the main cytolytic enzymes in blood serum and liver tissue also increased (Table 22.1). The induction of this enzymatic activity can be a consequence of both hepatocyte cell damage and an increase of enzyme production by liver tissue. During a reversible inflammatory process characterized by increased membrane permeability, cytosol enzymes such as alanine-aminotransferase (ALAT) were initially released. But under necrotic conditions the enzymatic activity of mitochondria, that is aspartate-aminotransferase (ASAT) activity, increased. The dynamics of enzymatic activity serves as circumstantial evidence of breaching of hepatocyte membrane integrity and indicates exhaustion of liver functional abilities.

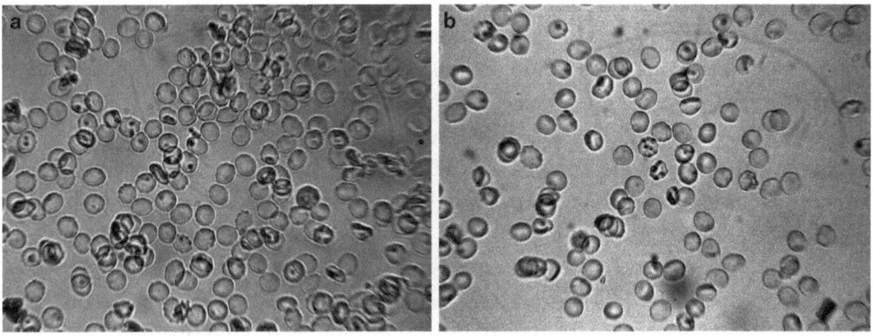

Fig. 22.1 Erythrocytes of rats with sub-chronic poisoning by heavy metal salts, animal group 2 (**a**), and after treatment, animal group 3 (**b**). Light microscopy magnification × 40

Table 22.1 Changes in biochemical parameters of blood, liver and cytolytic enzyme activity caused by heavy metal poisoning and after combined therapy course

Index	Group 1 - control (no HM)	Group 2 - combination of metals $P_{1\text{-}2}$	Group 3 - Therapy hepamal+pectin sorbent $P_{2\text{-}3}$	$P_{1\text{-}3}$
Total protein, g L^{-1}	74.2±2.3	45.3±2.0	67.0±2.9	
		<0.01	<0.01	>0.05
Albumin, g L^{-1}	40.3±2.0	21.3±1.8	30.0±1.5	
		<0.05	<0.05	<0.05
MM, a. u.	0.08±0.004	0.12±0.008	0.1±0.002	
		<0.01	<0.02	<0.02
Total bilirubin, μmol L^{-1}	2.40±0.27	4.5±0.7	1.3±0.5	
		<0.05	<0.02	>0.05
Direct bilirubin, μmol L^{-1}	0.67±0.04	1.9±0.4	0.75±0.2	
		<0.05	<0.05	>0.05
AsAT activity in blood, U L^{-1}	194±10.7	258±25	180.2±4.5	
		<0.05	<0.001	>0.05
ALAT activity in blood, U L^{-1}	63.3±2.8	91.0±6.7	50.3±3.4	
		<0.02	<0.02	<0.05
Liver tissue activity: AsAT, U g^{-1}	200±27	389±35	267±14	
		<0.02	<0.05	<0.05
ALAT, U g^{-1}	300±27	611±30	333±41	
		<0.05	<0.01	>0.05

HM intoxication resulted in marked depression of liver mono-oxygenase enzyme activity, responsible for detoxification of foreign substances. P-450 and B5-cytochrome content decreased by more than 36% in Group 2 animals, which indicates reduction of the compensation abilities of the organism and depression of liver detoxification mechanisms (Table 22.2). These changes took place along with considerable activation of lipid peroxidation (LPO) process and breach of antioxidative protection system. There was 40% increase in malonic dialdehyde (MDA) content. The total antioxidative activity (AOA) of blood serum reduced twofold, catalase and glutathione reductase activity reduced by 31% and 2.1 times respectively, which confirms exhaustion of antioxidative abilities of the organism. Thus, sub-chronic poisoning with heavy metals was accompanied by a marked stress of biotransformation processes in the liver and aggravation of free-radical oxidation processes, leading to depression of liver detoxification mechanisms.

Disorder of protein metabolism could be noticed in 13% decrease of total protein content in blood serum. The observed hypoproteinemia was stipulated by 25% decrease of albumin fraction. The index showing correlation between the level of "middle molecules" and total protein was 65% higher in Group 2 indicating prevalence of protein degradation processes over their synthesis. The revealed disorders indicated the development of liver failure syndrome. Profound disorders were also registered in lipid metabolism. We determined the intensification of lipolysis by increase in the concentration of the main lipid fractions in blood serum. The level

Table 22.2 Changes in metabolic activity caused by poisoning with heavy metal salts and after therapeutic treatment

	Group 1 - control	Group 2 - combination of metals	Group 3 - Therapy hepamal + pectin sorbent	
Index	(no HM)	P_{1-2}	P_{2-3}	P_{1-3}
Cytochrome P450, nmol mg^{-1} of protein	0.80±0.01	0.51±0.03	0.84±0.07	
		<0.001	<0.02	>0.05
Cytochrome B5, nmol mg^{-1} of protein	0.63±0.01	0.40±0.03	0.66±0,05	
		<0.001	<0.02	>0.05
MDA, µmol L^{-1}	2.5±0.02	3.5±0.1	2.22±0.1	
		<0.001	<0.01	>0.05
AOA,%	31.4±0.8	15.7±0.9	30.8±0.5	
		<0.001	<0.001	>0.05
Catalase, a. u.	25.2±3.2	17.3±0.6	24.6±1.2	
		<0.05	<0.02	>0.05
Glutathione reductase, a. u.	14.0±2.4	6.5±2.2	17.3±2.9	
		<0.05	<0.05	>0.05

of free fatty acids increased 1.7 times and concentration of triglycerides – 1.65 times. Cholesterol and ß-lipoprotein content increased by 31% and 1.8 times, respectively.

The morphological analysis of liver showed the existence of necrotic and dystrophic processes, disorder of liver architectonics and micro-circular disorders. Sub-chronic poisoning resulted in discomplexation of hepatocytes, hyperchromia and polychromia, and degeneration (vacuolization) of hepatocyte nuclei. Profile expansion of granular endoplasmatic net (GEN) was significant in some hepatocytes as well as decreased glycogen content, and reduced space of Disse confirming development of liver disease. Profile expansion of GEN was accompanied by a moderate increase in pore number of the liver nuclear membrane. Increase of lysosome content in hepatocyte cytoplasm was noticeable. It was often accompanied by Golgi complex hypertrophy of the smooth endoplasmic net (SEN). In this case glycogen rosettes became smaller and isolated granules of these inclusions could be found. At the same time with increasing SEN profile numbers in the cell cytoplasm, large vacuoles with flake-like content, or homogeneous and transparent in SEM images appeared. Their dimensions were comparable with the nuclear dimensions. These changes were often accompanied by overfilling of sinusoids with homogeneous content, accumulation of erythrocytes and other blood cells. Some hepatocytes contained smaller lipid granules than above described formations with homogeneous or flake-like content. There was a marked expansion of the bile ducts. Electronically dense corpuscles of lysosome type were often found at vascular hepatocyte poles not far from the ducts.

The most typical ultrastructural changes in hepatocytes were sharp swelling of mitochondria with pronounced enlightenment of their matrix and reduction of cristae that are important morphological symptoms of their damage (Fig. 22.2). They were accompanied by appearance of mitochondria of odd shapes, horseshoe shaped

The course of treatment also resulted in considerable positive changes in morphological and functional states of mitochondrial membranes. The passive permeability of their inner membranes for univalent cations decreased down to normal level, and transport rate of Ca^{2+} ions normalized to physiological level of healthy animals. The swelling rate of mitochondria in sucrose medium increased, though remained slightly lower when compared with healthy animals. The results obtained allow us to assume that the rehabilitation of CsA-sensible pore function and membrane potential was achieved.

22.4 Conclusions

The penetration of toxicants from the environment into inner medium of the organism (etiological factor) stimulates the initiation of pathological metabolic reaction cascades. Initially the LPO process, one of the key links in pathogenesis of exogenous poisonings, is activated. LPO activation stimulates membrane destabilization and change of membrane-related enzyme activity, including oxygenase. Our data are in accordance with the results of a number of investigations [8–11]. The acceleration of biotransformation process in liver creates a background for failure of compensatory detoxication mechanisms in liver [12], which leads to formation of a vicious circle. The damaging process of cell membranes has developed in liver; the deviations in metabolic processes of liver have led to a disorder of its functional activity and stipulated the beginning of liver failure. Negative effect of heavy metals at subcellular level was revealed in destabilization of mitochondrial membranes, disorder in passive ion transport through their inner membranes and made the work of the hydrogen "pump" non-efficient leading to the electrochemical gradient collapse. The situation was worsened by the fact that K^+-ion transport into mitochondrial matrix is naturally accompanied by swelling and edema of mitochondria. In turn, it provokes expansion of mitochondrial membrane and, as a consequence, creates a more serious disorder of its barrier functions. As a result, the cytolytic hepatitis with the symptoms of liver failure occurs.

The efficiency of complex treatment in many cases depends on the protection level of the structure and function of cell membranes. For correction of these disorders a complex of measures, including antioxidative and enterosorption preparations, was used. By chemical binding of heavy metals pectin enterosorbent ensures fast elimination of the primary source of intoxication.

The main effect of efferent action of Hepamal preparation is inhibition of LPO processes, increase of antioxidative ability of the organism and stimulation of enzymes of the organism's detoxication system. These activities are stipulated by natural vitamin complexes (A, E, PP, C, ß-carotenes, folic acid) present in Hepamal, which have high antioxidative potential, whereas flavonoids and terpenoids, also present in the preparation, stimulate both detoxication phases.

The proposed treatment scheme permits to solve the main tasks of detoxication: (1) clean the organism from of exo- and endogenous toxicants, and (2) block the cascade of pathological reactions. Positie results of the treatment are manifested by normalization of structure and function of natural detoxication organs, rehabilitation of liver morphology (both hepatocytes and its stromal components), structure and membrane functions of liver mitochondria.

References

1. Katznelson BA, Makeev OG, Degtyareva TD et al (2007) Experimental trial of the complex of means of biological protection of human organism from carcinogenic effect of a combination of exotoxins. Toksikologicheskii Vestnik (Russian "Toxicological Reports") 3:15–20
2. Lugovskoy SP, Legkostup LA (2002) Mechanism of biological action of lead on digestive system. Sovremennye Problemy Toksikologii (Russian "Modern Problems of Toxicology") 2:45–50
3. Skachkov MB, Skachkova MA, Vereshchagin NN, Korneev AG (2002) The mechanism responsible for predisposition to acute respiratory diseases in high man-made loaded areas. Gigiena i Sanitariia (Russian "Hygiene and Sanitary Journal") 5:39–42
4. Fowler BA (1992) Mechanisms of kidney cell injury from metals. Environ Health Perspect 100:56–63
5. Martel J, Marion M, Denizenu F (1990) Effect of cadmium on membrane potential in isolated rat hepatocytes. Toxicology 60:161–172
6. Giri SN, Hollinger MA (1995) Effect of cadmium on lung lysosomal enzymes in vitro. Arch Toxicol 69(5):341–345
7. Tsujimoto Y, Shimizu S (2002) The voltage-dependent anion channel: an essential player in apoptosis. Biochemie 84:187–193
8. Petrov VV, Podosinovikova PP, Kubraskaya LG, Dolgo-Saburov VB (2004) Contribution of the pro-oxidant factor to the mechanism of heavy metals and manganese toxicity. Toksikologicheskii Vestnik (Russian "Toxicological Reports") 1:12–15
9. Coban T, Beduke Y, Iscan M (1996) In vitro effect of cadmium and nickel on glutathione, lipid peroxidation and glutathione-S-transferase in human kidneys. Toxicol in Vitro 10:241–245
10. Gaetke LM, Chow CK (2003) Copper toxicity, oxidative stress and antioxidant nutrients. Toxicology 189:147–163
11. Irshad M, Chaudhuri PS (2002) Oxidant-antioxidant system: role and significance in human body. Indian J Exp Biol 40(11):1233–1239
12. Haonzi D, Lekahal M, Morean A et al (2000) Cytochrome P450-generated reactive metabolites cause mitochondrial permeability transition, cuspate activation and apoptosis in rat hepatocytes. Hepatology 32:303–311

Chapter 23
Clinical Signs of the Development of Acute Hepatocellular Insufficiency and Ways to Prevent it, in Patients with Liver Cirrhosis After Porto-Systemic Shunting

R.A. Ibadov, N.R. Gizatulina, and A.Kh. Babadzanov

Abstract The present study assesses the significance and evaluates the efficacy of hyperbaric oxygenation to treat liver cirrhosis in patients with porto-systemic shunting (PSS). Optimal tactics of a combination of hyperbaric oxygenation with porto-systemic shunting for radical correction of portal hypertension was elaborated. For the first time, morpho-functional changes in liver and peripheral blood under influence of hyperbaric oxygenation (HBO) in patients with liver cirrhosis after porto-systemic shunting have been investigated. The detoxification function of liver presented by the monooxygenase system in patients with liver cirrhosis after using several variants of splenorenal anastomosis was studied. Clinical efficacy of HBO for porto-systemic shunting was determined.

Keywords Hyperbaric oxygenation • Liver cirrhosis • Hepatic monooxygenase system

23.1 Introduction

It is known that the development of complications in postoperative period and their severity mostly depend on patient's adaptation capabilities to cope with the anaesthetic stress. Complications associated with anesthesia can be aggravated by the influence of other concomitant pathology, including the progression of liver tissue hypoxia [1–4].

We investigated homeostasis in patients with liver cirrhosis in the pre- and postoperative period, which has allowed us to reveal clinical pathological mechanisms of complications developed in the postoperative period and to study the effect of hyperbaric oxygenation to prevent these complications.

R.A. Ibadov (✉), N.R. Gizatulina, and A.Kh. Babadzanov
V.Vakhidov Republican Specialised Center of Surgery, Tashkent, Uzbekistan
e-mail: tmsravshan@mail.ru

S. Mikhalovsky and A. Khajibaev (eds.), *Biodefence*, NATO Science for Peace and Security Series A: Chemistry and Biology, DOI 10.1007/978-94-007-0217-2_23,

One of the basic systems participating in biotransformation and detoxification of various elements of endogenous and exogeneic origin is the monooxygenase system, located in smooth endoplasmic reticulum, and which maintain physical-chemical homeostasis of cells in various organs [5, 6]. It is important to monitor the activity of the hepatic monooxygenase system, as it plays the crucial role in biotransformation of xenobiotic toxins introduced from outside [7]. The purpose of this study was to compare the efficiency of the hepatocyte detoxification system in patients with micro- (MiLC) and macronodular liver cirrhosis (MaLC) at the porto-systemic shunting stage and after hyperbaric oxygenation (HBO).

23.2 Experimental

Our studies were based on the results of observation and treatment of 102 liver cirrhosis patients admitted to our Centre. All patients were operated in scheduled order to perform a spleenorenal anastomosis (SRA) at stable remission of the cirrhotic process. There are various types of porto-systemic shunting with removal or preservation of spleen. In 45 patients a total proximal spleenorenal anastomosis (PSRA) was performed, in 57 patients various types of selective, super-selective and partial shunting were performed. To assess the influence of HBO on metabolic processes in liver, biochemical investigations of liver membrane structures and blood parameters describing the liver detoxification function were performed. To prove oppression of liver oxygen-relayed systems in cirrhosis, we studied membrane structures in the liver biopsy material (1.5–2y), which had been taken during surgery, and functional activity in the microsomal fraction of monooxygenase system was determined.

The microsomal fraction of liver was obtained by centrifugation using ultracentrifuge VAC-601 (Germany), isolated in solution containing 0.25 M sucrose, 0.15 M KCl, 0.05 M Tris HCl buffer, at pH 7.4. Cytochrome P-450 in the microsomal fraction was assessed as described in [8] using a double-beam spectrophotometer Specord UV–vis M-40. Detection of cytochrome b_5 in microsomal proteids was carried out spectrophotometrically at 424 nm according to [9], utilising the ability of haemoproteid to be reduced in the presence of NADPH. The concentration of cytochrome was calculated from the difference in absorbance between 409 and 424 nm, using molar extinction coefficient $\varepsilon = 163\ \mathrm{mM^{-1}\,cm^{-1}}$. Results were expressed in nm/mg of the microsomal proteid.

Since 1995, to improve rehabilitation in our Centre, the hyperbaric oxygenation method has been used in the postoperative period in patients with liver cirrhosis. HBO was carried out in a single barocamera BLKS-3-01 in pure oxygen (purity 99.5%) at pressure of 1.6–2.0 kg-force $\mathrm{cm^{-2}}$. The duration of a session was 40–60 min, and 8–10 sessions were required for one course of treatment. All patients had a determined individual indication for HBO.

23.3 Results and Discussion

In patient groups with micro- and macronodular liver cirrhosis a significant monooxygenase system depression (MOS) of hepatocytes was seen when compared with the control group. The concentration of cytochrome P-450 in a terminal site of NADPH-cytochrome P-450 was dependent on the hepatocyte electrotransport system and in patients with MiLC appeared to be reduced to 46.5% ($p<0.05$), and in patients with MaLC to 65.5% ($p<0.05$), concentration of cytochrome b_5 reduced to 33.3% ($p<0.05$) and 59.2% ($p<0.05$) respectively. The activity of NADPH-cytochrome C reductase was considerably suppressed, being reduced in the group of the patients with MiLC to 31.2% ($p<0.05$) and patients with MaLC to 58.7% ($p<0.05$). In patients with liver cirrhosis a substantial depression of MOS activity in hepatocytes was observed. Clinically these changes are characterised by activation of the cirrhotic process with the subsequent development of acute hepatic insufficiency in the early postoperative period. Out of 19 patients who were diagnosed intra-operatively with MiLC, four (21.0%) had a marked activation of the cirrhotic process with two cases of hepatic encephalopathy. Out of 73 patients with MaLC activation of the cirrhotic process was observed in 41 (56.1%) cases with 15 cases of hepatic encephalopathy.

The revealed differences in levels of MOS depression between patient treatment groups with liver cirrhosis highlight the necessity for the selective approaches to employ HBO method. Taking into account the specificity of disturbances in MOS of hepatocytes, this should increase the efficiency of liver cirrhosis treatment. Due to objective reasons it is not always possible to estimate the influence of HBO on monooxygenase system depression of hepatocytes in the postoperative period. Therefore, to evaluate the degree of MOS of a liver we analysed the patients' urine for amidopyrine-4-amino-antipyrine and N-acetyl-4-amino-antipyrine metabolites. The results have shown that before the operation there was a significant decrease of extraction of amidopyrine metabolites with urine in all patients. In patients with MiLC the level of 4-AAP metabolite in daily urine was 3.62 times lower, and in the patients with MaLC 7.36 times lower than in the control group; the level of N-ac-4AAP metabolite in patients with MiLC was reduced by the factor of 3.0, and in the patients with MaLC 5.74 times lower than in the control group. Because the level of 4-AAP is determined by activity of amidopyrine N-demethylase, which catabolises in the course of monooxygenase reaction with cytochrome P-450, we established correlation factors between the concentration of 4-AAP in urine and activity of amidopyrine N-demethylase with the level of cytochrome P-450 in the isolated microsomal fractions in patients with micro- and macronodular liver cirrhosis. The analysis of results has revealed that the correlation factor r between 4-AAP concentration in urine and cytochrome P-450 was $r=+0.753$ ($p<0.02$) in patients with MiLC and $r=+0{,}872$ ($p<0.01$) in patients with MaLC. The correlation factor r between N-AP concentration in urine and cytochrome P-450 was $r=+0.632$ ($p<0.01$) in patients with MiLC and $r=+0.779$ ($p<0.01$) in patients with MaLC. Therefore, the correlation between changes in 4-AAP, N-AP and P-450 allows us to consider them as closely related processes, and determination of 4-AAP in urine as a relevant test to assess the functional status of MOS in liver in pre- and postoperative periods, and after HBO in patients with liver cirrhosis. Comparative assessment of the levels of 4-AAP and N-ac-4AAP between groups of the patients after PSRA and SRA with spleen preservation has shown more favourable reduction of amidopyrine metabolites in urine after selective spleen-renal anastomosis was performed. Following PSRA the level of 4-AAP in patients with MiLC has decreased by 1.98 times, and in patients with MaLC - by 1.59 times in comparison with preoperative level. After SRA with spleen preservation the level of 4-AAP was reduced by 1.60 times in patients with MiLC and by 1.35 times in patients with MaLC in comparison with preoperative values (2.42 ± 0.06 and 1.19 ± 0.01 respectively).

The concentration of N-ac-4AAP in urine changed similarly in patients with liver cirrhosis after the operative procedures. In patients with MiLC, following PSRA procedure N-ac-4AAP level in urine reduced by 1.53 times, and in the patients with MaLC by 1.37 times when compared with preoperative values ($\text{MiLC} = 9.76 \pm 0.05$, $\text{MaLC} = 5.11 \pm 0.05$). The inclusion of HBO in the preoperative period with PSRA and SRA with spleen preservation appeared to improve the efficiency of recovery of functional activity in liver MOS, when compared with the group of patients with liver cirrhosis receiving traditional therapy. In patients who underwent PSRA + HBO and had an established diagnosis of MiLC, the level of isolated 4-AAP metabolites in the urine of adults was reduced by 2.02 times, and N-ac-4AAP by 1.98 times.

In patients with MaLC the amount of isolated 4-AAP and N-ac-4AAP metabolites in the urine of adults was reduced by 4.8 and 4.17 times respectively, in comparison with preoperative values. More essential increase of amidopirine metabolites in urine was marked in patients after SRA with spleen preservation, supplemented with HBO procedure. 4-AAP after SRA with a spleen preservation + HBO in patients with MiLC exceeded preoperative values in a similar group of patients by 2.63 times, and N-ac-4AAP by 2.48 times, in MaLC group by 6.0 and 5.01 times respectively. It is necessary to emphasise that the best outcomes showing increased liver metabolic activity were seen in patients with selective porto-systemic shunt in combination with HBO. These revealed the evident dependence of the liver monooxygenase hydroxylase system status change in patients with liver cirrhosis on the initial degree of intoxication and applied surgical intervention [10]. SRA + HBO treatment produced better results in comparison with the group of the patients who did not receive HBO.

23.4 Conclusions

1. Surgical correction of portal hypertension in combination with HBO in patients with liver cirrhosis produces a clear clinical effect, and positive changes of the structural and functional status of cellular membranes of microsomes and associated enzymatic complexes of cytochrome P-450 of hepatocytes.

2. To evaluate the efficacy of postoperative treatment in combination with HBO, assessment of the levels of 4-AAP and N-ac-4AAP in urine is recommended. This is a reliable method of assessing the liver detoxification function in patients with liver cirrhosis.
3. Based on our studies, it is possible to recommend HBO in postoperative period for patients with liver cirrhosis to increase the efficacy of the liver detoxification function. Depending on the type of the morphological form of liver cirrhosis, this would help to optimise the process of surgical treatment of patients with liver cirrhosis.

References

1. Aliev MM (1991) Pathogenetic aspects of surgical treatment of intrahepatic blockage of portal blood circulation in children. MD Thesis (in Russian). Moscow, p 45
2. Nazyrov FG, Akilov KhA, Ibadov RA (1997) Influence of hyperbaric oxygenation on some parameters of homeostasis at patients with liver cirrhosis after operative treatment. Bull Gen Pract 2:5–7
3. Azizov KhA (1998) Surgical treatment of the patients with a liver cirrhosis in conditions portal hypertension decompensation with ascite syndrome. MD Thesis (in Russian) Tashkent, Uzbekistan, p 45
4. Aruin LI, Anykin T (1988) Influence of surgical treatment of liver cirrhosis with portal hypertension on morphological changes of a liver. In: Problems of surgical treatment of patients with liver cirrhosis with portal hypertension. Medicine Publ, Moscow, pp 18–19
5. Arzakov AI (1975) Microsomal oxygenation. Nauka (Science) Publ, Moscow, p 328
6. Albert A (1973) Selective toxicity: the physico-chemical basis of therapy, 5th edn. Chapman and Hall, London, p 400
7. Musabayev A, Spicina A, Ibadova G, Ibadov R (1996) Clinical pathogenic substantiation of intravascular laser therapy in complex management of patients with acute and chronic hepatitis. Int Islamic Med J Baku Azerbaijan 2:33–36
8. Omura O, Sato R (1964) The carbon monoxide-binding pigment of liver microsomes I. Evidence for its hemoprotein nature. J Biol Chem 230(7):2370–2378
9. Garfinkel D (1958) Studies on pig liver microsomes I. Enzymic and pigment composition of different microsomal fractions. Arch Biochem Biophys 77:493–509
10. Ziegler DI (1988) Flavin-containing monooxygenases: catalytic mechanism and substrate specificities. Drug Metab Rev 19(1):1–32

Chapter 24
Application of Innovative Technologies in Diagnostics and Treatment of Acute Pancreatitis

A.M. Khadjibaev, K.S. Rizaev, and K.H. Asamov

Abstract Laparoscopic methods of diagnostics and treatment of acute pancreatitis were applied to 52 patients, of whom 28 had edematous, non-destructive form of the disease, and others had destructive form of acute pancreatitis. A definite merit of the proposed method is transition from diagnostic laparoscopy to a therapeutic one, which makes it possible to perform the necessary surgical procedures with lesser risk than in the case of laparotomy. Of 38 patients subjected to curative laparoscopy, four had to undergo an open operation due to progression of purulent-septic complications. In order to remove the endogenous toxicosis, various methods of detoxification have been applied in 22 patients. In 14 cases, one or two sessions of plasmapheresis were performed. Biochemical markers used for determining the level of toxemia were "middle molecules". In six cases, against the background of intensive care, oral sorption (enterosorption) was administered 2–3 days after operative intervention. On the basis of the clinical results, indications and contraindications for the use of diagnostic laparoscopy and laparoscopic operation have been formulated.

Keywords Laparoscopy • Acute pancreatitis • Destructive cholecystitis • Plasmapheresis • Oral sorption

24.1 Introduction

Incidence of acute pancreatitis is steadily rising from year to year and according to world statistics, varies from 200 to 800 patients per million of population [1]. Some 15–20% of patients experience destructive, necrotic progression of acute pancreatitis [1, 2]. "Early toxemic" and "late septic" complications of destructive pancreatitis are still

A.M. Khadjibaev (✉), K.S. Rizaev, and K.H. Asamov
Scientific Centre of Emergency Medicine of the Ministry of Public Health of the Republic of Uzbekistan, Tashkent, Uzbekistan
e-mail: bokhodir@mail.ru

S. Mikhalovsky and A. Khajibaev (eds.), *Biodefence*, NATO Science for Peace and Security Series A: Chemistry and Biology, DOI 10.1007/978-94-007-0217-2_24,

the prime cause of death in this category of patients [3–5]. For example, in the Russian Federation, postoperative lethality in cases of acute pancreatitis without differentiation of its clinical form, reached 22.9–23.6% in 1996–1997, whereas the figure for Moscow city was 26.0% in 1998 [6]. This data is in agreement with statistics from other countries, which quote mortality rates from pancreatic necrosis varying between 20 and 45% [1, 7]. Difficulties with diagnostics of acute pancreatitis and contradictory views regarding its pathogenesis and choice of treatment further complicate the problem.

Modern methods of endosurgery may offer improvement in diagnostics and treatment of this category of patients. The aim of our research was to study laparoscopic methods of diagnostics and treatment of acute pancreatitis.

24.2 Experimental

During the period between 2001 and 2009, we carried out diagnostic laparoscopy of 936 patients with acute diseases of the abdominal cavity organs. Out of 52 patients diagnosed with acute pancreatitis, 28 had the edematous form, in 12 cases pancreatic fat necrosis was diagnosed, eight patients had hemorrhagic and four had a mixed form of acute pancreatitis. We established that 14 patients had other complications such as zymogenic peritonitis, infiltrates and retroperitoneal spread of the process. Taking into account the spreading of purulent-infiltrating process along retroperitoneal cellular tissue, conversion was performed in 14 patients, whereas for the remaining 38 patients we arranged for various laparoscopic interventions (laparoscopic sanitation and draining of the abdominal space and peritoneal omental sac (35 cases), laparoscopic draining of choledochitis using Pikovskiy's method and catheterization of the round ligament of liver for introduction of medicine [8–11]).

24.3 Results and Discussion

Among the patients with confirmed acute pancreatitis, 28 had edematous, non-destructive form of the disease, manifesting itself through moderate edema and hyperemia of the hepatoduodenal ligament, with singular steatonecroses. Exudates in the abdominal space were either absent or manifested through low serous transudate. Semiotics of destructive acute pancreatitis is notable in multiple symptoms. Pancreatogenic peritonitis is defined by either serous (14 diseased), or hemorrhagic (eight diseased) exudate. Hemorrhagic exudate gives evidence of zymogenic autolytic destruction of the pancreas and surrounding tissues. Pancreatogenic origin of exudates is confirmed by high (more than 2,048 activity units) level of diastase in the peritoneal fluid. Additive bile in peritoneal exudate that we observed in 13 patients, as well as impregnation of hepatoduodenal and round ligaments with bile, is attributable to zymogenic aggression, which disturbs barrier function of passages and causes permeation of bile by means of diapedesis.

The destructive form of acute pancreatitis is distinctive due to infiltration of hepatoduodenal, round and gastrocolic ligaments and mesenterium of transverse colon, which are identified during visual examination and instrumental palpation. Unlike singular patches in the edematous form of acute pancreatitis, the destructive process is characterized by multiple foci of steatonecroses which are identified in omentum, ligaments, mesenterium, visceral and abdominal peritoneum. A definite merit of the proposed method is transition from diagnostic laparoscopy to therapeutic one, which makes it possible to perform the necessary surgical procedures with lesser risk than in the case of laparotomy. Laparoscopic draining of the abdominal space was conducted for all patients with confirmed pancreatogenic peritonitis. The volume of drained exudate in some of the patients exceeded 1,500 mL per day. The duration of draining was 7 ± 1 days. Evacuation of toxic and aggressive exudate contributed to the reduction of clinical and laboratory manifestations of endotoxemia. Draining of the peritoneal omental sac was conducted either through the foramen of Winslow or gastrocolic ligament.

Laparoscopic catheterization of the round ligament of liver was conducted in 16 patients. Catheterization of the cellular tissue of the round ligament was performed by its centesis with a thin trocar at the point of projection of the ligament on the anterior abdominal wall and guiding of the catheter with 1–2 mm diameter to the depth of 5–7 cm. With subsequent introduction into the cellular tissue of the round ligament in a single step or by drops of 0.25% solution of novocaine, broad-spectrum action antibiotics, spasmolytic, antihistamine and anti-enzymatic preparations and cytostatic drugs in quantities determined by the severity of the disease. The duration of catheterization was 6 ± 1 days.

In overcoming zymogenic aggression, we attribute a significant role to the decompression of bile passages, which has been carried out in 12 patients by means of laparoscopic suspension (five patients) or endermic transhepatic cholecystostomy (seven), and in six patients by choledoch draining using the Pikovskiy's method.

External draining of the gall bladder was conducted using two methods: (1) direct draining of gall bladder through its bottom and (2) applying suspended cholecystostome. Direct draining was performed directly through the wall of the gall bladder using a drainage tube with 3–5 mm diameter so that it formed 2–3 spirals in the cavity of gall bladder, which prevented it from falling out. When using the second method, draining was conducted through the liver pulp and posterior wall of the gall bladder. The duration of drainage of biliary tracts was 16 ± 1 days.

Of 38 patients subjected to curative laparoscopy, four had to undergo an open operation due to progression of purulent-septic complications. The scope of the operation included extensive laparotomy, cholecystectomy with choledoch draining operation (in the event of bile hypertension), abdominisation of gastric cavity, lancing of abscesses, initial necrosequestrectomy of gastric cavity and extraperitoneal cellular tissue, draining of peritoneal omental sac and abdominal space, formation of omentobursostoma for subsequent programmed laparotomies. In our opinion, the reason for repeated operative interventions was that we underestimated the volume of pancreas injury by necrotic process in the event of laparoscopic revision, and two patients died.

In order to remove the endogenous toxicosis, we have applied various methods of detoxification in 22 patients. In 14 cases, one or two sessions of plasmapheresis were performed. Biochemical markers used for determining the level of toxemia were "middle molecules". In six cases, against the background of intensive care, oral sorption (enterosorption) was administered 2–3 days after operative intervention.

On the basis of the clinical results, indications for diagnostic laparoscopy are as follows:

- peritoneal syndrome, including ultrasonic detection of free liquids in the abdominal space;
- when there is a need to differentiate the diagnosis from other diseases of abdominal space organs.

Contraindications for the use of laparoscopy are:

- unstable circulatory dynamics (i.e. endotoxic shock);
- after multiple operations of abdominal space (pronounced cicatricial process of anterior abdominal wall and huge ventral hernias).

The objectives of a laparoscopic operation can be either diagnostic or curative.

1. Diagnostic objectives:

   (a) confirmation of the diagnosis of acute pancreatitis and respectively, exclusion of other diseases of the abdominal space, first of all acute surgical pathology, such as mesenteric ischemia. The symptoms of acute pancreatitis are:

   - edema of the root of mesenterium of the transverse colon;
   - transudate with high amylase activity, 2–3 times exceeding the activity of hemodiastase;
   - availability of steatonecroses;

   (b) indirect symptoms of pancreatic necrosis:

   - hemorrhagic nature of zymogenic transudate (pink, crimson, cherry-colored, brown);
   - generalized locus of steatonecroses;
   - extensive hemorrhagic suffusion of retroperitoneal cellular tissue, extending beyond the pancreas zone;

2. Curative objectives:

   - removal of peritoneal exudate and drainage of abdominal space;
   - cholecystostomy is recommended in case of progressive biliary hypertension with hyperbilirubinemia exceeding 100 μML^{-1} and not earlier than 24 h from the beginning of intensive care;
   - in the event of combined acute pancreatitis and destructive cholecystitis, in addition to the aforementioned activities, cholecystectomy with choledoch draining is recommended.

24.4 Conclusions

Establishing the correct diagnosis within the shortest time possible, timely arrangement for curative procedures during laparoscopy and operations with minimal trauma to tissues of patients with acute surgical diseases of abdominal space organs, assist quick rehabilitation of patients and lead to a 2–3-fold reduction in hospital bed time. Laparoscopic intervention in patients with acute pancreatitis is an efficient diagnostic tool as well as a surgical procedure. Laparotomy is recommended in the treatment of patients with complications of acute destructive pancreatitis with purulent peritonitis, destructive cholecystitis and purulent parapancreatitis.

References

1. Savelyev VS, Kubishkin VA (1993) Pancreatic necrosis: State of the problem and prospectives. Khirurgiia 6:22–29
2. Savelyev VS, Filimonov MI, Gelfand BR, Burnevich SZ, Sobolev PP (1996) Assessment of efficiency of contemporary methods of treatment of destructive pancreatitis. Annals of Surgical Hepatology 1:58–61
3. Kubishkin VA (1996) Draining operations in the event of acute pancreatitis. Khirurgiia 1:29–32
4. Ashrafov AA, Aliev SA (1995) Diagnostics and treatment of acute pancreatitis (in Russian). In: Materials of the first Moscow congress of surgeons. Moscow, pp 188–189
5. Materials of the ninth all-Russian congress of surgeons (2000). Volgograd, Russia, pp 330
6. Atanov YuP (1998) Laparoscopic semiotics of necrotic pancreatitis. Bulletin of Surgery 6:33–37
7. Briskin BS, Rybakov GS, Demidov AD, Suplotova AA (1998) Place and role of video-laparoscopy in treatment of patients with acute pancreatitis. Endoscopic Surgery 1:8–9
8. Lashchevker VM, Mishchenko NV (1998) Indications for conducting urgent operations concerned with pancreatolysis and its optimal dimensions. In: Materials of the second congress of aurgeons of the Ukraine: collection of scientific papers. Donetsk, Ukraine. Clinical Surgery pp 122–123
9. Sakhautdinov VG, Galimov OV, Prazdnikov EN (1999) Laparoscopic interventions in the event of acute destructive pancreatitis. Endoscopic Surgery 1:6–7
10. Strizheletzkiy VV, Borisov AE, Rutenberg GM, Mikhailov AP, Rumyantzev IP, Akimov VP, Zhemchuzhnaya TYu (1998) Laparoscopic techniques in emergency surgery (opportunities and results)... In: Materials of the First All-Russian Congress on Endoscopic Surgery. Endoscopic Surgery 1:51
11. Gurevich AP, Markevich YuV, Ershov DV, Gribov SI, Yurchenko SA (1998) Place of laparoscopy in emergency surgery. In: Materials of the First All-Russian Congress on Endoscopic Surgery. Endoscopic Surgery 1:16

Chapter 25
A Novel Skin Substitute Biomaterial to Treat Full-Thickness Wounds in a Burns Emergency Care

R.V. Shevchenko, P.D. Sibbons, J.R. Sharpe, and S.E. James

Abstract A novel porcine collagen-based paste dermal substitute to treat full-thickness wounds has been investigated. A thin split-thickness skin graft or autologous cultured keratinocytes have been combined with dermal replacement biomaterial and applied to full-thickness wounds in a porcine wound chamber preclinical experimental model. The data obtained suggest that: (1) dermal substitute biomaterials may improve wound re-epithelialisation when combined with cultured autologous keratinocytes and (2) porcine collagen paste is able to support split-thickness skin graft survival as well as autologous cultured keratinocyte proliferation. These results demonstrate that the novel porcine collagen paste has a potential as a dermal substitute to treat acute full-thickness wounds and an application for the burns emergency care treatment.

Keywords Permacol • Integra • Skin substitute • Dermal substitute • Cultured keratinocytes • Collagen • Animal model

R.V. Shevchenko (✉) and S.E. James
School of Pharmacy and Biomolecular Sciences, University of Brighton, Brighton, BN2 4GJ, United Kingdom
e-mail: R.V.Shevchenko@brighton.ac.uk

J.R. Sharpe
Blond McIndoe Research Foundation, Queen Victoria Hospital, East Grinstead, RH19 3DZ, Sussex, United Kingdom

P.D. Sibbons
Northwick Park Institute for Medical Research, Harrow, HA1 3UJ, Middlesex, United Kingdom

S. Mikhalovsky and A. Khajibaev (eds.), *Biodefence*, NATO Science for Peace and Security Series A: Chemistry and Biology, DOI 10.1007/978-94-007-0217-2_25,

25.1 Introduction

Military warfare actions or peace time disasters such as fires, mining accidents or industrial and domestic gas explosions may often result in significant thermal skin damage. This is routinely treated using autologous skin grafting techniques; however in the case of major skin loss these approaches could be inapplicable due to limited availability of skin sources. If dermis is restored with the help of artificial biomaterials [1], extra-thin split-thickness skin grafts (SSG) could be harvested instead of full-thickness SSGs to epithelialise the wounded sites. An alternative approach which allows for the immediate definitive wound closure by epithelialisation is the use of cultured keratinocytes. These are most commonly applied as confluent sheets or cell suspensions. Both approaches have been recently reviewed [2, 3]. Although techniques of cultured cell application may be a life-saving treatment for some patients, the resulting epithelial cover is very thin, fragile and lacks some essential skin properties such as elasticity and strength. This is thought to be due to the lack of dermis [4–7], which is destroyed in full-thickness burns and cannot be regenerated; thus collagenous scar tissue is formed. Various skin substitutes such as epidermal, dermal and composite biomaterials have been described and compared in a number of reviews [8–14].

Previously we investigated the use of an in-house prepared collagen paste, a modification of Permacol® Injectable, as a dermal substitute [15]. The ability of the porcine collagen paste to integrate successfully into full-thickness experimental wounds was shown. These results suggested that paste could be used as a successful alternative to existing dermal substitute biomaterials; however, additional studies where material would be combined with epidermal sources were required. The current study has sought to answer two important questions: would an autologous split-thickness skin graft survive being placed over collagen paste contributing to permanent wound closure and would cultured autologous keratinocytes survive and proliferate when combined *in vivo* with collagen paste in a porcine full-thickness wound model.

25.2 Materials and Methods

Porcine collagen paste was prepared as described previously [15] by cryomilling porcine acellular crosslinked collagen sheet Permacol™. The biomaterial was implanted into acute full-thickness experimental wounds to provide a dermal support for epithelial treatment by either extra-thin split-thickness skin grafts or cultured autologous subconfluent sprayed keratinocytes (Fig. 25.1). Six female Large White pigs were used to recreate full-thickness wound chamber experimental model [16]. Wound biopsies were collected on days 0, 3, 6, 14 and 21. Tissue samples were processed for histological and immunohistochemical analysis. Levels of the graft "take", epithelialisation, host cellular infiltration, inflammation, neovascularisation, formation of granulation tissue and basement membrane, and collagen deposition were assessed either qualitatively or quantitatively using image analysis

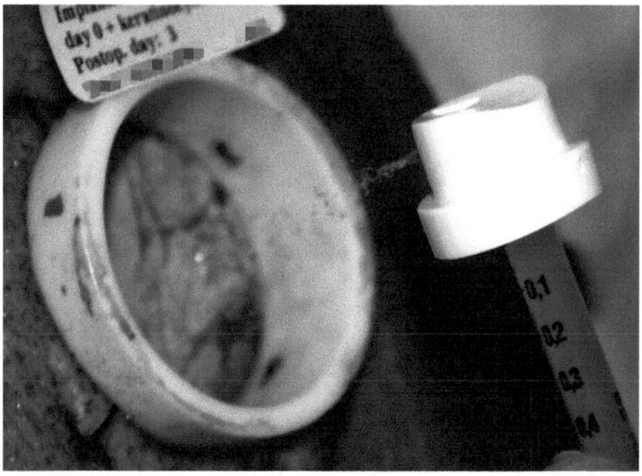

Fig. 25.1 Spraying cultured autologous keratinocytes over Permacol paste dermal substitute biomaterial to achieve epithelialisation of the full-thickness wound

software. The data obtained were analysed statistically using one-way analysis of variance (ANOVA) or Student's *t*-test as appropriate. The differences between test groups were considered to be statistically significant at $p<0.05$.

25.3 Results and Discussion

The biomaterials tested exhibited successful integration, confirming results of previous studies, and the partial wound epithelialisation was achieved by day 21 where either split-thickness skin graft or cultured keratinocytes were applied over dermal substitute biomaterial (Figs. 25.2 and 25.3).

25.3.1 Epithelialisation by a Split-Thickness Skin Graft Applied Directly to Full-Thickness Wounds

Split-thickness skin grafts applied directly to the wound bed survived and integrated into the wound when applied as early as day 0. Skin grafts applied on day 0 exhibited a steady reduction of traceable epithelial areas from 88% on day 6 to 64% by day 21 post grafting. However, grafts applied on day 6 sustained greater and quicker contraction. Clinical observations on day 10 revealed similar areas of epithelialisation for grafts applied on days 0 and 6 (83.7%, SD = 13.6 and 83.0%, SD = 10.7), but drastic reduction in "day 6" graft area was seen on days 14 (51.7%, SD = 27.3) and 17 (42.9%, SD = 4.8), which stabilised by day 21 at 42.7%, SD = 6.0. Epithelial area of the skin graft applied on day 0 made up 64.3% (SD = 19.1) of the wound area by day 21.

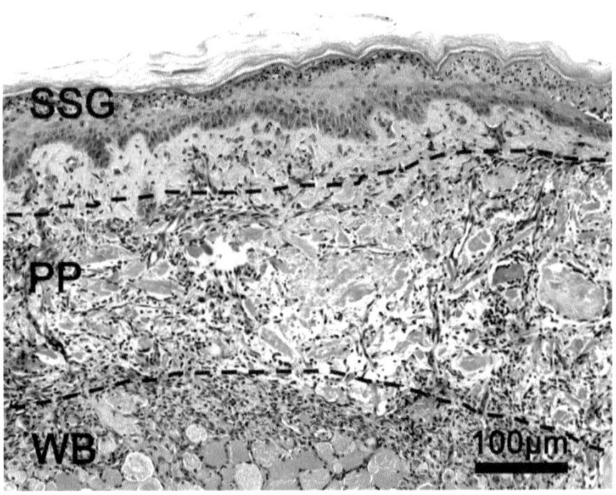

Fig. 25.2 Survival of a split-thickness skin graft applied over Permacol™ paste. SSG day 0, assessed 6 days post grafting, haematoxylin and eosin, x100. Epithelium of a split-thickness skin graft (SSG) was viable and well-structured. Dermal component of the graft was intimately attached to the well-cellularised Permacol™ paste (*PP*) with minimal signs of the inflammatory reaction. Dermal substitute biomaterial integrated into the full-thickness wound via granulation tissue in growth present at the paste and wound bed (*WB*) interface

25.3.2 Epithelialisation by a Split-Thickness Skin Graft Combined with Permacol™ Collagen Paste

Split-thickness skin grafts applied over collagen paste dermal substitute biomaterial on days 0, 3, and 6 showed consistent rates of integration and ability to survive (Fig. 25.2). By day 14 post implantation of collagen paste the wounds grafted with SSG on days 0 and 3 had epithelial cover 48.7–49.3% (SD = 15.9–33) of wound area, representing area of skin graft "take". The wounds grafted on day 6 after Permacol™ paste implantation had a reduction in epithelial cover down to only 16.2% (SD = 5.8) of wound area.

Extra-thin skin grafts applied over collagen paste on days 0 and 3 allowed epithelialisation of up to 40–49% of the wound, which was considerably lower when compared with grafts applied directly over the wound bed (70–90%). However the possibility to restore simultaneously both epidermal and dermal skin layers is very attractive from the clinical point of view, as the application of collagen paste combined with SSG does not require a delay dictated by spontaneous separation of the pseudoepidermal layer as is the case with skin substitute Integra®. A single-stage operating procedure obviates the need for more traumatic multiple operations. Harvesting thinner SSG reduces scarring of the donor site, leads to faster healing and is therefore suitable for early serial SSG re-harvesting [17]. An ability to use thinner skin grafts may also contribute to reduction of complications associated with donor sites. Positive outcomes may include lower rates of lethality due to the earlier definitive wound closure, minimisation of

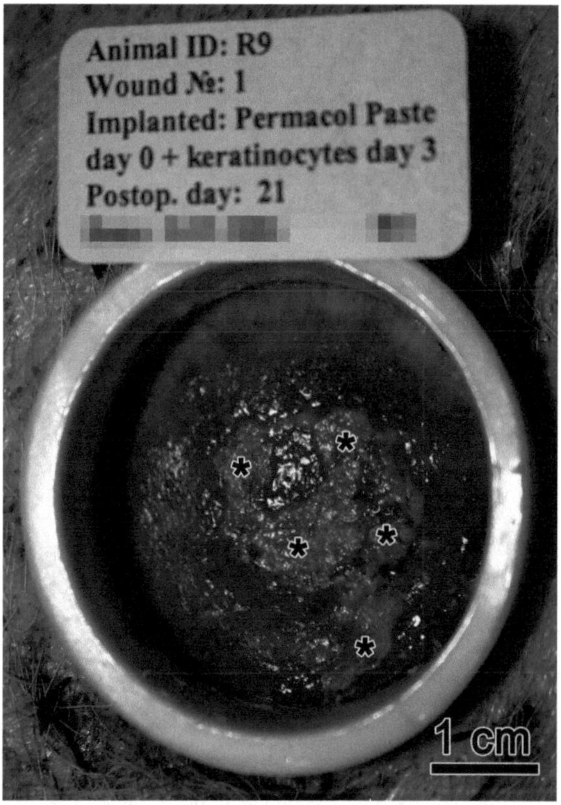

Fig. 25.3 Epithelium derived from cultured autologous keratinocytes sprayed over Permacol™ paste, 21 days postgrafting. Epithelial layer appeared as a thin opaque whitish non-reflective patch (*) on the darker background of the granulating wound

scarring, reduced levels of wound contamination with microorganisms, reduced pharmacological load on the patient, and lower cost of treatment associated with a shorter stay in a hospital [17, 18].

25.3.3 Epithelialisation by Sprayed Cultured Autologous Keratinocytes Applied Directly to Full-Thickness Wounds

Wounds grafted with sprayed cultured autologous keratinocytes did not show significant levels of epithelial cover. As measured by image analysis software, the area of epithelialisation derived from sprayed keratinocytes did not exceed 2% (SD = 0.2–2.2) of the wound size at any time point (Fig. 25.4). Histological sections on day 21 post grafting revealed small patchy areas of keratinocytes located at the surface of the granulation tissue, the epithelial layer appeared to be hyper-proliferative, lacking cornified layer and rete ridges. The keratinocyte layer bonding to underlying granulation tissue seemed to be poor as evidenced by intervening cavities filled with exudate and erythrocytes. Epithelial origin of cells was confirmed with positive immunofluorescent anti-Cytokeratin-14 staining specific for keratinocytes.

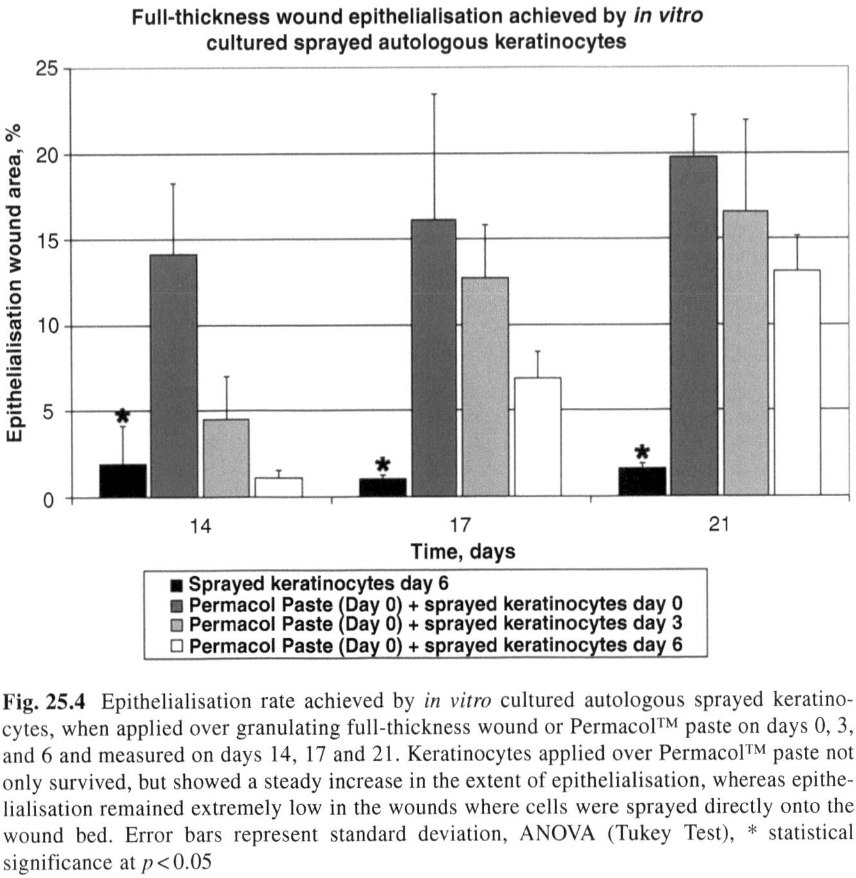

Fig. 25.4 Epithelialisation rate achieved by *in vitro* cultured autologous sprayed keratinocytes, when applied over granulating full-thickness wound or Permacol™ paste on days 0, 3, and 6 and measured on days 14, 17 and 21. Keratinocytes applied over Permacol™ paste not only survived, but showed a steady increase in the extent of epithelialisation, whereas epithelialisation remained extremely low in the wounds where cells were sprayed directly onto the wound bed. Error bars represent standard deviation, ANOVA (Tukey Test), * statistical significance at $p<0.05$

Surprisingly, keratinocytes dispersed over full-thickness wounds without dermal substitute biomaterial support did not initiate wound epithelialisation. This is in line with the work of Orgill and co-authors [19] who reported only a 4% take of cultured epithelial cells grafted over granulating wounds. This may be attributed to rapid formation of granulation tissue and inability of dispersed cultured keratinocytes to form a confluent epithelial layer under constant mechanical disturbance from the underlying tissue. However, keratinocyte take rates were significantly higher when they were grafted over dermal substitute biomaterials [19, 20].

25.3.4 Epithelialisation by Sprayed Cultured Autologous Keratinocytes Combined with Permacol™ Collagen Paste

Our experiments indicate that cultured subconfluent autologous keratinocytes, when applied via aerosol in dermal substitute-grafted full-thickness wounds, have the ability to survive and proliferate *in vivo* thus contributing to definitive wound epithelialisation. Cultured autologous sprayed keratinocytes showed the progression of epithelialisation over the entire study period (Fig. 25.4).

Keratinocytes, when applied over collagen paste on days 0, 3 and 6, not only survived but showed a steady increase in the extent of epithelialised area over the 21-day period as measured by image analysis software. Keratinocytes applied over collagen paste on day 0, resulted in epithelial area of 14.1% (SD=4.1) at day 14, 16.1% (SD=7.3) on day 17 and 19.8% (SD=2.4) at day 21. This was significantly higher when compared with epithelialisation levels of wounds grafted directly with cultured keratinocytes (1.9%, 1.0%, and 1.7% respectively). Keratinocytes applied over collagen paste on day 6 showed definitive closure of the wounds with epithelial areas of 1.1% (SD=0.4) on day 14; 6.8% (SD=1.6) on day 17; and 13.1% (SD=2.1) on day 21. Progression of epithelialisation was noticeable and comparable with that seen in wounds treated with collagen paste and cultured keratinocytes on days 0 and 3. Clinical observations of the collagen paste grafted with sprayed cultured keratinocytes on day 0 and assessed on day 3 did not find any epithelial layer formation whereas histological assessment of tissue stained with anti-Cytokeratin-14 revealed clearly visible clusters of keratinocytes which started to spread over the collagen paste. Histological analysis also revealed complete penetration of the entire thickness of the collagen paste with host cells which appeared to be of mesenchymal origin, e.g. dermal fibroblasts, as they were positively stained with antibody to vimentin. Wounds grafted with cultured keratinocytes over collagen paste on days 0, 3 and 6 did not exhibit noticeable differences in epithelial cover when results were normalised for the grafting time lag. Histological quality of the formed epithelium was also comparable: by day 21 wounds showed formation of well-structured epithelium with minor hyperproliferation and mild rete ridges. Epithelial origin of cells was confirmed by anti-Cytokeratin-14 immunostaining; immunofluorescent staining for collagen VII revealed basement membrane formation between epithelial layer and neodermis.

Although low in area, reconstituted epidermis in our work demonstrated typical epithelial structure which is important for the protective function of skin [21]. Rete ridges in re-epithelialised wounds were mild, however a defined basement membrane was clearly seen on day 21 in wounds grafted with collagen paste and cultured keratinocytes on days 0, 3 and 6. This was not the case in the wounds where keratinocytes were grafted directly to the wound bed and a dermal-epidermal junction area was not clearly defined. This observation suggests that dermal substitute collagen paste may positively contribute to the longevity and quality of epithelial attachment of the epidermis derived from cultured subconfluent autologous keratinocytes, since the basement membrane plays a major role in keratinocyte attachment to the underlying layers of the skin [22].

Take rates of up to 47% have been reported by other researchers if cells were grafted over dermal substitute biomaterial [19]. Other studies where sprayed keratinocytes were combined with alternative dermal substitute Integra®, in a similar porcine chamber experimental model, revealed epithelialisation of 20–25%, 21 days post grafting [20], which is in agreement with results of our experiments. It is reasonable to construe that the low percentage of epithelialisation achieved in the current experiments, when compared with traditional SSG grafting techniques, might preclude this method from clinical application. However, in cases of deep extensive burns with insufficient donor sites there may be no alternative approach to reduce morbidity and mortality but to use cultured skin substitutes or *in vitro* expanded keratinocytes. Clinical studies with cultured skin substitutes have shown a potential to close 20.5% of total body surface area (TBSA) deep burns when compared with 52% TBSA closure with SSG 28 days post grafting [23]. This is an excellent achievement since the ratio of closed to donor areas was 66:1 for cultured skin substitute and 4:1 for each SSG harvest; therefore the use of cultured cells reduced requirements for extensive skin harvesting and resulted in earlier wound closure.

25.4 Conclusions

In an aftermath of large scale natural or man-made disasters there is likely to be lack of donor sites for SSG harvest to treat extensive burns. Use of isolated keratinocytes which can be actively propagated *in vitro* [24] and applied *in vivo* along with dermal substitutes may potentially solve the problem of epithelial deficiency and scarring complications, thus reducing the rates of morbidity and mortality in burns critical care.

Results of our experiments suggest that: (1) dermal substitute biomaterials may contribute to the improved wound re-epithelialisation when combined with cultured autologous keratinocytes and (2) porcine collagen paste is able to support split-thickness skin graft survival as well as autologous cultured keratinocyte proliferation.

This makes the novel collagen paste a suitable alternative to current dermal substitutes to treat acute full-thickness wounds with a potential to be widely used in a burns emergency care.

Acknowledgments We would like to thank the Blond McIndoe Research Foundation and the Mark Hanna Fellowship for funding this research; staff at the Blond McIndoe Research Foundation, Northwick Park Institute for Medical Research and the University of Brighton for their support; Ms. C. Gray at NPIMR for technical operative assistance, and Dr P. Sibbons for providing the Permacol® Injectable material used in this study.

References

1. MacNeil S (2007) Progress and opportunities for tissue-engineered skin. Nature 445(7130):874–880
2. Wood FM, Kolybaba ML, Allen P (2006) The use of cultured epithelial autograft in the treatment of major burn injuries: a critical review of the literature. Burns 32(4):395–401
3. Atiyeh BS, Costagliola M (2007) Cultured epithelial autograft (CEA) in burn treatment: three decades later. Burns 33(4):405–413

4. Chakrabarty KH, Dawson RA, Harris P, Layton C, Babu M, Gould L, Phillips J, Leigh I, Green C, Freedlander E, Mac NS (1999) Development of autologous human dermal-epidermal composites based on sterilized human allodermis for clinical use. Br J Dermatol 141(5):811–823
5. Boyce ST, Kagan RJ, Yakuboff KP, Meyer NA, Rieman MT, Greenhalgh DG, Warden GD (2002) Cultured skin substitutes reduce donor skin harvesting for closure of excised, full-thickness burns. Ann Surg 235(2):269–279
6. Bannasch H, Momeni A, Knam F, Stark GB, Fohn M (2005) Tissue engineering of skin substitutes. Panminerva Med 47(1):53–60
7. Wood FM, Kolybaba ML, Allen P (2006) The use of cultured epithelial autograft in the treatment of major burn wounds: eleven years of clinical experience. Burns 32(5):538–544
8. Burke JF, Yannas IV, Quinby WC Jr, Bondoc CC, Jung WK (1981) Successful use of a physiologically acceptable artificial skin in the treatment of extensive burn injury. Ann Surg 194(4):413–428
9. Hansen SL, Voigt DW, Wiebelhaus P, Paul CN (2001) Using skin replacement products to treat burns and wounds. Adv Skin Wound Care 14(1):37–44
10. Jones I, Currie L, Martin R (2002) A guide to biological skin substitutes. Br J Plast Surg 55(3):185–193
11. Supp DM, Boyce ST (2005) Engineered skin substitutes: practices and potentials. Clin Dermatol 23(4):403–412
12. Anthony ET, Syed M, Myers S, Moir G, Navsaria H (2006) The development of novel dermal matrices for cutaneous wound repair. Drug Discov Today: Ther Strateg 3(1):81–86
13. Bar-Meir E, Mendes D, Winkler E (2006) Skin substitutes. Isr Med Assoc J 8(3):188–191
14. Ehrenreich M, Ruszczak Z (2006) Update on tissue-engineered biological dressings. Tissue Eng 12(9):2407–2424
15. Shevchenko RV, Sibbons PD, Sharpe JR, James SE (2008) Use of a novel porcine collagen paste as a dermal substitute in full-thickness wounds. Wound Repair Regen 16(2):198–207
16. Kangesu T, Navsaria HA, Manek S, Shurey CB, Jones CR, Fryer PR, Leigh IM, Green CJ (1993) A porcine model using skin graft chambers for studies on cultured keratinocytes. Br J Plast Surg 46(5):393–400
17. Papini R (2004) Management of burn injuries of various depths. BMJ 329(7458):158–160
18. Cubison TC, Pape SA, Parkhouse N (2006) Evidence for the link between healing time and the development of hypertrophic scars (HTS) in paediatric burns due to scald injury. Burns 32(8):992–999
19. Orgill DP, Butler C, Regan JF, Barlow MS, Yannas IV, Compton CC (1998) Vascularized collagen-glycosaminoglycan matrix provides a dermal substrate and improves take of cultured epithelial autografts. Plast Reconstr Surg 102(2):423–429
20. Currie LJ, Martin R, Sharpe JR, James SE (2003) A comparison of keratinocyte cell sprays with and without fibrin glue. Burns 29(7):677–685
21. Micali G, Lacarrubba F, Bongu A, West DP (2001) The skin barrier. In: Frenkel RK, Woodley DT (eds) The biology of the skin. The Parthenon Publishing Group, London, pp 219–232
22. Woodley DT, Chen M (2001) The basement membrane zone. In: Frenkel RK, Woodley DT (eds) The biology of the skin. The Parthenon Publishing Group, London, pp 133–152
23. Boyce ST, Kagan RJ, Greenhalgh DG, Warner P, Yakuboff KP, Palmieri T, Warden GD (2006) Cultured skin substitutes reduce requirements for harvesting of skin autograft for closure of excised, full-thickness burns. J Trauma 60(4):821–829
24. Rheinwald JG, Green H (1975) Serial cultivation of strains of human epidermal keratinocytes: the formation of keratinizing colonies from single cells. Cell 6(3):331–343

gynaecology, ENT (ear, nose and throat) diseases, and dentistry. FarGALS is used as an antiseptic and wound treatment medication. It shows bactericidal properties against a wide range of microorganisms such as Gram positive and Gram negative bacteria, aerobic and anaerobic bacteria, including; *Pseudomonas aeruginosa*, *Helicobacter pylori* and *Candida* type fungi. Our investigations showed that FarGALS can be used as an anti-microbial agent in the treatment of purulent-necrotic processes; it has strong anti-inflammatory properties and a high necrolytic effect, which allows fast cleaning of purulent wounds.

The aim of this work was to investigate the potential use of FarGALS for prophylaxis and treatment of pyrogenic inflammatory lung disease in patients supported by long-term AVL.

26.2 Experimental

The database of our investigation comprises the results of bacteriological tests from trachea, mouth, washing material from bronchi of 52 patients, who underwent various surgical interventions and were on the AVL in the ICU during the period of 2008–2009 (Table 26.1).

These patients were divided into two groups: the 1st, main group comprised 20 patients who received nebuliser therapy with FarGALS (1:4 dilution); and the 2nd, control group of 32 patients who received standard nebuliser therapy [7, 8]. The average age of patients was 39.4 ± 15.4 years.

The microorganisms were identified using various bacterium growth media ("HiMedia", India). The sensitivity of microorganisms to antibiotics, such as cephalosporin, aminoglycoside, tetracycline and fluorochinolone, was evaluated by diffusion in the agar gel.

In total 306 samples of clinical materials were investigated, of which 132 contained various types of microorganisms (Table 26.2).

Table 26.1 Number of patients subjected to different types of intervention

	Group					
	Main		Control		Total	
Intervention type	abs.	%	abs.	%		%
Mitral valve replacement	4	20.0	10	31.3	14	26.9
Coronary artery bypass grafting	6	30.0	6	18.8	12	23.1
Descending aorta prosthesis operation	2	10.0	4	12.5	6	11.5
Myasthenia gravis	2	10.0	4	12.5	6	11.5
Lower lobectomy	2	10.0	4	12.5	6	11.5
Jejunum resection complicated with peritonitis	4	20.0	4	12.5	8	15.4
Total	20	100	32	100	52	100

Table 26.2 Microorganisms identified in clinical samples

	Sample					
	Mouth		Bronchi		Trachea	
Microorganism	abs.	%	abs.	%	abs.	%
Pseudomonas aeruginosa	2	1.5	6	4.5	20	15.2
Klebsiella pneumoniae	7	5.3	2	1.5	29	22.0
Acinetobacter spp.	2	1.5	0	0.0	12	9.1
Staphylococcus aureus	7	5.3	4	3.0	4	3.0
Staphylococcus spp.	4	3.0	2	1.5	0	0.0
rp.p.Candida	22	16.7	2	1.5	7	5.3
Total	44	33.3	16	12.1	72	54.5

26.3 Results and Discussion

Analysis of different types of samples showed the presence of microorganisms in 56 samples taken from the main group: 16 from mouth (28.6%), 6 from bronchi (10.7%) and 34 from trachea (60.7%), whereas in the control group microorganisms were found in 76 samples, of which 28 were taken from mouth (36.8%), 10 from bronchi (13.2%) and 38 from trachea (50.0%).

The most common microorganisms found in the samples were *Klebsiella pneumoniae* – 28.8%, *Candida fungus* – 23.5% and *Pseudomonas aeruginosa* – 21.2% (Fig. 26.1).

The antibioticogram analysis showed that in the long term AVL conditions, the microflora were resistant to the majority of antibiotics used and the application of these drugs were ineffective in about 50% cases, which led to the development of different broncho-pulmonary complications. The identified microorganisms showed mild resistance to amikacin, meropenem and polymyxin and total resistance to cephalosporins with exception of *Staphylococcus spp.* (Table 26.3).

High sensitivity of *Staphylococcus spp.* to different antibiotics can be explained by its relatively low presence in the general population. This microorganism has been found only in 4.5% of population and its resistance did not develop. Other agents with higher presence have high antibiotic resistance. The mean resistance of *Klebsiella pneumoniae* to different antibiotics was 74.8±22.5%; *Pseudomonas aeruginosa* – 68.4±26.7%; *Acinetobacter spp.* – 77.9±21.8%; and *Staphylococcus aureus* – 72.0±20.1%.

The analysis of the anti-microbial activity of FarGALS showed high sensitivity of the tested cultures (Gram+ve, Gram -ve and mycoses) to this drug. Clinical improvement in patients infected with Gram-negative microorganisms and treated with FarGALS was evident in 2–3 days, much earlier than in control group. The occurrence of broncho-pulmonary complications was lower in the main group. In this study, one patient developed AVL associated pneumonia and the second patient had purulent bronchitis, which corresponds to 10% of the group, whereas in control group 25% of patients developed such complications. Overall, the clinical improvement was 5–6 days in the main group versus 8–10 days in control group.

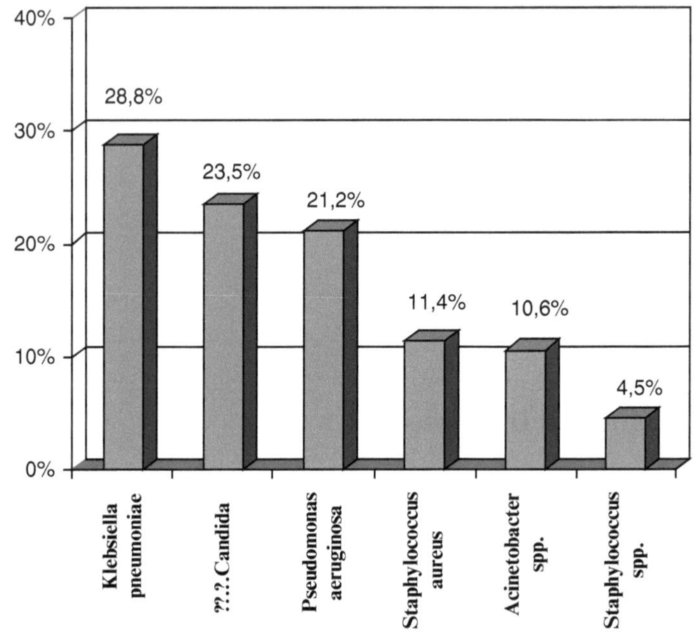

Fig. 26.1 Distribution of microorganisms found in the clinical samples

Table 26.3 Resistance of the extracted microflora to the medication

Antibiotic/ micro-organism	*P. aeruginosa*	*K. pneumoniae*	*Acinetobacter spp.*	*S. aureus*	*Staphylococcus spp.*	*Candida*
Amikacin	29.0%	34.0%	37.0%	54.0%	17.0%	*
Gentamicin	78.0%	81.0%	87.0%	82.0%	32.0%	*
Meropenem	24.0%	49.0%	54.0%	*	*	*
Ofloxacin	59.0%	62.0%	64.0%	32.0%	15.0%	*
Ciprofloxacin	68.0%	76.0%	81.0%	68.7%	33.0%	*
Cefotaxime	95.0%	100.0%	100.0%	92.0%	38.0%	*
Ceftazidime	96.0%	98.0%	100.0%	87.0%	66.6%	*
Ceftriaxone	89.0%	92.0%	94.0%	84.0%	17. 0%	*
Cefoperazone	78.0%	81.0%	84.0%	76.4%	7.0%	*
Polymyxin	6.0%	6.5%	4.0%	*	*	*
Nitroxolin	*	*	*	*	*	22.0%
Terbinafine	*	*	*	*	*	33.0%
Amphotericin	*	*	*	*	*	34.0%
Fluconazole	*	*	*	*	*	43.0%
FarGALS	0.2%	0.4%	0.7%	0.0%	0.0%	0.0%

Note: * Natural resistance

26.4 Conclusions

Gram-positive, gram-negative bacteria and fungi showed high sensitivity to a novel anti-microbial agent FarGALS. Its use in nebuliser therapy of patients with purulent postoperative lung diseases, who stay on artificial ventilation of lungs for a long time, reduced frequency of broncho-pulmonary complications from 25 to 10%. The use of FarGALS led to clinical improvement in 2–3 days, and overall improvement in 5–6 days, which is significantly faster than in the control group, which was treated with standard nebuliser therapy.

This study confirmed high activity of FarGALS for polyresistant microorganisms.

References

1. Skyler JS, Weinstock RS, Pascin P, Yale JF, Barrett E, Gerich JE, Gerstein HC (2005) Use of inhaled insulin in a basal/bolus insulin regimen in type 1 diabetic subjects A 16-month randomized, comparative trial. Diab Care 28(7):1630–1635
2. Frutos-Vivar F, Esteban A (2003) When to wean from a ventilator: an evidence-based strategy. Cleve Clin J Med 70(5):383–398
3. Cook D (2000) Ventilator-associated pneumonia: perspectives on the burden illness. Intensive Care Med 26(S1):31–37
4. MacIntyre NR, Cook DJ, Ely WE, Epstein SK, Fink JB, Heffner JE, Hess D, Hubmayer RD, Scheinhorn DJ (2001) Evidence-based guidelines for weaning and discontinuing ventilatory support. Chest 120(6):375–395
5. Kollef MH (2000) Ventilator-associated pneumonia: the importance of initial empiric antibiotic selection. Infect Med 17:278–283
6. Bajenov LG, Mustamov AN, Ekubjanov FT, Bajenova SS, Shanieva ZA (2008) Antimicrobal activity of the new biotechnological drug - ForGALS and its clinical use. Bull Int Sci Surg Assoc 3(1):23–25
7. Smaldone GC, McKenzie J, Cruz-Rivera M, Hoag JE (2000) Budesonide inhalation suspension is chemically compatible with other nebulizing formulations. Chest 118(4):98S
8. Boe J, Dennis JH, Driscoll BR (2001) European Respiratory Society guidelines on the use of nebulizers. Eur Respir J 18:228–242

Chapter 27
Oxidant and Antioxidant Status of Patients with Chronic Leg Ulcer Before and After Low Intensity Laser Therapy

M.E.E. Batanouny, S. Korraa, and A. Kamali

Abstract Low level (intensity) Laser Therapy (LLLT) has been shown to have biostimulatory effects on wounds however, the precise mechanism remains unclear. Recently antioxidants have been reported to play a significant role in the wound healing process. Twenty two patients suffering from chronic leg ulcers were exposed to three sessions per week of 632.8 nm He–Ne laser irradiation at energy density of 0.5–2 $J\,cm^{-2}$. Malondialdehyde (MDA) was measured in serum, while protein carbonyls (PC), DNA-fragmentation, and activity of glutathione peroxidase (GPX), superoxide dismutase (SOD) and catalase (CAT) enzymes were measured in the tissue biopsies of these patients before and after the 8th session of laser irradiation during the course of treatment of chronic leg ulcer. Results showed that laser irradiation decreased the ulcer size in 63% of the treated patients and 34% exhibited complete recovery. Biochemical investigations revealed an increase in the levels of serum GPX, SOD and CAT, however, serum MDA was decreased. Positive correlations between the rate of ulcer healing and decrease of serum MDA/SOD, MDA/GPX and MDA/CAT ratios respectively were observed. This study shows that low intensity laser therapy is of great benefit in the treatment of chronic leg ulcers and sheds light on the oxidant/ antioxidant status as a possible mechanism of enhancing ulcer healing whilst using this clinical modality.

S. Korraa (✉)
National Institute of Laser Enhanced Sciences, Cairo University, Gama street 1, Giza, Cairo, Egypt
e-mail: soheirskorraa@hotmail.com

M.E.E. Batanouny
Department of General and Vascular Surgery, Cairo University, Giza, Cairo, Egypt
National Institute of Laser Enhanced Sciences, Cairo University, Gama street 1, Giza, Cairo, Egypt

A. Kamali
National Center for Radiation Research and Technology, Ahmad El Zomor Street, Nasr City, Cairo, Egypt

S. Mikhalovsky and A. Khajibaev (eds.), *Biodefence*, NATO Science for Peace and Security Series A: Chemistry and Biology, DOI 10.1007/978-94-007-0217-2_27,

Keywords Antioxidants • Catalase • Chronic leg ulcer • Glutathione peroxidase • Low intensity laser • Helium-neon laser • Lipid peroxidation • Malondialdehyde • Superoxide dismutase

27.1 Introduction

Chronic ulcers are a significant health problem in young and elderly individuals that culminates in disability, decreased productivity, and loss of independence [1, 2]. The economic costs associated with chronic wounds are enormous for the healthcare system as well as for patients [3]. The healing process is slow and often incomplete and patients not responding to conservative therapy become candidates for amputation [4].

The technology of Low Level Laser Therapy (LLLT) was introduced into clinical medicine more than three decades ago. This form of treatment has great appeal due to its novelty, ease in use, relatively cost-efficient and low morbidity profile [5]. LLLT has been shown to improve remarkably the process of wound healing in humans [5–8] and animal models [9–11]. *In vitro* studies demonstrated that LLLT has a stimulating effect on cell mitosis [12] and proliferation and migration of fibroblasts [13], keratinocytes [14, 15] and endothelial cells [16]. LLLT enhances NO secretion [17] and cytokine production [18, 19] and may lead to increased dermal angiogenesis [20].

In spite of the above evidence, there is still a question mark concerning the enhancing effects of low energy laser irradiation on chronic wounds, although several studies showed that LLLT remarkably improves the process of skin wound healing in humans [3–6]. Conversely, some recent studies indicated that LLLT does not enhance the process of wound healing [21, 22], thus raising an issue of LLLT efficiency that needs further investigation.

Most skin lesions heal rapidly and efficiently within a week or two. However, ulcers are among conditions associated with abnormal wound healing due to abnormalities in cell migration and proliferation, inflammation, synthesis and secretion of extracellular-matrix proteins and cytokines, and/or remodeling of the wound matrix have been described [23]. Increased activity of fibrogenic cytokines such as transforming growth factor ß1, insulin-like growth factor 1, and interleukin-1, and exaggerated responses to these cytokines have also been noted [24, 25]. In addition, abnormal epidermal – mesenchymal interactions and mutations in regulatory genes such as p53 have recently been proposed to help explain abnormal healing [26, 27]. Whatever is the case in chronic ulcers, the inflammatory phase does not resolve in chronic wounds, as it persists over a long period of time with subsequent continuous damage and perpetuation of inflammation [28].

Inflamed tissue associated with an oxidative stress as a consequence of a disbalance in the pro-oxidant/antioxidant homeostasis in chronic wounds is thought to drive a deleterious sequence of events that finally results in the non-healing state [29]. Experimental studies showed that wounds of delayed healing type are accompanied by increased levels of markers of oxidative damage and decreased levels of markers of anti-oxidative activity, mainly glutathione peroxidase (GPX), superoxide dismutase (SOD) and catalase (CAT) enzymes, vitamin E and glutathione [30, 31]. It is well established that during a diseased state the generation of reactive oxygen species (ROS) exceeds the capacity of endogenous antioxidant defences. This leads to a disturbance of the oxidant/antioxidant balance in favour of the former [32], whose magnitude depends on the ability of the tissues to detoxify the generated ROS [33] and consequently damaging cellular lipids, proteins and DNA inducing lipid peroxides, protein carbonyls and DNA damage [34]. It has been emphasised that the proteolytic environment of the inflamed wound could be the cause of the impaired wound healing response [35], and the shift in the oxidant/antioxidant balance is the mechanism encountered by LLLT induced healing [36, 37].

The aim of the present study was to evaluate the effect of LLLT on oxidative markers in serum and tissue biopsies of healing ulcers before and after the 8th session of an LLLT course of chronic leg ulcer treatment. Oxidative damage was assessed in terms of lipid peroxidation reflected by serum malondialdehyde (MDA) level, protein oxidation was measured in terms of tissue protein carbonyls (PCb), and DNA damage was measured in terms of DNA fragmentation. Antioxidative activity was estimated by measuring activity of SOD, GPX and CAT enzymes.

27.2 Experimental

27.2.1 Patients

Twenty two chronic leg ulcers patients, not amenable to surgical interface or reconstruction and not responding to conventional treatment, were included in this study. The patients were of the middle class population of mean age 48.5 ± 14.6 years. Their ulcers were unresponsive to conservative treatment for a duration that ranged between 3 to 17 years (mean of 14.67 ± 4.66 years).

27.2.2 Clinical Evaluation

Before commencing the sessions the patients were assessed by physical examination and full medical history including age, sex, occupation, residence, special habits of medical importance with particular emphasis on the history of the underlying disease including: duration of ulcer, mode of onset, ulcer pain, history of deep vein thrombosis or varicose veins, trauma, lump, varicosities, contact dermatitis and symptoms suggestive of ischaemia. Photographic reference of ulcer and ulcer area measurements were carried out at the commencement of treatment and during the follow up laser therapy, which continued for 6 months.

27.2.3 Laser Irradiation

Irradiation was carried out using the Levelaser M 300 (CSO-Med, Mogliano Vento, Italy) at the outpatient Clinic of the National Institute of Laser Enhanced Sciences (NILES) – Cairo University. This apparatus is equipped with an automated computer, which after setting the required power density and the required scanning area, automatically calculates the required time of exposure and the laser beam falls vertically over the required area for the duration of the calculated time. Irradiation was carried out with a 10 mW He-Ne laser (wavelength 632.8 nm) at energy fluence of 0.5–2 $J\,cm^{-2}$ thrice a week and their treatment continued for an average period of 20 weeks.

27.2.4 Biochemical Assessment

Samples of blood and tissue biopsies were taken just before treatment and after the 8th session of laser therapy. Biochemical tests were carried out on 22 male patients, who agreed by an informed consent to provide tissue biopsies and blood samples. The samples were used for measuring tissue and serum markers of oxidative stress (tissue DNA fragmentation [38], tissue PCb [39] and serum lipid peroxidation in terms of MDA concentration [40]) along with tissue antioxidant enzymatic activity of GPX [41], SOD [42] and CAT [43]. The biochemical parameters of the patients' blood were compared to those of the cohort of 20 age and socioeconomic matching healthy controls (mean age 47 ± 12.3 years). The biopsy samples were compared with 15 surgical appendages from hernia surgery or plastic surgery.

27.3 Results

27.3.1 LLLT Effects on Clinical Healing of Chronic Leg Ulcers

After laser therapy there was a significant decrease in the mean size of ulcer (Figs. 27.1–27.3) compared to its level before laser therapy (14.40 ± 1.98 vs 17.34 ± 2.28, $p < 0.01$). The total number of ulcers which showed complete healing was 23 (34%). An incomplete healing was found in 42 cases (63%) and two ulcers deteriorated (3%).

27.3.2 Serum Malondialdehyde

Serum MDA level was significantly higher among patients with chronic leg ulcer compared to normal controls (5.23 ± 1.4 vs 2.2 ± 0.8 $\mu mol\,L^{-1}$, $p < 0.001$). It was significantly decreased after laser therapy (5.23 ± 1.4 vs 3.35 ± 1.4 $\mu mol\,L^{-1}$, $p < 0.01$). The difference between the high and low healing response groups before laser therapy was not significant (6.1 ± 1.6 vs 4.7 ± 1.1 $\mu mol\,L^{-1}$, $p > 0.05$), but after LLLT

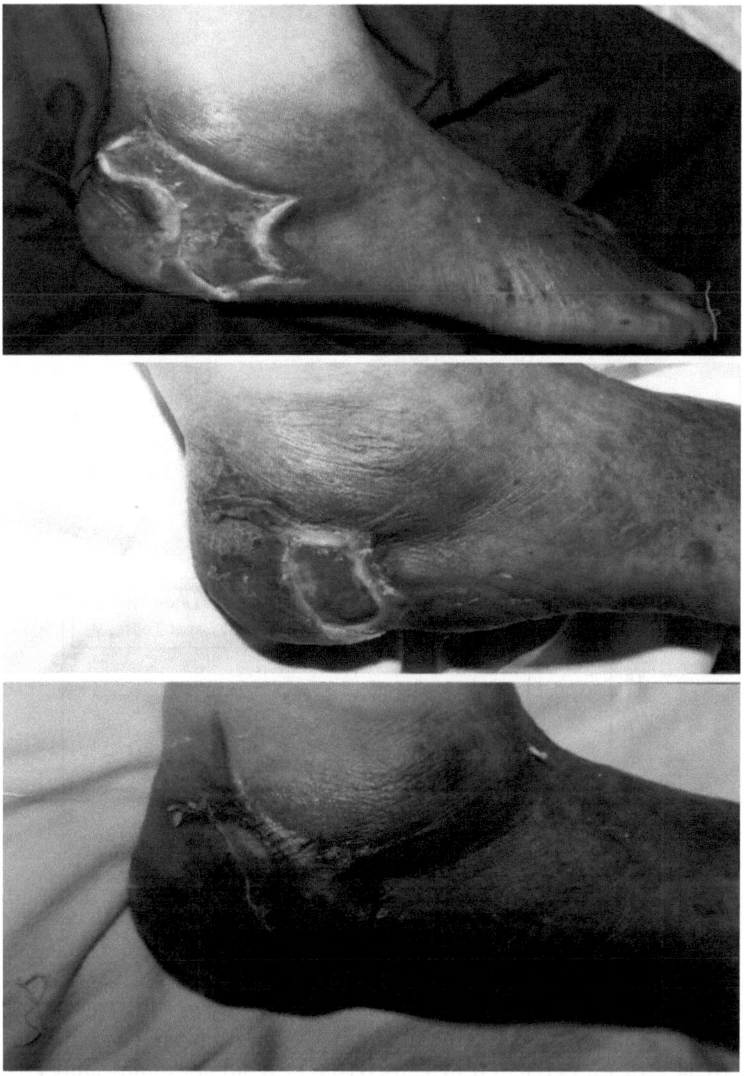

Fig. 27.1 Chronic leg ulcers of a 60 years old male patient before and after laser therapy, three sessions per week at energy fluence of 0.5 $J cm^{-2}$, He–Ne laser. Duration of ulcer was 16 months

it became significantly higher in patients with low healing response (5.2 ± 1.4 vs 2.7 ± 0.49 $\mu mol L^{-1}$, $p<0.0001$) as demonstrated in Fig. 27.4.

27.3.3 Tissue Protein Carbonyls

PCb (Fig. 27.4) (percentage/total protein) was significantly higher among patients with chronic leg ulcer when compared to normal controls ($0.85 \pm 0.14\%$ vs

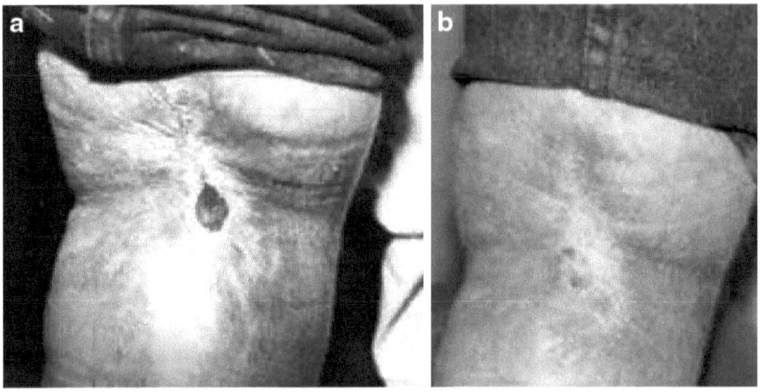

Fig. 27.2 Chronic leg ulcers on the lateral lower half of the leg of a 45 years old male patient before (a) and after laser therapy (b). Duration of ulcer was 2 years and the ulcer size before treatment was 5 cm^2. This patient received three sessions per week of 0.5 $J\,cm^{-2}$ He–Ne laser LLLT and complete healing was achieved in the 12th session

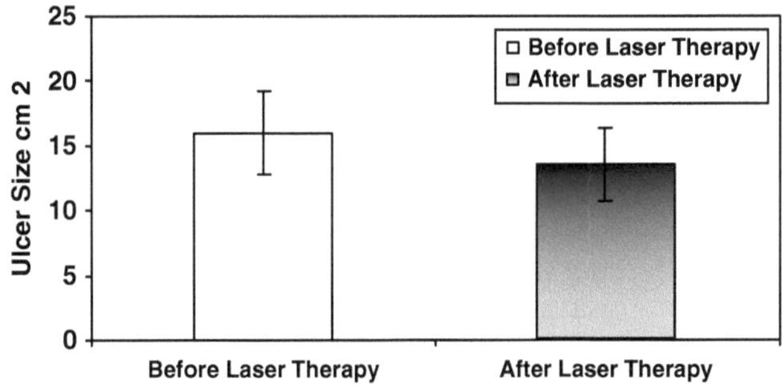

Fig. 27.3 Decrease in mean size of ulcer after laser therapy

0.32 ± 0.03%, $p < 0.001$). It significantly decreased after laser therapy compared to controls (0.54 ± 0.23% vs 0.32 ± 0.03%, $p < 0.001$) and compared to its level before LLLT (0.54 ± 0.23% vs 0.85 ± 0.14%, $p < 0.01$). PCb did not significantly change in the group of patients with low healing response after LLLT (0.95 ± 0.15% vs 0.85 ± 0.06%, $p > 0.05$), and became significantly lower in patients with high healing response (0.38 ± 0.06% vs.0.8 ± 0.01%, $p < 0.0001$).

27.3.4 Tissue DNA Fragmentation

Tissue DNA fragmentation (Fig. 27.4) was significantly higher among patients with chronic leg ulcer when compared to normal controls (2.2 ± 0.3% vs 0.45 ± 0.02%, $p < 0.001$). It significantly decreased after LLLT compared to its level

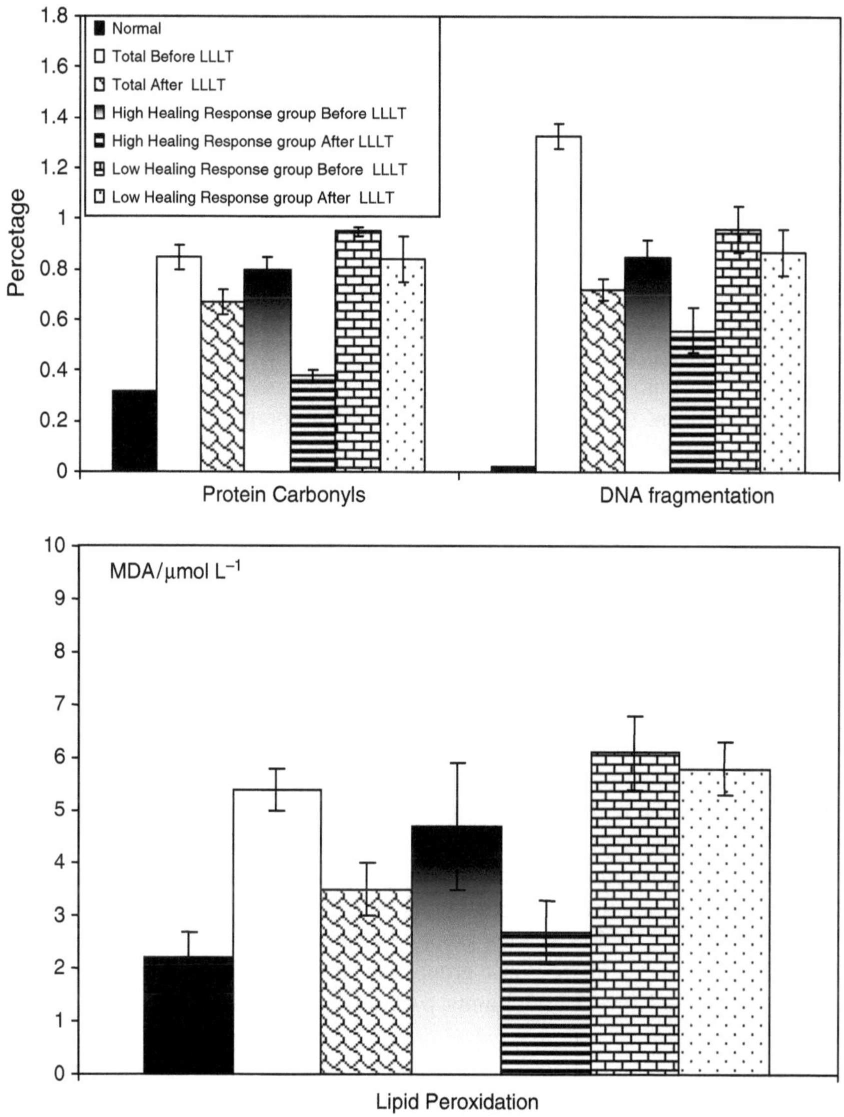

Fig. 27.4 Level of tissue protein carbonyls, DNA fragmentation and serum MDA in normal and chronic leg ulcer patients before and after LLLT: total, in low and high response groups

before LLLT (0.94±0.06% vs 2.2±0.3%, $p<0.01$) and compared to controls (0.94±0.06% vs 0.45±0.02%, $p<0.001$). The difference between the high and low healing response groups before laser therapy was not significant (1.2±0.6% vs 1.7±1.1%, $p>0.05$) before LLLT and after LLLT it became significantly lower in patients with high healing response (0.87±1.4% vs 0.56±0.49%, $p<0.0001$) compared to the low response group.

27.3.5 Tissue Superoxide Dismutase

The level of SOD was significantly lower in sera of patients with chronic leg ulcer before laser therapy compared to normal controls (3.35 ± 1.10 vs 6.7 ± 1.1 units, $p < 0.0001$). After laser therapy SOD levels were increased showing no significant difference in its value when compared to normal controls (6.4 ± 1.0 vs 6.7 ± 1.1 units, $p > 0.05$). Before laser therapy there were no significant differences between both the low healing response group and the high response healing group (5.0 ± 1.0 vs 5.6 ± 1.2 units, $p > 0.05$). After laser therapy, SOD also showed significantly higher levels in sera of patients showing high healing response, when compared to those who showed low healing response (6.9 ± 0.87 vs 5.5 ± 0.5 units, $p < 0.001$). Meanwhile, chronic leg ulcer patients who showed high healing responses exhibited no significant difference in SOD level when compared to normal controls (6.9 ± 0.9 vs 6.6 ± 1.1 units, $p > 0.05$) (Fig. 27.5).

27.3.6 Tissue Catalase

Compared to normal controls the level of CAT was significantly lower in sera of patients before laser therapy (5.0 ± 1.4 vs 8.9 ± 3.2 units, $p < 0.001$). There was a strong significant increase of CAT levels in sera of chronic ulcer patients after laser therapy (10.7 ± 4.6 vs 5.0 ± 1.4 units, $p < 0.001$). It exceeded CAT levels in controls with no significant difference (13.2 ± 3.1 vs 8.9 ± 3.2 units, $p > 0.05$). CAT level after laser therapy in the high response group was significantly higher than that in the control group. This level exceeded significantly the control level in patients exhibiting high healing response (13.2 ± 3.1 vs 8.9 ± 3.2, $p < 0.001$). After laser therapy CAT activity was significantly higher in the sera of the high healing response group when compared to the low healing group (13.2 ± 3.2 vs 4.4 ± 1.0 units, $p < 0.0001$). However, the low healing response group also showed significant increase of CAT after LLLT (4.0 ± 1.0 vs 5.8 ± 1.2 units, $p < 0.001$) (Fig. 27.5).

27.3.7 Tissue Glutathione Peroxidase

Compared to normal controls, the level of GPX was significantly lower in sera of chronic leg ulcer patients before laser therapy (219 ± 39 vs 268 ± 72 units, $p < 0.01$) There was a significantly strong increase in the levels of GPX in sera of chronic ulcer patients after laser therapy (293 ± 64 vs 219 ± 39 units, $p < 0.01$). It even exceeded the GPX level in the normal control group (293 ± 64 vs 268 ± 72 units, $p > 0.05$). Patients exhibiting high healing response had the highest level compared to the control group (318 ± 51 vs 268 ± 72 units, $p < 0.01$) or the low healing group after LLLT (318 ± 51 vs 247 ± 62 units, $p < 0.01$). Nevertheless GPX level became

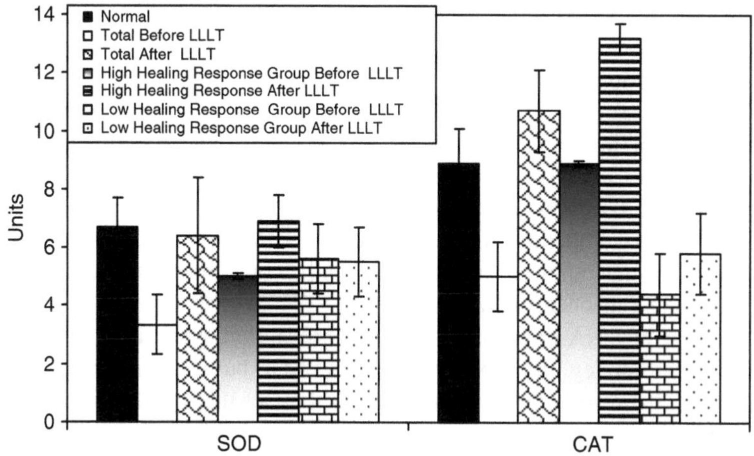

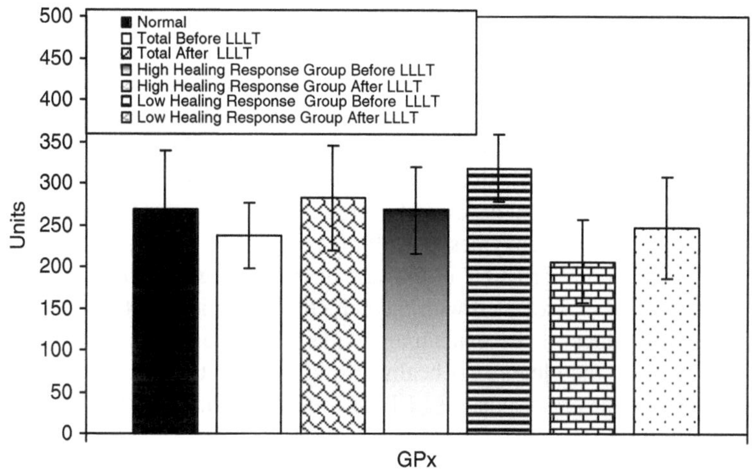

Fig. 27.5 Level of tissue antioxidant enzymes SOD, CAT and GPX in control (normal) and chronic leg ulcer patients before and after LLLT among total, low and high response groups

significantly higher in the low response group after laser therapy compared to its level before laser therapy (247 ± 62 vs 206 ± 50 units, $p < 0.05$) (Fig. 27.5).

27.4 Discussion and Conclusions

Delayed re-epithelialisation and persistent epithelial defects are typical features of chronic ulcers which hardly heal [31, 37]. It has been proposed that excessive and uncontrolled proteolytic activity is an important pathogenesis factor for chronic wounds [44]. Proteolysis is caused mainly by the oxidative stress accompanying an inflammatory response, which leads to oxidation of biomolecules such as proteins [44]. Oxidatively modified proteins are not repaired and must be removed by proteolytic degradation [44, 45]. The elevated PCb level in the tissue of chronic leg ulcer patients before laser treatment and its significant decrease after treatment, indicate that an inflammatory process was brought under control after LLLT. Further evidence supporting this relationship is provided by the observation that while tissue PCb levels in patients with high healing response significantly decreased after laser therapy, its level in patients with low healing response did not significantly change after the treatment. It can be concluded that LLLT stimulates the antioxidative mechanism *in vivo* [46].

Percentage of DNA fragmentation was significantly higher at the tissue edge of wounds of chronic leg ulcers before and after LLLT, but it significantly decreased post LLLT. This result could be attributed to the fact that regulation of apoptotic phenomena during wound healing may be important in scar establishment and development of pathological scarring [47]. It has been suggested that the cleavage of nuclear DNA into high molecular weight fragments is associated not only with apoptosis but also accompanies changes in the functional activity of non-apoptotic cells [48]. This conclusion is supported by the fact that chronic venous leg ulcers are characterised by excessive or prolonged inflammation, which is accompanied by an increase in ROS released from polymorphonuclear leukocytes and proteinases, along with increased connective tissue degradation and lipid peroxidation, further enhancing the hostile pro-oxidant microenvironment [29, 32, 33]. During the chronic inflammatory phase the level of necrotic DNA increases due to the presence of lysing and proteolytic enzymes [49, 50]. Concurrently, the decrease in the level of lipid peroxidation after LLLT in the sera of these patients is due to the chronically inflamed tissue associated with the depletion of antioxidant enzymes, which leads to a disturbance of the oxidant/antioxidant balance in favour of the former [29, 32, 33]. Once the ulcers start healing, lipid peroxidation decreases due to the decrease in inflammatory response. LLLT has been demonstrated to be a non-stressful treatment *in vitro* [51].

The results of the present study confirm that LLLT enhances the induction of antioxidant enzymes SOD, CAT and GPX. The activity of antioxidant enzymes in those patients who responded to laser therapy returned to the normal level, which was significantly higher than their activity in patients whose ulcers did not respond to laser therapy. It was shown experimentally that the activity of antioxidant enzymes decreased in the wound environment. This decrease is probably related to the process of wound healing, as it allows blood granulocytes and tissue macrophages to perform their function in cleansing the wounded area in the form of phagocytic cells, which engulf pathogens and other cellular debris, concomitantly liberating substantial amounts of ROS needed for this function [29]. Once this inflammatory phase is completed the wounded area recovers its oxidant/antioxidant balance, and re-epithelialisation and matrix remodelling processes proceed [31, 32]. In a previous study, after experimental wounding a 40–60% decrease in the level of antioxidant enzymes SOD, GPX and CAT was observed [46]. In the present study the recovery in the level of antioxidant enzymes was 54.0–66.4% for SOD,

72.4–74.7% for GPX and 41.0–46.7% for CAT. The increase in activity of antioxidant enzymes is opposite to their decrease observed in self healing wounds without use of laser therapy [37]. Thus it can be concluded that chronic leg ulcer patients lack the stimulatory mechanism needed to normalise their antioxidant enzymes after wounding and that laser therapy enhances this mechanism. Accordingly, the significant increase in the level of serum SOD, GPX and CAT antioxidant enzymes observed in patients of this study after LLLT is most probably the cause of the significant decrease in the level of serum MDA, PC and DNA fragmentation observed post treatment with laser therapy.

The activity of SOD has been shown previously to increase in the skin of animals exposed to LLLT [52]. This observation agrees with the results of our study but the increase of response is different, which may be due to the difference in the laser dose [53–55]. LLLT has been shown to increase the level of SOD and lower the increase in lipid peroxidation associated with experimental ischemia and reperfusion, and human acute edema [56, 57]. Laser therapy reduced the incidence and severity of chemotherapy-induced mucotitis in bone marrow transplantation patients [58]. SOD has also been shown to enhance the stimulatory effects of nitric oxide by eliminating superoxide anion, the scavenger of nitric oxide [55, 59]. Nitric oxide has been shown to enhance the microcirculation in laser-irradiated arterioles [60], and to enhance cell proliferation and gene expression in many cell systems including smooth muscles [61]. The shift in oxidant/antioxidant balance induced by He–Ne laser leading to increased levels of superoxide dismutase which consequently leads to enhancing NO stimulatory functions, could be the cause of the wound healing effect induced by laser therapy in this study [61].

The increase in levels of tissue CAT is compatible with previous results which showed that LLLT induced an increase in CAT activity of irradiated isolated cardiomyocytes compared to controls. It was suggested that laser therapy efficacy in chronic wounds and ulcers can be attributed to the activation of CAT in tissue fluids [62]. He–Ne laser has been shown to cause photoactivation and structural modifications of catalase enzymes that positively correlated with its functional properties in cell free system [63].

Before treatment a negative correlation between the percentage of wound healing and oxidant/antioxidant ratios of MDA/SOD, MDA/GPX and MDA/CAT was observed. These ratios were $r = -0.2$, $r = -0.5$ and $r = -0.54$ respectively. During recovery and the 8th session the oxidant/antioxidant ratios increased significantly to $r = -0.87$, $r = -0.49$ and $r = -0.82$ respectively. The latter finding together with the significant decrease in the oxidant/antioxidant ratio observed in those patients who responded to treatment compared to those who did not respond to laser therapy, indicates that LLLT induces a shift of the oxidant/antioxidant ratio towards the latter.

It is concluded that chronic leg ulcer patients probably lack the mechanisms that normalise their levels of antioxidant enzymes, which normally decrease at early stages of wound healing in order to allow blood granulocytes and tissue macrophages to perform their function in cleansing the wounded area. Consequently re-epithelialisation and matrix remodeling processes are delayed. LLLT stimulates antioxidant enzyme production and consequently reduces the oxidative stress at the wound site thus restoring the oxidant/antioxidant balance, allowing re-epithelialisation and matrix remodeling processes. Overall LLLT has an antioxidant and an anti-inflammatory effect on chronic leg ulcers.

References

1. Hamer C, Cullum N, Roe B (1994) Patients' perceptions of chronic leg ulcers. J Wound Care 3:99–101
2. Ebbeskog B, Ekman SL (2001) Elderly persons' experiences of living with venous leg ulcer: living in a dialectal relationship between freedom and imprisonment. Scand J Caring Sci 15: 235–243
3. Bosanquet N (1992) Costs of venous ulcers: from maintenance therapy to investment programmes. Phlebology 7(suppl 1):44–46
4. Pelham F, Keith M, Smith A, Williams D, Powell G (2007) Pressure ulcer prevalence and cost in the U.S. population. J Am Med Dir Assoc 8(3):B20
5. Sugrue M, Carolan J, Leen E, Feeley T, Moore D, Shanik G (1990) The use of infrared laser therapy in the treatment of venous ulceration. Ann Vasc Surg 4(2):179–181
6. Król P, Franek A, Hu ka-Zurawi ska W, Bil J, Swist D, Polak A, Bendkowski W (2001) Laser's biostimulation in healing or crural ulcerations. Pol Merkur Lek 11(65):418–421
7. Schindl A, Heinze G, Schindl M, Pernerstorfer-Schön H, Schindl L (2002) Systemic effects of low-intensity laser irradiation on skin microcirculation in patients with diabetic microangiopathy. Microvasc Res 64(2):240–246
8. El Batanouny M, Shokeir H, Zayed A, Korraa S, Kamali A (2004) Enhanced healing effects of low energy irradiation on chronic leg ulcers of different etiologies. Dermatology and Andrology 24(1-4):11–22
9. Yasukawa A, Hrui H, Koyama Y, Nagai M, Takakuda K (2007) The effect of low reactive-level laser therapy (LLLT) with helium-neon laser on operative wound healing in a rat model. J Vet Med Sci 69(8):799–806
10. Maiya G, Kumar P, Rao L (2005) Effect of low intensity helium-neon (He-Ne) laser irradiation on diabetic wound healing dynamics. Photomed Laser Surg 23(2):187–190
11. Yu W, Naim J, Lanzafame R (1997) Effects of photostimulation on wound healing of diabetic mice. Lasers Surg Med 20(1):56–63
12. Lubart R, Wollman Y, Friedmann H, Rochkind S, Laulicht I (1992) Effects of visible and near-infrared lasers on cell cultures. J Photochem Photobiol B 12:305–310
13. Evans D, Abrahamse H (2008) Efficacy of three different laser wavelengths for in vitro wound healing. Photodermatol Photoimmunol Photomed 24(4):199–210
14. Colin W, Steiniechner B, Dyson M (1993) The effect of low level laser therapy on the proliferation of keratinocytes. Laser Therapy 5:65–73
15. Haas R, Isseroff R, Wheeland R, Rood P, Graves P (1990) Low energy helium-neon laser irradiation increases the motility of cultured human keratinocytes. J Invest Dermatol 94:822–826
16. Chen C, Hung H, Hsu S (2008) Low-energy laser irradiation increases endothelial cell proliferation, migration, and eNOS gene expression possibly via PI3K signal pathway. Lasers Surg Med 40(1):46–54
17. Gavish L, Perez LS, Reissman P, Gertz SD (2008) Irradiation with 780 nm diode laser attenuates inflammatory cytokines but upregulates nitric oxide in lipopolysaccharide-stimulated macrophages: implications for the prevention of aneurysm progression. Lasers Surg Med 40(5):371–378
18. Yu H, Chang K, Yu C, Chen J, Chen G (1996) Low-energy helium-neon laser irradiation stimulates interleukin-1 alpha and interleukin-8 release from cultured human keratinocytes. J Invest Dermatol 107(4):593–596

19. Novoselova E, Cherenkov D, Glushkova O, Novoselova T, Chudnovski V, Iusupov V, Fesenko E (2006) Effect of low-intensity laser radiation (632.8 nm) on immune cells isolated from mice. Biofizika 51(3):509–518
20. Schindl A, Schindl M, Schindl L, Jurecka W, Honigsmann H, Breier F (1999) Increased dermal angiogenesis after low intensity laser therapy for a chronic radiation ulcer determined by a video measuring system. J Am Acad Dermatol 40:481–484
21. Kopera D, Kokol R, Berger C, Haas J (2005) Does the use of low-level laser influence wound healing in chronic venous leg ulcers? J Wound Care 4(8):391–394
22. Kokol R, Berger C, Haas J, Kopera D (2005) Venous leg ulcers: no improvement of wound healing with 685-nm low level laser therapy: Randomized, placebo-controlled, double-blind study. Hautarzt 56(6):570–575
23. Tredget E, Nedelec B, Scott P, Ghahary A (1997) Hypertrophic scars, keloids, and contractures: the cellular and molecular basis for therapy. Surg Clin North Am 77:701–730
24. Babu M, Diegelmann R, Oliver N (1992) Keloid fibroblasts exhibit an altered response to TGF-beta. J Invest Dermatol 99:650–655
25. Zhang K, Garner W, Cohen L, Rodriguez J, Phan S (1995) Increased types I and III collagen and transforming growth factor-beta 1 mRNA and protein in hypertrophic burn scar. J Invest Dermatol 104:750–754
26. Saed G, Ladin D, Olson J (1998) Analysis of p53 gene mutations in keloids using polymerase chain reaction-based single-strand conformational polymorphism and DNA sequencing. Arch Dermatol 134:963–967
27. Machesney M, Tidman N, Waseem A, Kirby L, Leigh I (1998) Activated keratinocytes in the epidermis of hypertrophic scars. Am J Pathol 152:1133–1141
28. Wlaschek M, Scharffetter-Kochanek K (2005) Oxidative stress in chronic venous leg ulcers. Wound Repair Regen 13(5):452–461
29. Henson P, Johnston R (1987) Tissue injury in inflammation, oxidants, proteinases and cationic proteins. J Clin Invest 79:669–674
30. Cerutti C (1986) Prooxidant states and tumor promotion. Science 227:375–381
31. Shukla A, Rasik A, Patnaik M (1997) Depletion of reduced glutathione, ascorbic acid, vitamin E and antioxidant defense enzymes in healing cutaneous wounds. Free Radic Res 26(2):93–101
32. Rasik A, Shukla A (2000) Antioxidant Status in delayed type of wounds. Int J Exp Pathol 81(4):257–263
33. Gutteridge J (1995) Lipid peroxidation and antioxidants as biomarkers of tissues damage. Clin Chem 41(12):1819–1828
34. Wiesman H, Halliwell B (1996) Damage to DNA by reactive oxygen species and nitrogen species: role of inflammatory disease and progression to cancer. Biochem J 313:17–29
35. Schmidtchen A (2000) Degradation of antiproteinases, complement and fibronectin in chronic leg ulcers. Acta Derm Venereol 80(3):179–184
36. Vaalomo M, Mattila L, Johansson N, Kariniemi A, Karjalainen Lindsberg M, Kahari V, Saarialho-Kere U (1997) Distinct populations of stromal cells express collagenase-3 (MMP-I3) and collagenase-1 (MMP-I) in chronic ulcers but not in normally healing wounds. J Invest Dermatol 109:96–101
37. Lauer G, Sollberg S, Cole M, Flamme I, Sturzebecher J, Mann K, Krieg T, Eming S (2000) Expression and proteolysis of vascular endothelial growth factor is increased in chronic wounds. J Invest Dermatol 115:12–18
38. Ioannou Y, Chen F (1996) Quantification of DNA fragmentation in apoptosis. Nucleic Acid Res 24(5):992–993
39. Reznick A, Packer L (1994) Oxidative damage to proteins: spectrophotometric method for carbonyl assay. Methods Enzymol 233:357–363
40. Yagi K (1982) Assay for serum lipid peroxide level and its clinical significance. In: Yagi KJ (ed) Lipid peroxide in biology and medicine. Academic, New York, pp 223–242
41. Minami M, Yoshikawa H (1979) A simplified assay method of superoxide dismutase activity for clinical use. Clin Chim Acta 92:337–342
42. Plagia D, Valentine W (1967) Studies on the quantitative and qualitative characterization of erythrocyte glutathione peroxidase. J Lab Clin Med 70:158–169

43. Johansson L, Borg H (1988) A spectrophotometric method for the determination of catalase activity in small tissue sample. Anal Biochem 174(1):331–336
44. Harris IR, Yee KC, Walters CE, Cunliffe CE, Kearney IN, Wood EJ et al (1995) Cytokines and protease levels in healing and non-healing chronic venous leg ulcers. Exp Dermatol 4:342–349
45. Gohel MS, Windhaber RAJ, Tarlon JF, Whyman MR, Poskitt KR (2008) The relationship between cytokine concentrations and wound healing in chronic venous ulceration. J Vasc Surg 48(5):1272–1277
46. Kim G, Pack S, Lee S (2000) Hairless mouse epidermal antioxidants and lipid peroxidation assessed by He– Ne laser. Lasers Surg Med 27:420–426
47. Buttke T, Sandstorm PA (1994) Oxidative stress as a mediator of apoptosis. Immunol Today 15:7–10
48. Fujimura M, Morita-Fujimura Y, Narasimhan P, Copin J, Kawase M, Chan P (1999) Copper-zinc superoxide dismutase prevents the early decrease of apurinic/apyrimidinic endonuclease and subsequent DNA fragmentation after transient focal cerebral ischemia in mice. Stroke 130:2408–2415
49. Andriessen M, van Bergen B, Spruijt K, Go I, Schalkwijk J, van de Kerkhof P (1995) Epidermal proliferation is not impaired in chronic venous ulcers. Acta Derm Venereol 75(6):459–462
50. Takahashi A, Aoshiba K, Nagai A (2002) Apoptosis of wound fibroblasts induced by oxidative stress. Exp Lung Res 28(4):275–284
51. Abou Hashieh I, Tardieu C, Franquin JC (1997) Helium neon laser irradiation is not a stressful treatment: A study on heat-shock protein (HSP70) level. Lasers Surg Med 20:451–460
52. Tarnuzzer RW, Schultz GS (1996) Biochemical analysis of acute and chronic wound environment. Wound Rep Reg 4:321–325
53. Parlato G, Cimmino G, Devendittis E, Monfrecola G, Bocchini V (1983) Superoxide dismutase activity in the skin of rats irradiated by He–Ne laser. Experientia 39(7):750–751
54. Vladimirov IuA, Klebanov GI, Borisenko GG, Osipov AN (2004) Molecular and cellular mechanisms of the low intensity laser radiation effect. Biofizika (Moscow) 49(2):339–350
55. Romm A, Sherstnev M, Volkov V, Valdimirove Iu (1986) Action of laser irradiation on the peroxide chemiluminescence of wound exudates. Biull Eksp Biol Med (Moscow) 102(10): 426–428
56. Karageuzyan K, Sekoyan E, Karagyan A, Pogosyan N, Manucharyan G, Sekoyan A, Tunyan A, Boyajyan V, Karageuzyan M (1998) Phospholipids pool, lipid peroxidation, and superoxide dismutase activity under various types of oxidative stress of the brain and the effct of low-energy infrared laser. Biochemistry (Moscow) 63(10):1226–1232
57. Vin'cova G, Ionin A, Ionin G (1999) The treatment of post Traumatic uveitis with low-intensity laser radiation. Vestn Oftalmol (Moscow) 115(5):209–211
58. Barasch A, Peterson D, Tanzer J, D'Ambrosio J, Nuki K, Schubert M, Franquin J, Clive J, Tutschka P (1995) Helium-neon laser effects on conditioning-induced oral mucositis in bone marrow transplantation patients. Cancer 76(12):2550–2556
59. Park JW, Qi WN, Liu JQ, Urbaniak JR, Folz RJ, Chen LE (2005) Inhibition of iNOS attenuates skeletal muscle reperfusion injury in extracellular superoxide dismutase knockout mice. Microsurgery 25(8):606–613
60. Chen C, Korshunov V, Massett M, Yan C, Berk B (2007) Impaired vasorelaxation in inbred mice is associated with alterations in both nitric oxide and super oxide pathways. J Vasc Res 44(6):504–512
61. Klebanov G, Poltanov E, Chichuk T, Osipov A, Vladimirov Y (2005) Changes in superoxide dismutase activity and peroxynitrite content in rat peritoneal macrophages exposed to He–Ne laser. Biochemistry (Moscow) 70(12):1335–1340
62. Sasaki Y, Seki J, Giddings JC, Yamamoto J (1996) Effects of NO-donors on thrombus formation and microcirculation in cerebral vessels of the rat. Thromb Haemost 76(1):111–117
63. Aryukhov G, Basharina O, Pantak A, Sveklo L (2000) Effect of helium-neon laser on activity and optical properties of catalase. Biull Eksp Biol Med (Moscow) 129(6):633–636

Part V
Extracorporeal Methods of Treatment

Chapter 28
Advances and Problems of Biospecific Hemosorption

V.V. Kirkovsky and D.V. Vvedenski

Abstract Hemosorption over activated carbon is a recognized method of treatment of exo- and endogenous intoxications. However activated carbons are non-selective adsorbents and remove physiologically important metabolites along with toxins. Novel biospecific sorbents based on polyacrylamide with incorporated bioligands have been designed to eliminate target high molecular weight biotoxins. Biospecific adsorbents with immobilized ovomucoid (Ovosorb), L-tryptophan and Polymyxin E (Lyposorb) were produced. Hemosorption with biospecific sorbents significantly improved clinical results and conditions of patients with acute pancreatitis (Ovosorb), severe asthma (L-tryptophan) and abdominal sepsis (Lyposorb).

Keywords Efferent therapy • Anti-protease sorbents • Immunosorbents • LPS • Ig-E • Hemosorption

28.1 Introduction

Hippocrates, the "father" of scientific medicine, considered that "The medicine is the art of addition of lacking and withdrawal of excessive. And who does this better is considered to be the best doctor". Progress of modern pharmacology, wide application of products of chemical industry, consumption of drugs and genetically modified products, and inflow of other xenobiotics through the bowel, skin and lungs often lead to functional, metabolic, and then morphological alterations of the body functions. Therefore many scientists work on developing devices and methods which allow efficient removal of chemical and biological toxins and xenobiotics from the human body.

V.V. Kirkovsky (✉) and D.V. Vvedenski
Laboratory of Hemo and Lymphosorption, Minsk State Medical Institute,
83, Dzerzhinsky Prospect, Minsk 220798, Republic of Belarus
e-mail: kirkovskv.v@mail.ru

S. Mikhalovsky and A. Khajibaev (eds.), *Biodefence*, NATO Science for Peace and Security Series A: Chemistry and Biology, DOI 10.1007/978-94-007-0217-2_28,

This direction in medical practice has been in existence since ancient times. Even without sufficient knowledge of pathogenesis of different diseases various approaches aimed at extracting pathogenic substances from human body, such as vomiting and use of laxatives, treatment of wounds with substances possessing adsorption properties have been long used.

More recently, with the rapid development of molecular biology and medicine, new devices and techniques aimed at correction of homeostasis have been developed.

There are several possible approaches to correct homeostasis abnormalities:

- to decrease the damaging effect of pathogenic substances using inhibitors of enzymes, antibiotics, antioxidants, immunoglobulins, and serum albumin;
- to force transport of pathogen substances from the depot site or from organs, providing their neutralization and excretion using macro- and microhemodynamics correction drugs, and serum albumin;
- to intensify natural detoxication process using diuretics, immunocorrection, hepatoprotection, photo-, ozone-, and hypochlorite induced blood modification;
- to eliminate pathogenic metabolites and toxins from the organism using extracorporeal techniques of plasmapheresis, hemodialysis, and hemosorption (hemoperfusion).

Success of extracorporeal treatment methods in medical practice has allowed scientists to found a new direction in medicine named «efferent medicine» [1]. These methods proved to be easy to use, highly efficient and cost effective, which ensured their fast development in medical institutions in Belarus.

In the former USSR a very successful hemosorbent based on uncoated carbons, which has satisfactory compatibility with blood, has been created. Its clinical use has allowed scientists to develop original treatment modes.

Hemosorption with uncoated carbon can provide elimination of substances with a wide range of molecular weights from blood and, what is especially important, hydrophobic metabolites can also be eliminated from the surface of blood cells and unbound from proteins. Unfortunately, this requires a tight contact of blood cells with uncoated carbon, which adversely affects cells reducing their number. Other undesirable side effects include sorption of physiological substances, activation of inflammatory mediators and blood coagulation. Development of hemosorbents with high hemocompatibility and ability to selectively eliminate target metabolites and toxins from blood is a significant task for clinical medicine. In this paper modern approaches towards design of biospecific hemosorbents are described.

28.2 Anti-Protease Sorbents

The protease-inhibitor system imbalance is the key element of alterations in purulent inflammatory diseases such as purulent peritonitis and destructive pancreatitis. This imbalance is the result of a massive release of cellular proteases, activation of cellular proteolytic systems, and decrease of protease inhibitors concentration. Application of the multivalent protease inhibitors such as aprotinin and its analogues in this case is theoretically sound, however these drugs may damage the protease-mediated regulation of various physiological processes.

Pathogenesis of systemic abnormalities during pancreatitis is associated with a high concentration of pancreatic proteases in the blood, which reduce activation of the blood proteolytic systems. Alteration of the balance between proteases and their natural inhibitors is a trigger of endogenous intoxication syndrome, which controls disease severity and the clinical outcome. Therefore, drugs which act as inhibitors of proteases are an important component of a complex treatment of acute pancreatitis.

A high fatality rate associated with this disease suggests that the effectiveness of conservative and surgical treatment is not sufficient in the case of acute pancreatitis. New methods of extracorporeal detoxification using hemoperfusion over carbon sorbents has made it possible to improve the outcome of pancreatitis treatment. However, hemosorption leads to only a transient decrease in blood proteolytic activity and does not correct the imbalance in the protease-inhibitor system, and the carbon hemosorbents are nonspecific. The development and application of anti-protease hemosorbents with specific bioligands therefore has potential in pancreatitis treatment.

We have developed an efferent method for correction of hyperproteasemia, which is based on elimination of active proteases from blood by means of biospecific hemosorption. A new generation of biospecific anti-protease hemosorbents have been developed with the use of ovomucoid immobilized in a polyacrylamide gel. Ovomucoid is a highly glycosylated protein abundant in hen's egg white, with a molecular weight of 28 kD [2]. The ovomucoid ligand inhibits serine proteases very effectively. Here we present medical and biological studies and results of clinical trials of the anti-protease hemosorbent "Ovosorb"→which has been previously tested in dogs and a small number of patients [3, 4].

431 randomly chosen patients treated for destructive pancreatitis in surgical departments of Minsk, Belarus, hospitals, were studied. The diagnosis was based on the clinical symptoms and amylase level (>1,000 $U{\cdot}L^{-1}$) and was verified during laparoscopy or laparotomy. All patients were treated with conservative and surgical methods. Direct hemosorption (HS) was used after an adequate correction of circulatory injury was reached. HS was carried out for 100 min, at the blood flow rate of 60–80 $mL{\cdot}min^{-1}$, and general intravenous hyalinization (Heparin, Gedeon Richter, Hungary, 0.5 $mg{\cdot}kg^{-1}$ of body mass) was performed. The vein-venous mode of hemoperfusion was used with subclavian, basilic or femoral veins. The anti-protease sorbent "Ovosorb" (80 mL) was used in an extracorporeal plastic column.

The time interval between successive HS sessions (from 4 h to 2 days) and the number of sessions were determined in each specific case in accordance with the character and extent of generalization of the inflammatory process in the pancreas and abdominal cavity, severity of endogenous intoxication, and therapeutic effect of the previous sessions.

or became more intensive. Any purulent complications in or around the pancreas were not recorded either. Thus, the fatality rate in the group of patients under study constituted 6.2%. At the same time, the fatality rate in group of patients treated by hemosorption with conventional activated carbon sorbents was much higher (24.7%).

The present study shows effectiveness of the biospecific antiprotease hemosorbent “Ovosorb” in the treatment of critically ill patients with destructive pancreatitis. Effectiveness of “Ovosorb” is mediated mostly via reduction of endogenous intoxication, functional and metabolic disorders.

We suggest that the extracorporeal elimination of proteases from blood and decrease in the level of toxic and biologically active peptides stimulate endogenous detoxification systems and improve functioning of the compensatory systems in the organism.

The clinical effect of “Ovosorb” can be attributed to its effect on reduction of proteolytic activity in plasma and, as a result, restoration of the balance between proteases and their inhibitors. Immediately after hemoperfusion, in spite of decrease of the trypsin-like activity, the activity of protease inhibitors in plasma remained at its initial low level. This fact is in line with our knowledge on the rates of biosynthesis of these proteins.

28.3 Sorbent for IgE-Dependent Pathology

Recently the number of allergic diseases has grown considerably. The traditional methods of treatment of allergic patients are often ineffective; therefore it is necessary to develop new methods for treatment of such patients. It is well known that the high blood level of IgE is the key element in pathogenesis of most allergic diseases. Taking into account this fact, IgE elimination from blood may lead to improvement in the conditions of allergic patients.

We developed a hemosorbent for selective and effective IgE elimination from blood. We studied its treatment action and proposed a method of hemosorbent application in patients with drug-resistant allergic and combined bronchial asthma.

As a biospecific ligand the anti-IgE sorbent L-tryptophan was used. Polyacrylamide gel was chosen as a matrix. We carried out experiments to study sorption properties of this sorbent with the plasma of patients after plasmapheresis with high IgE level (500 $IU \cdot L^{-1}$ and higher). Plasma perfusion through the column with this hemosorbent decreased IgE levels in plasma by 40%. Taking into account the obtained rather encouraging experimental data, the developed immunosorbent was used for direct hemosorption to treat patients with allergic and combined variants of bronchial asthma.

There were two groups of patients suffering from the severe form of asthma. Treatment of patients in the first group included standard drug therapy and biospecific hemosorption for anti-IgE. The patients in second (control) group were treated only with drug therapy. The treatment of each patient in the first group included three sessions of hemosorption with 2–3 days intervals. The hemosorption was performed by vein-to-vein mode using a peristaltic pump. An anticoagulant heparin was introduced at the level of 125 ± 25 IU kg^{-1} of body mass. The hemosorbent was packed in a specially designed single-use unit. The perfusion volume was 1.5–2.0 l of the whole circulating blood volume. There were no significant adverse effects noted after hemosorption.

As a result, treatment of patients in the basic group, using biospecific hemosorption with anti-IgE sorbent decreased the IgE level in plasma by 50%. This decrease correlated with significant improvement of clinical symptoms and laboratory indices of patients. Patients in the control group had no significant clinical or laboratory signs of improvement.

In summary, it can be concluded that the developed biospecific anti-IgE hemosorbent may be widely used to treat patients with severe forms of allergic and combined bronchial asthma, as well as in situations where high IgE level plays a critical role and its reduction may benefit a patient.

28.4 Efferent Methods in the Complex Treatment of Septic Pathology

In recent decades a significant growth of septic diseases has been seen in developed countries. In spite of continuous development of treatment methods and increased use of antibiotics, septic complications remain the most frequent cause of patient death. According to a number of authors, septic conditions in more than 50% of complications are caused by gram-negative flora. A gram-negative infection is characterized by an extremely fast development of such severe complications as a septic shock, multiple organ failure, disseminated intravascular clotting, and respiratory distress syndrome of adults. According to a number of researchers the mortality rate caused by gram-negative infections is higher than caused by gram-positive infections.

The main cause of septic complications is gram-negative flora, and in particular bacterial endotoxin lipopolysaccharide (LPS). LPS is the constant structural component of the cell wall of gram-negative bacteria. Its molecular weight varies from 10,000 to 20,000 Da, but it can also form much larger aggregates in blood [8]. The LPS molecule consists of three parts. According to the majority of authors, it is the presence of a hydrophobic domain lipid A in the LPS molecule that initiates cytokine cascade, and activates cellular systems (monocyte-macrophages, endothelial cells, lymphocytes, granulocytes, fibroblasts) and the complement system.

Endocrine and paracrine effects of cytokines and secondary mediators lead to vasodilation and hypotension, hyperactivation of coagulation systems, endothelium damage, increase of leukocyte adhesion as a result of reduced perfusion and hypoxia.

Endotoxemia correlates with severity of gram-negative sepsis. Nowadays, one of the recognized effective treatment methods is the use of Polymyxin B, which links and inactivates LPS both in a bacterium wall and in a free form, however its application is hindered by neuro- and, especially, nephrotoxicity of this antibiotic even in therapeutic concentrations.

The experience of application of various efferent methods of endotoxin elimination has led to the idea of creating selective anti-LPS hemosorbents with Polymyxin B as the bioligand. The covalently immobilized Polymyxin B does not cause side effects characteristic of free Polymyxin B and keeps its therapeutic effects. G.W. Duff in 1982 demonstrated for the first time the sorption efficiency of Polymyxin B-immobilized sorbent *in vitro* [9]. In 1984 K. Hanasawa with co-workers developed PMX-F - a fibrous polystyrene based hemosorbent with immobilized Polymyxin B that could be used directly for blood perfusion [10]. In 1994 PMX-F sorbent was officially approved for patient treatment in Japan. Currently, there are several polymyxin immobilized (PMX-F) sorbents produced commercially for clinical use, such as "Alteca" – "LPS Absorber" (Sweden), "Toray Industries Inc." (Japan), etc. However these sorbents have poor hemocompatibility and are very expensive.

The purpose of the given work was to study clinical efficiency of hemosorbent Lyposorb®, developed by the group of researchers from Belarus.

The biospecific hemosorbent Lyposorb is composed of polyacrylamide hydrogel with fixed polymyxin antibiotic groups of Polymyxin E (PMX). Polymyxin E, or colistin, is effective against most gram-negative bacteria. The polyacrylamide matrix was chosen due to its stability, biological inertness, and a possibility of the bioligand introduction at a polymerization stage; it is also relatively inexpensive to produce.

72 sessions of vein-venous extracorporeal hemoperfusion using the hemosorbent Lyposorb were carried out in 40 patients with abdominal sepsis and peritonitis of various genesis.

The level of endotoxin (LPS) in blood was determined by turbidimetric immunoassay. Turbidimetric immunoassay of LPS was carried out before and after the hemosorption.

Patients with abdominal sepsis received usual drug therapy combined with biospecific hemosorption with Lyposorb. All patients were urgently operated. After operative procedure patients were transferred to intensive care unit for recovery, where all the necessary treatment and observations were carried out during critical postoperative period.

Extracorporeal affine sorption was carried out by vein-venous method with the use of a peristaltic pump. Heparin was used as anticoagulant in a dose 80 ± 20 IU kg^{-1}. Gram-negative bacteremia was revealed in all cases. Continuous monitoring of systemic hemodynamics indicators, gas composition of blood, general and biochemical analyses of blood, and blood coagulation parameters was carried out. In all patients the phenomenon of an accruing hypotension which demanded application of dopamine in doses exceeding 5 mL $kg^{-1} min^{-1}$ was observed. The majority of patients required artificial ventilation support.

Blood perfusion through a column with a biospecific hemosorbent at a flow rate of 50–70 ml min^{-1} after 30 min achieved a significant decrease in LPS level from 66.7 ± 3.1 to 30.5 ± 2.2 pg·mL^{-1} ($P < 0.01$). By the end of hemoperfusion sessions stabilization of systemic hemodynamics was observed (Table 28.2), which permitted

Table 28.2 Characteristics of hemodynamics during hemosorption with Lyposorb

Characteristics	Before hemosorption	After hemosorption	P
Average arterial pressure (mm Hg)	75±3	90±1.6	<0.01
Pulse pressure (mm Hg)	42±2	60±1.5	<0.01
Heart rate (impact min^{-1})	118±5	101±3	= 0.258
Central venous pressure (mm Hg)	8±3	8±4	= 0.76
Cardiac spike ($L\,min^{-1}\,m^{-2}$)	4.4±1.0	4.6±1.4	= 0.38
Systemic vascular resistance index (dyn-s $cm^{-2}{\cdot}m^{-2}$)	1.41±0.57	1.5±0.5	= 0.02
Dopamine ($\mu g\,kg^{-1}\,min^{-1}$)	8.0±0.05	3.2±0.1	<0.01

to reduce or eliminate the use of vasopressin drugs. In some patients the effect of stabilization of hemodynamics was unstable; therefore PMX-hemosorption over Lyposorb was used 2–3 times with an interval of 4–6 h. By the end of hemoperfusion positive dynamics in the general condition, indicators of blood gas composition and biochemical parameters was achieved in all patients (Table 28.2).

Statistically significant decrease in level of endotoxin (LPS) after hemosorption with Lyposorb was noticeable.

Out of 40 operated patients 34 (85%) have survived, and after 28±8 days they were transferred from intensive care unit to general wards to continue treatment in therapeutic regime. After stabilization of hemodynamics, the correction of protease-inhibitor imbalance was performed by biospecific hemosorption with hemosorbent Ovosorb. To correct an electrolyte imbalance a prolonged kidney therapy using "Multifiltrate" device was performed.

It has been concluded that hemosorption with Polymyxin hemosorbent Lyposorb is an effective method of treatment of abdominal sepsis caused by gram-negative flora. HS eliminates endotoxins and stabilizes hemodynamics. The use of Polymyxin hemosorbent Lyposorb for hemosorption in the integrated therapy of patients with abdominal sepsis significantly improves results of treatment.

References

1. Lopukhin YuM (1987) Hemosorption and other efferent methods in medicine. Biomater Artif Cells Artif Organs 15(1):21–29
2. Besler M, Steinhart H, Paschke A (1997) Allergenicity of hen's egg-white proteins: IgE binding of native and deglycosylated ovomucoid. Food Agric Immunol 9:277–288
3. Plate NA, Kirkovsky VV, Antiperovich OF, Nicolaichik VV, Valueva TA, Sinilo SB, Moin VM, Lobacheva GA (1994) Biospecific haemosorbents based on proteinase inhibitor: II. Efficiency of biospecific antiproteinase haemosorbent 'Ovosorb' in complex treatment of experimental generalized purulent peritonitis and acute destructive pancreatitis in dogs. Biomaterials 15(4):285–288
4. Kirkovsky VV, Antiperovich OF, Valueva TA, Moin VM, Lobacheva GA, Berezkina OG (1994) Biospecific haemosorbents based on proteinase inhibitor: III. Biospecific antiproteinase

haemosorbent 'Ovosorb' in complex therapy of acute destructive pancreatitis. Biomaterials 15(5):334–336
5. Lahaye J, Nansé G, Bagreev A, Strelko V (1999) Porous structure and surface chemistry of nitrogen containing carbons from polymers. Carbon 37(4):585–590
6. Vanholder R, Van Laecke S, Glorieux G (2008) The middle-molecule hypothesis 30 years after: lost and rediscovered in the universe of uremic toxicity? J Nephrol 21(2):146–160
7. SU Patent, application no. 4,879,819/14
8. Raetz CR, Whitfield C (2002) Lipopolysaccharide endotoxins. Annu Rev Biochem 71:635–700
9. Duff GW, Waisman DM, Atkins E (1982) Removal of endotoxin by a Polymyxin-B affinity column. Clin Res 30(2):A565
10. Hanasawa K, Tani T, Oka T, Kodama M (1984) A new treatment for endotoxemia with direct hemoperfusion by polymyxin-immobilized fiber. Artif Organs 8(3):397–398

Chapter 29
Deliganding Carbonic Adsorbents for Simultaneous Removal of Protein-Bound Toxins, Bacterial Toxins and Inflammatory Cytokines

V.G. Nikolaev, V.V. Sarnatskaya, A.N. Sidorenko, K.I. Bardakhivskaya, E.A. Snezhkova, L.A. Yushko, V.N. Maslenny, L.A. Sakhno, S.V. Mikhalovsky, O.P. Kozynchenko, and A.V. Nikolaev

Abstract In this work structural and sorption properties of granulated carbonic sorbents obtained by deep pyrolysis of synthetic resins, are described. It has been shown that these sorbents possess high (up to 2.7 $cm^3 g^{-1}$) pore volume, low (up to 0.06 $g\,cm^{-3}$) bulk density, well developed supermicro- and mesoporosity and significantly fractal structure in the range from 75 to 900 Å. Upon contact with solutions of human serum albumin (HSA), they efficiently adsorb protein-bound ligands with association constants from 10^3 to 10^8 M^{-1}. These sorbents coded as HSGD (from HemoSorbent Granulated Deliganding) demonstrate adsorption capacity for unconjugated bilirubin, fatty and bile acids, phenols, CMPF, hippuric acid and indoxyl sulfate, which is tenfold higher than that for conventional granulated synthetic carbon hemosorbents. At the same time capacity of HSGD for freely soluble low molecular weight compounds, such as creatinine and methylene blue increases insignificantly. Simultaneously HSGD demonstrates high adsorption capacity for inflammatory cytokines TNF-α, IL-1, IL-6 that could be further enhanced by coating of the carbonic surface with native DNA or dextrane sulfate. Hemocompatibility of HSGD may be significantly increased by adding citrate to blood or by coating its surface with serum albumin. Finally, HSGD capacity coated with HSA for bacterial lipopolysaccharide (LPS) is by 15–20% higher than that of uncoated one. The use of certain molecular or pH-conformers of HSA for HSGD coating creates a diffusion

V.G. Nikolaev (✉), V.V. Sarnatskaya, A.N. Sidorenko, K.I. Bardakhivskaya, E.A. Snezhkova, L.A. Yushko, V.N. Maslenny, and L.A. Sakhno
R.E. Kavetsky Institute of Experimental Pathology, Oncology and Radiobiology, NAS of Ukraine, 45, Vasylkivska street, Kiev 03022, Ukraine
e-mail: aos@onconet.kiev.ua

S.V. Mikhalovsky
University of Brighton, Brighton, United Kingdom

O.P. Kozynchenko
MAST Carbon International Ltd., Henley Park, Guildford, Surrey GU3 2AF, England

A.V. Nikolaev
Moscow Physical Technical Institute, Moscow, Russia

S. Mikhalovsky and A. Khajibaev (eds.), *Biodefence*, NATO Science for Peace and Security Series A: Chemistry and Biology, DOI 10.1007/978-94-007-0217-2_29,

"transparent" layer that practically does not affect the adsorption capacity of the carbonic matrix towards protein-bound ligands.

It has been demonstrated that the deep pyrolysis technology used to produce HSGD can be applied to other carbonic sorbents made from granular synthetic, natural and fibrous raw materials.

Keywords Uremic toxins • Blirubin • Hemoperfusion • Activated carbon • Protein bound toxins

29.1 Protein Bound Uremic and Hepatic Toxins

The problem of purification of whole blood and blood plasma from protein-bound toxins is far from being resolved [1,2]. It is largely related to deliganding of human serum albumin (HSA), the main transporter molecule of hydrophobic ligands in blood plasma [3]. The affinity of different ligands to HSA molecules is measured by their association constant K, which has values mainly in the range of 10^2–10^9 M^{-1}. Compounds with $K=10^2$–10^3 M^{-1} are considered weakly bound, 10^4–10^5 M^{-1} - moderately bound, and 10^6–10^8 M^{-1} - strongly bound ligands. HSA may have more than one binding site available for the same toxin, with different binding affinity.

One should also consider that protein-bound toxins, due to their hydrophobicity can easily pass through a lipoprotein cell membrane acting directly on intracellular structures.

Table 29.1 contains examples of weakly, moderately and strongly bound uremic toxins, permeation of which through a dialysis membrane is hindered due to the size of albumin molecules associated with them. Although these toxins are small molecules, their complexes with HSA (MW 67,000 kD) are significantly larger and cannot diffuse through the membrane.

The most commonly used hydrophobic marker of hepatic insufficiency is unconjugated bilirubin ($K=10^8 \times M^{-1}$), which is tightly bound to HSA. If one could learn how to remove it effectively from HSA using carbonic sorbents, then these sorbents could be applied for removing other protein-bound ligands as well. Generally, bilirubin as a free molecule is efficiently adsorbed by activated carbons, but in the presence of a competing liquid sorbent HSA, the carbon capacity for bilirubin falls drastically (Fig. 29.1).

29.2 Calorimetry of Serum Albumin with Strongly Bound Ligands

It is recognized that an "albumin-high affinity ligand" complex can be regarded as a new biopolymer, the conformation and complexing properties of which determine the intramolecular energy distribution, which may be quite different from the initial

Table 29.1 Parameters of HSA-ligand complex formation with some uremic toxins

Uremic toxin	MW/D	n_1	$K_1/(10^5 \times M^{-1})$	n_2	$K_2/(10^3 \times M^{-1})$
3-carboxy-4-methyl-5-propyl-2-furanpropionate, CMPF	240	1	130.5	2	33.4
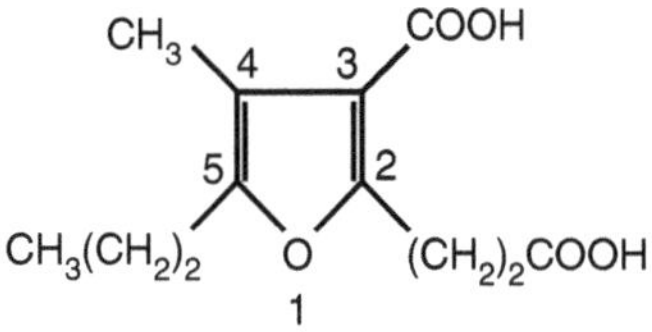					
Indoxyl sulfate	251	1	16.1	3	8.3
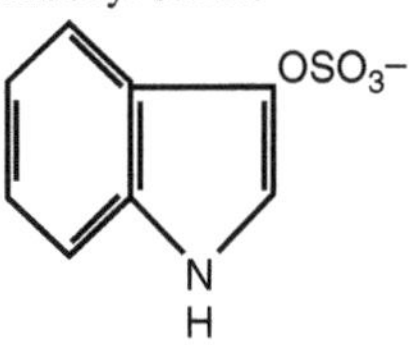					
Hippuric acid	179	1	0.1	7	0.3
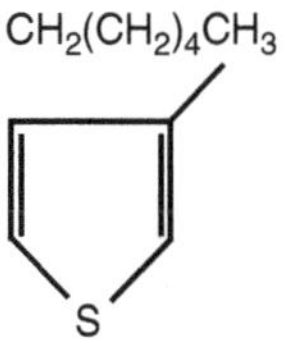					

MW molecular weight, n_1 number of ligands bound to higher affinity sites, n_2 number of ligands bound to weaker affinity sites

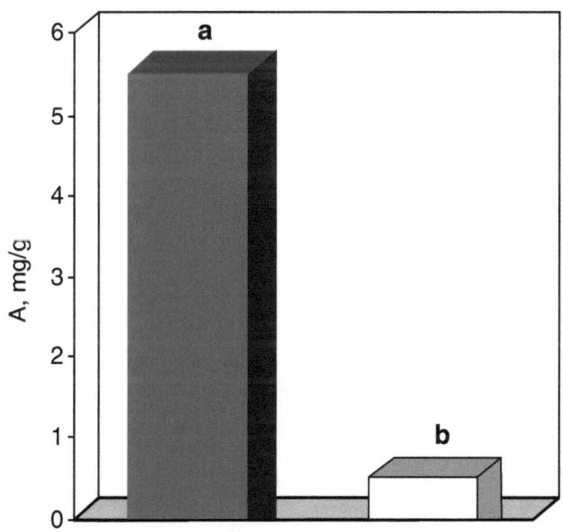

Fig. 29.1 SCN hemosorbent capacity towards unconjugated bilirubin adsorbed from (**a**) phosphate buffer solution and (**b**) 3% human serum albumin solution. SCN is one of the most efficient conventional hemosorbents based on activated carbon [4]

characteristics of pure (unloaded) HSA [5]. Properties of this "new polymer" can be studied using modern biophysical methods, in particular differential scanning calorimetry, which registers alterations of heat capacity of a biopolymer by the

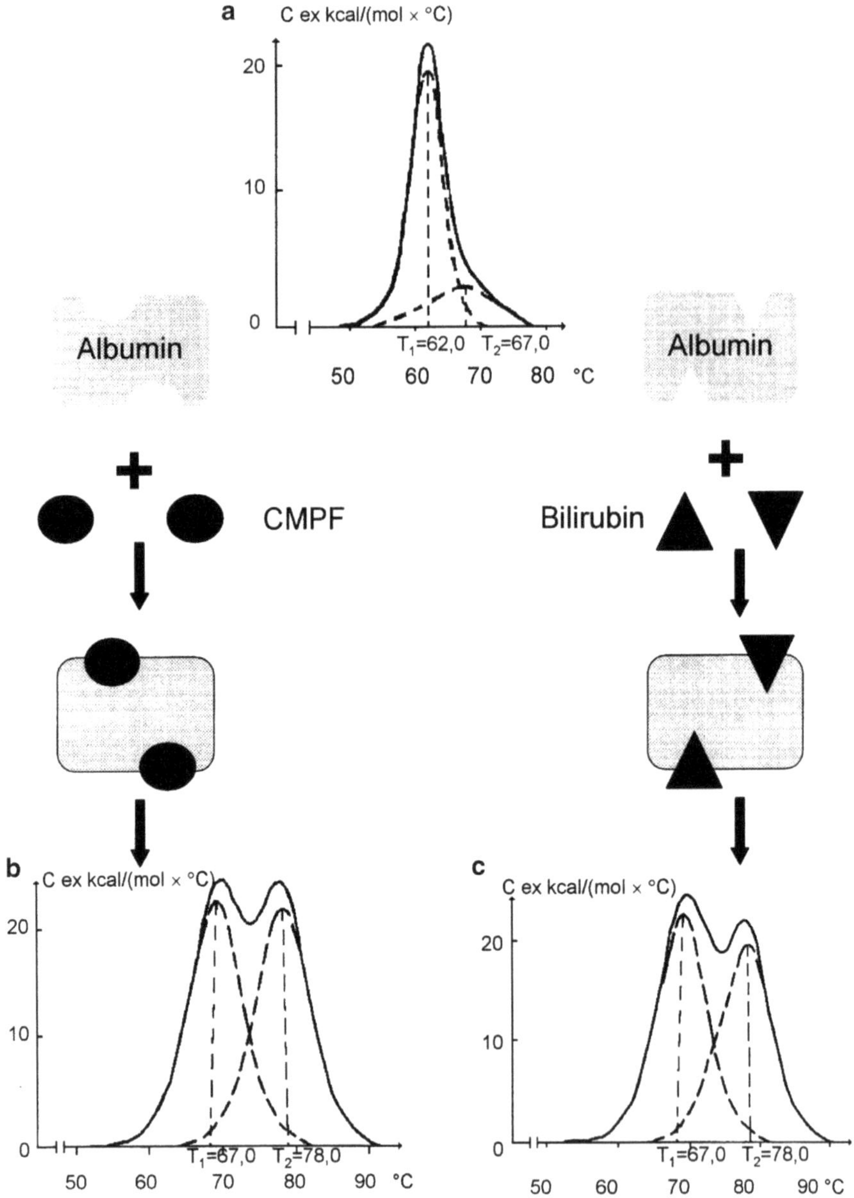

Fig. 29.2 Melting curves of HSA unloaded (**a**), loaded with CMPF (**b**) and loaded with unconjugated bilirubin (**c**)

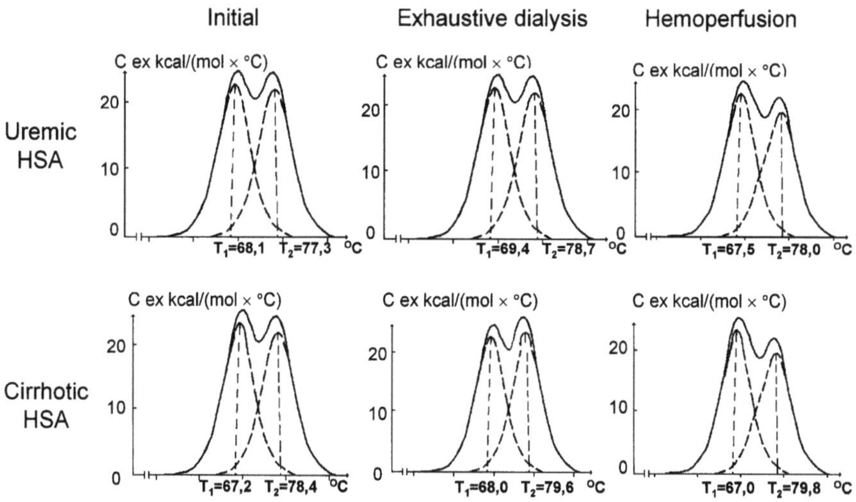

Fig. 29.3 Lack of notable influence of exhaustive dialysis and conventional DHP on the melting curves of HSA extracted from blood plasma of uremic and cirrhotic patients

process of its thermal denaturation [6]. Therefore, along with an increase of the number of internal bonds between the ligand molecules and the carrier molecule, melting temperature of the complex rises, and the shape of the melting curve becomes more complex.

The addition of bilirubin or uremic toxin CMPF, which are strongly bound to HSA, alters the shape of the melting curve of serum albumin producing a bimodal curve, and causes a shift of the temperature maximum of the first peak to the right (Fig. 29.2) [7,8].

Serum albumin is a natural transporter of hydrophobic metabolites; it binds toxic ligands reversibly, and if the ligand can be removed from the complex then the melting curve of unloaded albumin should return to that of pure protein. However this remains a difficult task, and neither exhaustive dialysis, nor the use of conventional carbonic sorbents, influence the shape of melting curves of albumin isolated from blood plasma of uremic patients and patients with hepatic insufficiency (Fig. 29.3) [9].

29.3 Structure of Carbon Sorbent HSGD

To solve this problem, we have developed a novel activated carbon hemosorbent HSGD (HemoSorbent Granulated Deliganding) produced by pyrolysis of nitrogen-containing synthetic (4-vinylpyridine-styrene-divinylbenzene copolymer) resins. The internal structure of smooth spherical granules of HSGD could be described as intertwined multilayer carbon nanotubes of different diameter (Fig. 29.4) [7].

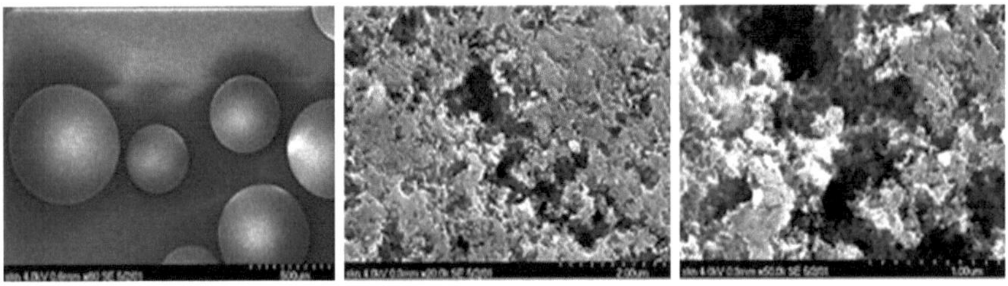

Fig. 29.4 External surface of HSGD hemosorbents at different SEM magnifications

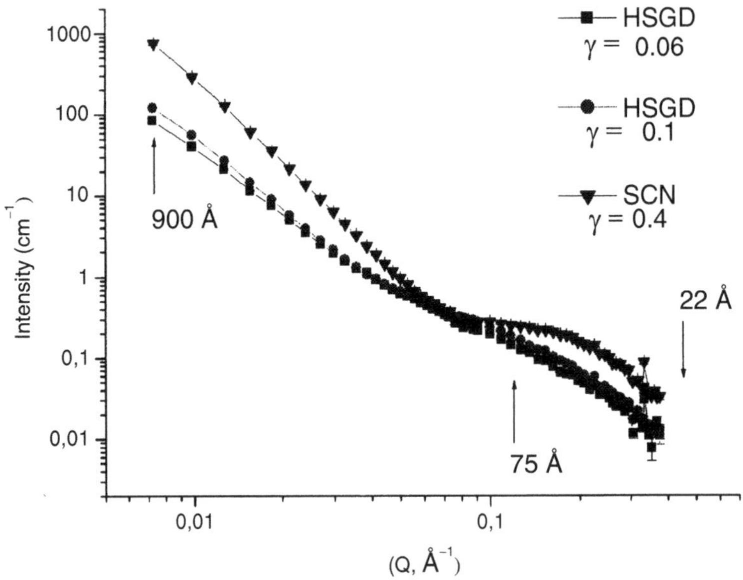

Fig. 29.5 SANS curves of HSGD carbons in comparison with a conventional activated carbon hemosorbent SCN. γ - adsorbent bulk density, $g\,cm^{-3}$

SANS (Small Angle Neutron Scattering) curves of HSGD distinctively differ from those for conventional activated carbon SCN, which is also produced from the same resin. For HSGD samples these curves have a linear shape as opposed to SCN sorbent. Absence of dominating structure size in the range from 75 to 900 Å provides evidence of significant mass-fractal structure of HSGD sorbents (Fig. 29.5).

The fractality index α obtained from analysis of SANS curves correlates with the adsorption capacity of carbon materials for unconjugated bilirubin adsorbed from HSA solution in micro-column single-pass experiments (Table 29.2) [10].

The pore size distribution in highly activated carbon HSGD measured with low temperature nitrogen adsorption shows absence of the curve maximum in the range of 75–900 Å (Fig. 29.6). In comparison with the pore distribution of SCN hemosorbent, HSGD has predominantly meso- and small macroporous structure, with some

Table 29.2 Correlation between fractality of carbonic sorbents (α) and their adsorption capacity towards unconjugated bilirubin (mg/g) from albumin-containing solution

α	Type of structure	Adsorption of bilirubin, mg g^{-1}
−3.51	Surface-fractal (SCN)	0.82
−2.99	Mass-fractal (HSGD)	5.20
−2.80	Mass-fractal (HSGD)	13.40
−2.39	Mass-fractal (HSGD)	98.70

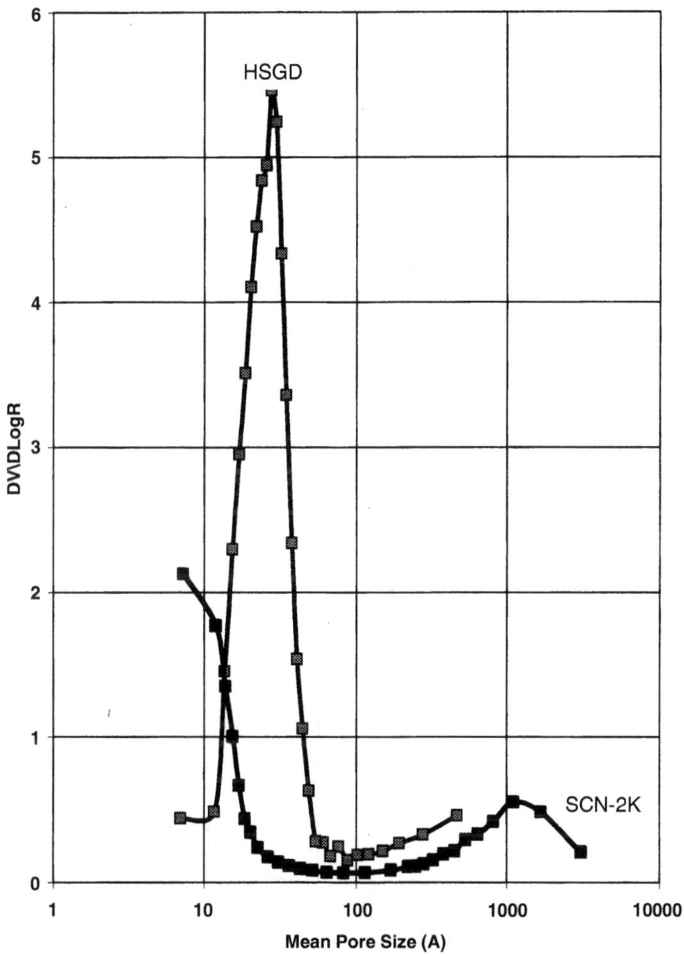

Fig. 29.6 Pore size distribution in SCN hemosorbent (S_{BET} 1,285 $m^2\,g^{-1}$, pore volume 1.08 $cm^3\,g^{-1}$) and highly activated HSGD hemosorbent (S_{BET} 3,000 $m^2\,g^{-1}$, pore volume 2.34 $cm^3\,g^{-1}$)

micropores in the range of 10–20 Å. Mesoporous structure of HSGD is very well developed compared to SCN. A benefit of such a structure for adsorption kinetics is the reduced distance for the diffusion of the ligand-carrier complex to reach the internal pore surface. The ligand is then removed from the albumin complex at the surface, allowing restoration of free albumin and binding the low molecular free ligand to the carbon surface. This process maintains practically zero concentration of free ligand in the biological system.

29.4 Deliganding Properties of HSGD Sorbent

The use of HSGD sorbents allows efficient purification of albumin from unconjugated bilirubin (Fig. 29.7). Upon contact of loaded albumin solution with HSGD the melting curve of albumin normalizes and the molecular ratio of ligand to carrier falls by 300 times (Fig. 29.7) [7]. Normalization of the melting curve of albumin after its purification with HSGD from a mixture of "hepatic toxins" is shown in Fig. 29.8.

The results of microcolumn experiments presented in Fig. 29.9 prove that perfusion through HSGD purifies HSA from a mixture of uremic toxins, which have high, medium and low affinity with albumin (Table 29.1) [11]. The results show that even after 4 h of perfusion the concentration of all three protein-bound uremic toxins remains low, and their clearance is respectively high [10].

Figure 29.10 displays notable normalization of melting curves of albumin after purification of blood plasma of uremic patients (a) and patients with liver cirrhosis (b), with the deliganding sorbent HSGD.

Figure 29.11 presents the kinetics of bilirubin removal from blood plasma of cirrhotic patients with hepato-renal syndrome. In this case, blood perfusion was

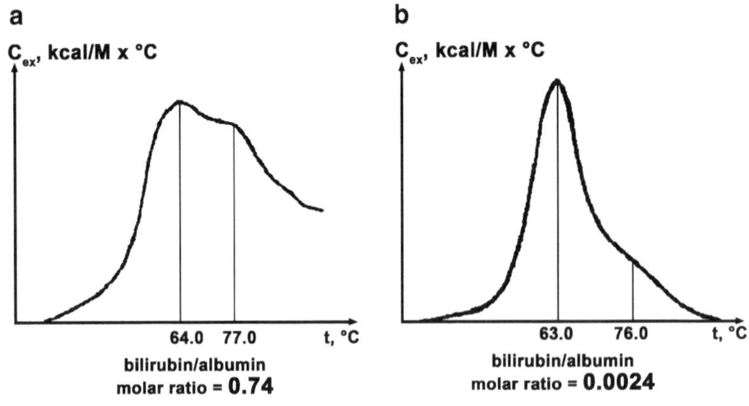

Fig. 29.7 Melting curves of HSA loaded with unconjugated bilirubin before (**a**) and after (**b**) contact with HSGD hemosorbent

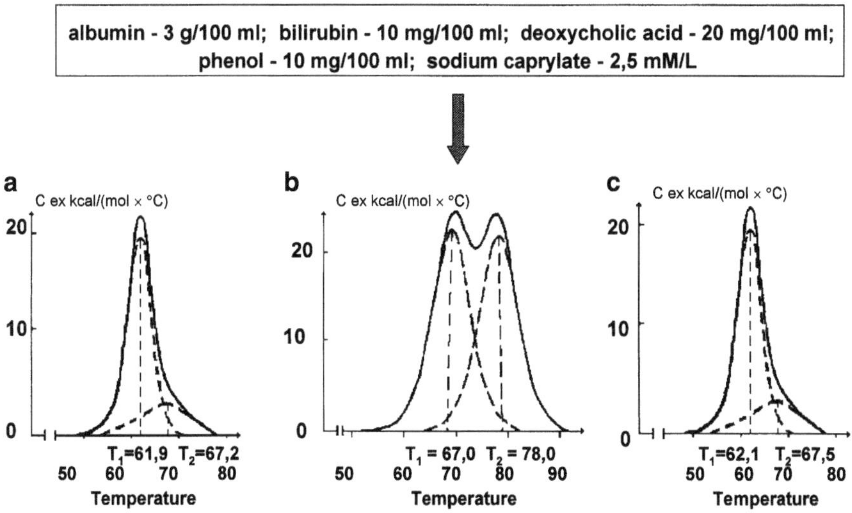

Fig. 29.8 Melting curves of pure HSA (**a**), HSA loaded with a mixture of "hepatic toxins" (**b**) and after purification of the loaded BSA on HSGD hemosorbent (**c**)

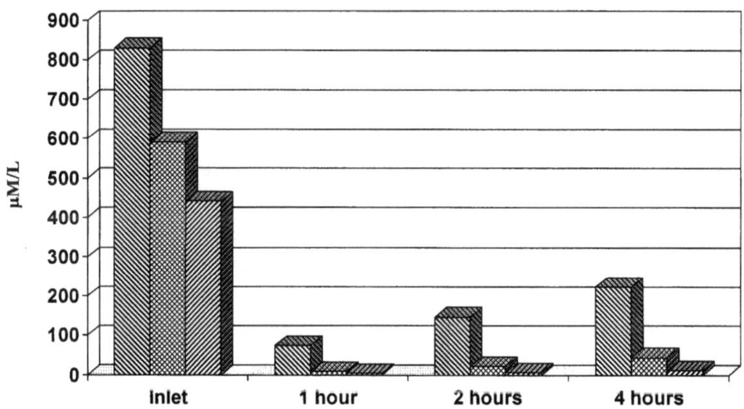

Fig. 29.9 Inlet and time-dependent outlet concentrations of uremic toxins CMPF (\\\\\), indoxyl sulfate (##) and hippuric acid (/////) during 4 h perfusion of HSA-containing mixture of these metabolites through HSGD microcolumn

conducted at flow rate of 35 $\mathrm{mL\,min^{-1}}$ for 5 h, which corresponds to 35 $\mathrm{mL\,min^{-1}} \times 300$ min = 10.5 L of blood passed through a column containing 10 g of deliganding sorbent HSGD. However, as any other activated carbon, HSGD sorbents may initiate the process of coagulation in heparinized blood. This process could be prevented by coating the sorbent surface with a hemocompatible polymer, such as serum albumin, or by replacing heparinization with citrate anti-coagulation [7].

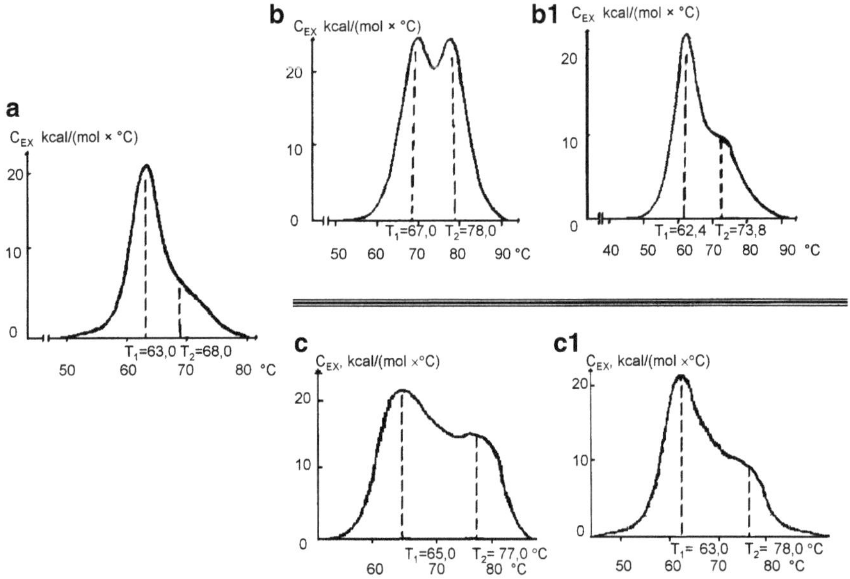

Fig. 29.10 Melting curves of HSA from healthy donors (**a**); extracted from blood plasma of cirrhotic (**b**) and uremic patients (**c**) before and after (b1, c1) contact with HSGD hemosorbent

29.5 Effect of Coating on Sorption Properties of HSGD

Previously we reported that coating of HSGD with defatted HSA led to a reduction of its sorption capacity by 20%, while the use of pH-conformers of HSA or caprylate-containing HSA preserved the sorption capacity of uncoated HSGD [12].

As follows from Fig. 29.12, in micro-column experiments HSGD hemosorbent coated with caprylate-containing HSA conformer preserves the same dynamics for bilirubin adsorption that is characteristic of uncoated carbon. It is worth noting that albumin coating of highly porous HSGD hemosorbent is comparable by weight with the carbon matrix, and consequently, one should regard it as carbon-albumin rather than carbon only adsorbent. It is known that albumin-containing adsorbents possess certain affinity for bacterial endotoxin [13], and the albuminized HSGD has shown higher sorption capacity towards LPS in comparison to uncoated carbon (Fig. 29.13). Capacity of both sorbents towards bacterial endotoxin LPS is sufficiently high.

29.6 HSGD Performance in Comparison with Other Carbon Hemosorbents

Figure 29.12 demonstrates that after 6-h perfusion both uncoated and coated samples of HSGD hemosorbent adsorb significant amounts (140 $mg\,g^{-1}$) of unconjugated bilirubin, and, according to the trend of adsorption kinetics shown, they have not

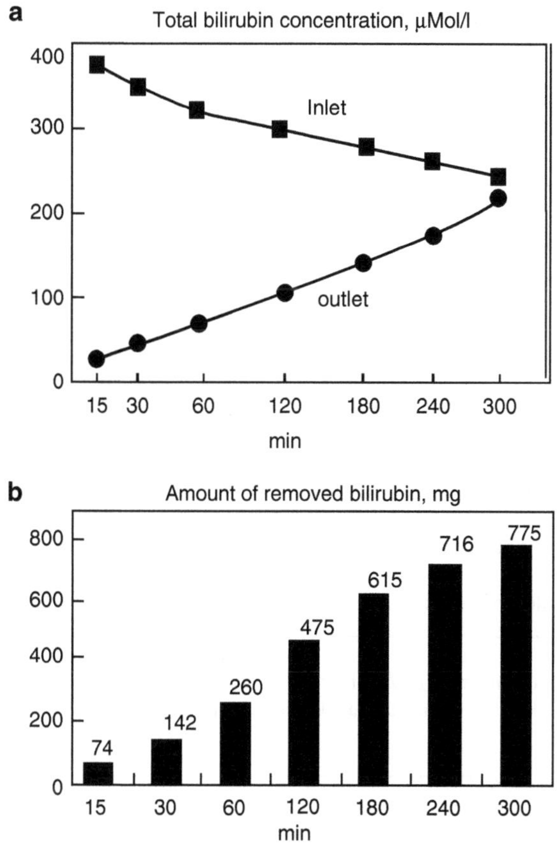

Fig. 29.11 Inlet and outlet concentration of total bilirubin (**a**) and cumulative (conjugated and unconjugated) bilirubin extraction (**b**) by hemoperfusion column containing 10 g of HSGD hemosorbent

reached the saturation point. Adsorption capacity of HSGD towards unconjugated bilirubin is by two orders of magnitude higher than that of carbon sorbents used in hemoperfusion columns commercially manufactured by Gambro (Sweden) and Asahi (Japan), which have capacities of 0.3 and 0.8 $mg\,g^{-1}$, respectively. These hemosorbents however, show capacities comparable to HSGD for creatinine adsorption: 55 $mg\,g^{-1}$ for HSGD vs 30 and 38 $mg\,g^{-1}$ for Gambro and Asahi, respectively.

In Table 29.3 the results of adsorption of pro-inflammatory cytokines by four types of hemosorbents in micro-column single-pass experiments are presented.

From Table 29.3 one may conclude that under experimental conditions, cellulose coated Adsorba 300C sorbent (Gambro) has negligible capacity towards cytokines or BSA. Sorption capacity of conventional SCN carbon hemosorbent is by an order of magnitude lower compared to both uncoated HSGD hemosorbent and HSGD coated with native DNA [14]. Capacity for BSA correlates to the capacity towards cytokines. Similar results were obtained upon coating of HSGD with dextrane

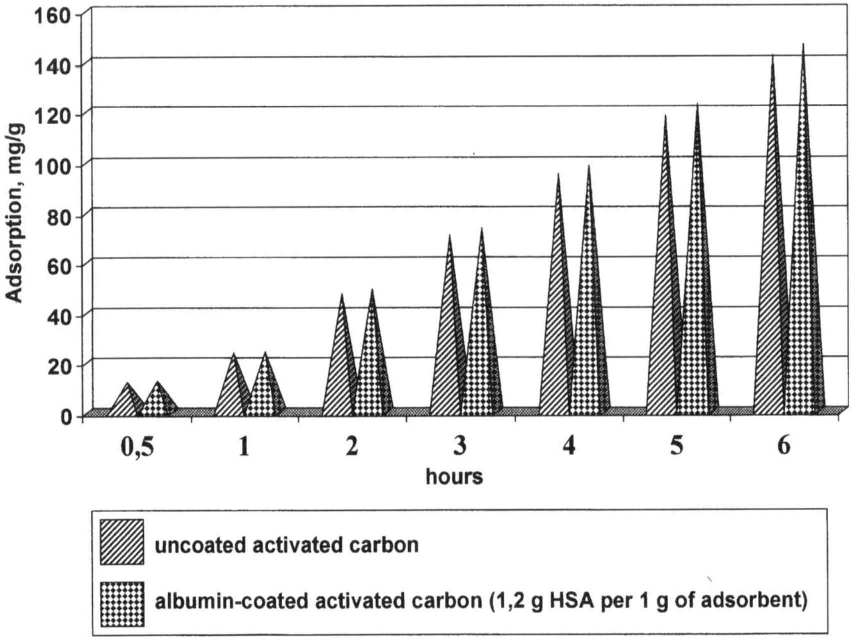

Fig. 29.12 HSGD coating with HSA conformer (≅ 13 moles of sodium caprylate per 1 mole HSA) does not affect the kinetics of unconjugated bilirubin adsorption

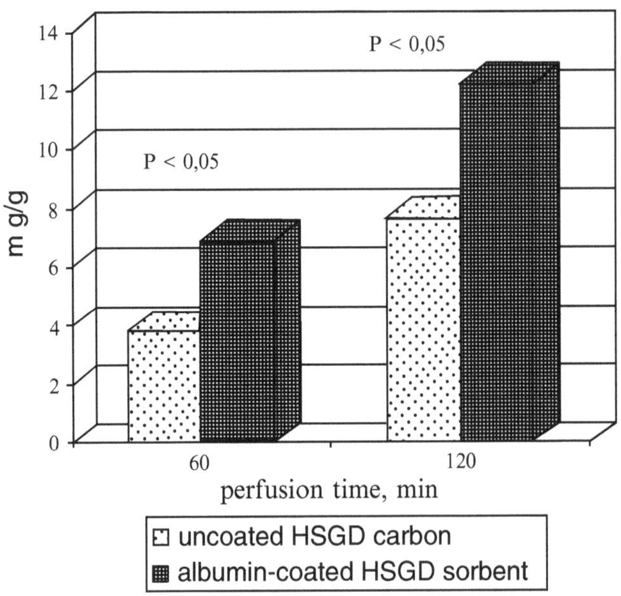

Fig. 29.13 Albumin coating enhanced LPS adsorption from its solution (550 μg/mL) in 3% HSA solution

Table 29.3 Adsorption of pro-inflammatory cytokines, $ng\,g^{-1}$ of sorbent, from 3% bovine serum albumin (*BSA*) solution. Inlet cytokine concentration is 1,000 $ng\,mL^{-1}$

Adsorbent	IL-6, $ng\,g^{-1}$	IL-1β, $ng\,g^{-1}$	TNF-α, $ng\,g^{-1}$	BSA, $mg\,g^{-1}$
Adsorba (Gambro)	0.41±0.08	0.06±0.02	2.78±0.30	0.50±0.15
SCN	5.09±0.50	4.10±0.45	2.98±0.25	12.00±1.15
HSGD	42.9±0.55	44.5±0.40	42.2±0.60	169±3.45
HSGD+DNA	45.04±0.65	45.7±0.35	44.7±0.55	96.0±2.78

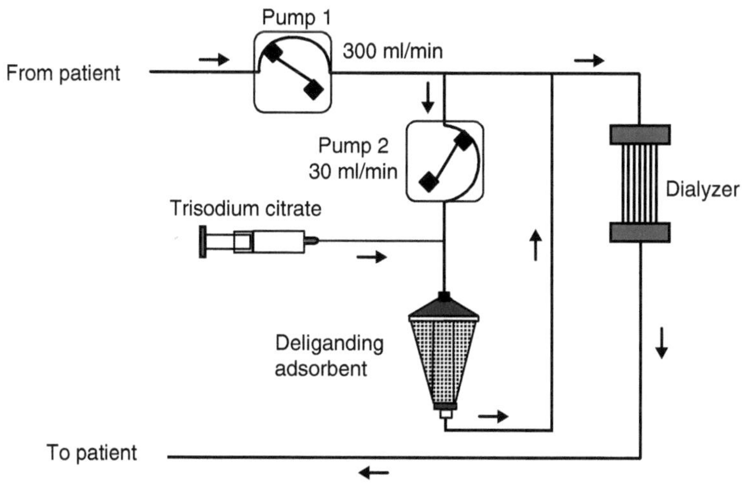

Fig. 29.14 Attachment of HSGD-unit to a conventional hemodialysis machine

sulphate [15]. High sorption capacity towards BSA in comparison with cytokines (mg vs ng) should be considered in the context of their concentrations in solution (30 g BSA vs 1 mg cytokine per liter). Despite BSA adsorption, its concentration in solution remains practically unaffected, and numerous laboratory and clinical observations have shown no substantial albumin loss during hemoperfusion.

Figure 29.14 demonstrates a schematic of connection of HSGD-containing unit to a hemodialysis machine. Here hydrodynamic stability of the column with uncoated deliganding sorbent is achieved via local citrate injection followed by removal of excessive citrate, and concentration of Ca^{2+} is restored in the connected dialyser.

Finally, it is important to note that it is possible to produce carbon sorbents with deliganding properties from different materials. In Table 29.4 this is demonstrated for granulated activated carbon Novocarb (MAST Carbon International, US Patent 20020176840A1, Nov. 2002) prepared by pyrolysis of phenol-formaldehyde resins, and coconut shell derived activated carbon ZL-150 (Huzhou Beigang Enterprises Group Corp., P.R. China).

Modified activated carbons Novocarb and ZL-150 retain adsorption capacity (per unit of weight) towards creatinine, a low molecular weight freely soluble uremic

Table 29.4 Sorption capacity (A) of original and modified activated carbons Novocarb and ZL-150 measured in batch experiments. Adsorption from 3% HSA solution

	Creatinine (MW = 113.1)	Unconjugated bilirubin (MW = 584)
A, mg g^{-1}Sample	mg g^{-1}	mg g^{-1}
Novocarb	52.5	0.56
Novocarb modified	52.7	4.71
ZL-150	45.5	0.80
ZL-150 MODIFIED	57.4	4.08

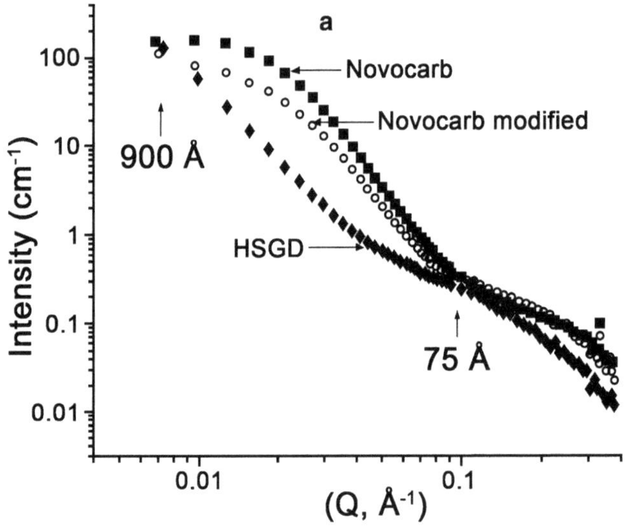

Fig. 29.15 SANS curves for the original and modified Novocarb samples in comparison with HSGD carbon

toxin, at the same level as original carbons. At the same time modified materials demonstrate a significant increase of adsorption capacity for strongly protein-bound ligands such as unconjugated bilirubin. The described transformation in the properties of carbon adsorbents is reflected in flattening of the SANS curve profile in the area of 75–900 Å (Fig. 29.15, compared to the nearly linear slope for HSGD in this area), and in pore size distribution. Modified Novocarb has a distinctive peak in the mesopore range (Fig. 29.16). Similar results were obtained for fibrous activated carbons.

In Table 29.5 sorption capacity of a fibrous carbon (activated carbon felt, MAST Carbon International), experimental deliganding carbon felt and mass-fractal (α = – 2.39) HSGD carbon towards methylene blue and unconjugated bilirubin, measured in batch experiments are compared.

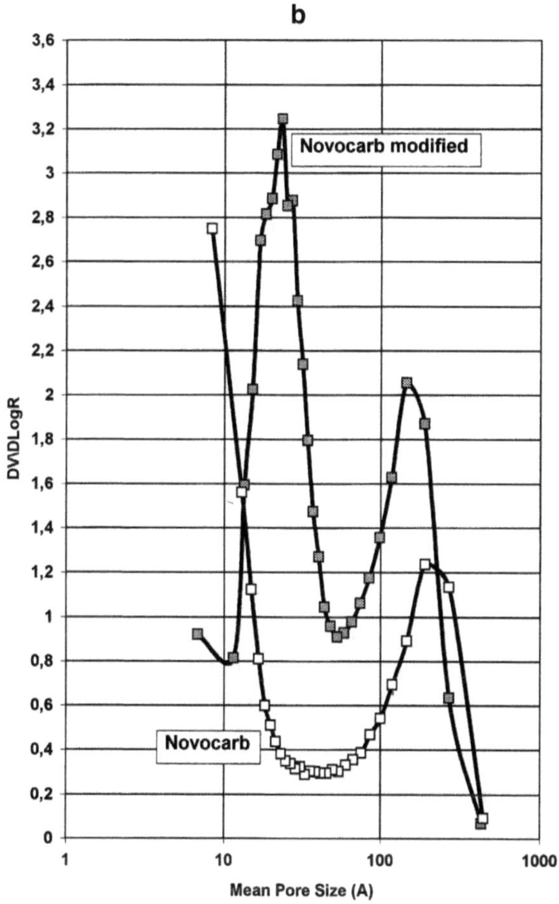

Fig. 29.16 Pore size distribution in the original and modified Novocarb samples

Table 29.5 Sorption capacity of activated carbons towards free (methylene blue) and protein-bound (unconjugated bilirubin) substances of two types of carbon fibrous materials in comparison with HSGD hemosorbent of high fractality

Carbon	Pore volume by benzene, $cm^3 g^{-1}$	Methylene blue (MW = 374 Da), $mg g^{-1}$	Unconjugated bilirubin (MW = 584 Da), $mg g^{-1}$
Activated carbon felt	0.51	386	0.33
Deliganding carbon felt	2.70	416	22.0
HSGD, $\alpha = -2.39$	2.40	743	20.8

29.7 Discussion

From the results presented in this work it can be concluded that deliganding carbon hemosorbents HSGD possess high capacity for protein-bound toxins and also show good sorption capability for bacterial toxins and pro-inflammatory cytokines. Characteristic structural features of these sorbents are their low bulk density, high fractality degree in the pore size range of 75–900 Å, well developed supermicro- and mesoporosity, with wide pore size distribution. These characteristics are the key to providing simultaneous removal of a number of very different toxins playing a major role in the development of clinical conditions like renal and hepatic insufficiency, multi-organ failure, abdominal sepsis, and septic shock. A possible explanation of such beneficial sorption properties is in correspondence of the pore structure of these sorbents to the wide range of molecular sizes of endogenous toxins causing development of severe endogenous intoxication.

29.8 Conclusions

It has been shown that HSGD hemosorbents obtained by pyrolysis of vinylpyridine copolymer styrenedivinylbenzene, possess high porosity (up to 2.4 $cm^3 g^{-1}$), high degree of fractality in the range of 75–900 Å, predominantly mesoporous structure and large sorption capacity for protein-bound toxins, bacterial toxins and pro-inflammatory cytokines, which is superior to conventional activated carbon hemosorbents. Deliganding properties typical of HSGD may also be developed for other granulated and fibrous activated carbons obtained from different natural and synthetic precursors.

Acknowledgements This work was supported by The Royal Society (UK) International Joint Project 2006/R2 'Development of New Adsorbents for Blood and Plasma Purification' and NATO Collaborative Linkage Grant SA(LST.CLG.978860) 'Biolisation of carbon adsorbent surface with ligand-induced conformers of human serum albumin.'

References

1. Ash SR (2006) Artificial organs: A new chapter in medical history. ASAIO J 52(6):e3–9
2. Weber V, Linsberger I, Hauner M et al (2008) Neutral styrene divinylbenzene copolymers for adsorption of toxins in liver failure. Biomacromolecules 9(4):1322–8
3. Peters TJR (1996) All about albumin. Biochemistry, genetics and medical applications. Academic Press Ltd, London
4. Nikolaev VG, Sarnatskaya VV, Sigal VL et al (1991) High-porosity activated carbons for bilirubin removal. Intl J Artif Organs 14:179–185
5. Privalov PL, Gill SJ (1998) Stability of protein structure and hydrophobic interaction. Adv Protein Chem 39:191–234
6. Privalov PL, Dragan AI (2007) Microcalorimetry of biological macromolecules. Biophys Chem 126(1–3):16–24

7. Sarnatskaya VV, Lindup WE, Walther P et al (2002) Albumin, bilirubin and activated carbon: New edges of an old triangle. Artifi Cells Blood Substit Immobil Biotechnol 2:113–127
8. Sarnatskaya VV, Lindup WE, Niwa T et al (2002) Effect of protein-bound uraemic toxins on the thermodynamic characteristics of human albumin. Biochem Pharmacol 63:1287–1296
9. Nikolaev VG, Sarnatskaya VV, Bardakhivskaya KI et al (2003) New approaches to adsorptive therapy of liver failure. Efferent Therapy 1:26–39
10. Sarnatskaya VV, Yushko LA, Nikolaev AV et al (2007) New approaches to the removal of protein-bound toxins from blood plasma of uremic patients. Arti Cells Blood Substit Biotechnol 35:287–308
11. Sarnatskaya VV, Lindup WE, Ivanov AI et al (2003) Extraction of uraemic toxins with activated carbon restores the functional properties of albumin. Nephron Physiol 95:10–18
12. Sarnatskaya VV, Yushko LA, Korneeva LN et al (2005) Biolization of activated carbons by human serum albumin conformers. Efferent Theraphy 11(3):10–20
13. Ullrich H, Jakob W, Frohlich D et al (2001) A new endotoxin adsorber: First clinical application. Ther Apher 5(5):326–34
14. Bardakhivska K, Gurina N, Mikhalovsky S et al (2004) Proinflammatory cytokines elimination with non-specific and biospecific carbonic adsorbents. Immunol and Allerg 3:34–35
15. Snezhkova E, Muller D, Bardakhivskaya K et al (2004) Synthetic activated carbon as a possible matrix for dextran-sulfate immobilization. Biomater Artif Cells Artif Organs 32(4):529–537

Chapter 30
Plasmapheresis and Laser Therapy in Complex Treatment of Myasthenia and their Influence on Erythrocytes and Endothelium

I.M. Baybekov, Sh.Z. Kasimov, J.A. Ismailov, B.A. Saidkhanov, and A.Kh. Butaev

Abstract The main factor in the pathogenesis of myasthenia gravis is the antibody mediated autoimmune response to acetylcholine receptors (AChR). Myasthenia is accompanied by significant increase in pathological forms of erythrocytes in peripheral blood. Plasmapheresis is the most effective way to eliminate antibodies from blood. However, plasmapheresis significantly increases the level of pathological forms of erythrocytes. Endovascular laser blood irradiation (ELBI) is one of the most effective methods of erythrocyte preservation and restoration. ELBI is conducted to decrease the level of pathological forms of erythrocytes and increase the level of discocytes – the normal form of erythrocytes. The investigation of low intensive laser irradiation (LILI) effect on blood vessel walls revealed that ELBI lasting longer than one hour causes alteration in endothelial cells. But endothelial cells recover very soon post ELBI. Laser therapy in combination with efferent methods of detoxification such as plasmapheresis allows elimination of antibodies from blood and restores the optimal ratio between discocytes and pathological forms of erythrocytes.

Keywords Plasmapheresis • Laser therapy • Myasthenia • Ultrastructure

30.1 Introduction

Myasthenia gravis is an autoimmune disease resulting from production of autoantibodies against AChR at the motor end plate, causing defects in neuromuscular transmission. Depending on the muscles affected a patient may develop dysphagia or respiratory failure [1]. The appearance of pathological forms of erythrocytes such as stomatocytes, echinocytes etc., in peripheral blood causes microcirculation disorders [2].

I.M. Baybekov (✉), Sh.Z. Kasimov, J.A. Ismailov, B.A. Saidkhanov, and A.Kh. Butaev
V.Vakhidov Republican Specialised Center of Surgery, Tashkent, Uzbekistan
e-mail: baibekov@mail.ru

S. Mikhalovsky and A. Khajibaev (eds.), *Biodefence*, NATO Science for Peace and Security Series A: Chemistry and Biology, DOI 10.1007/978-94-007-0217-2_30,

Efferent methods of detoxification such as haemosorption (haemoperfusion), plasma sorption (plasma perfusion) and plasmapheresis are the most effective ways to eliminate antibodies from the blood at myasthenia. Among these methods plasmapheresis is the preferred choice [3].

It is known that any sorption method used for blood purification increases the quantity of pathological forms of erythrocytes. Endovascular laser blood irradiation (ELBI) is the most effective method of preserving and restoring erythrocytes however, application of ELBI in the clinic is largely based on empirical evidence. The influence of ELBI on the main blood vessel's walls through which the irradiation is performed has not been clarified.

On the other hand, low intensive laser irradiation (LILI) was used for endovascular treatment of blood for different pathological conditions including myasthenia [4]. However the influence of the LILI on blood cells and particularly on erythrocytes has not been investigated.

In this work we have studied the endothelial microrelief alteration of main arteries and veins in the zones where the waveguide was placed. The variation of erythrocyte forms influenced by ELBI, their morphological changes induced by LILI using He-Ne laser (HNL) and UV Nitrogen laser (UVL) in vitro and in small animals (rabbits), and erythrocyte structure in patients with myasthenia before and after plasmapheresis have been investigated. The complex usage of ELBI together with plasmapheresis has been studied.

30.2 Material and methods

Chinchilia rabbits were used to study ELBI effect on microrelief of endotheliocytes [3, 4]. The waveguide connected to HNL –LG -75 (Russia) was inserted into the aorta or femoral vein under ether anaesthesia. The irradiation power on the end of the waveguide was 8 mW. The vessels underwent perfusion fixation after 10 min, 30 min, 1 h, 6 h and 1–2days following the completion of irradiation with 2.5% glutaraldehyde in phosphate buffer for 15 min. The vessel segments after perfusion were cut and fixed with 2.5% glutaraldehyde in phosphate buffer for 24 h. The segments were dehydrated using a series of water-acetone mixtures with progressively increasing acetone content and critical point dried using CO_2 in HCP-2 (Hitachi). Dried specimens were mounted on a metal brass stub with conductive paint and coated with gold in Eiko IB-3. Samples were examined in a Hitachi S-405A scanning electron microscope operated at 15 kV.

ELBI effect on the morphology of erythrocytes was studied in seven rabbits. ELBI was performed by introducing the waveguide into the lumen of the femoral vein under ether anesthesia. He-Ne laser LG-75 (HNL), Russia, and nitrogen ultraviolet laser LGI-21 (UVL) were used. The power of radiation at the end of waveguide was 2.5 mW, and irradiation was applied for one hour.

HNL and UVL direct effect on human erythrocytes was studied using fresh donor blood. The blood was placed into a quartz flask, and the end of the waveguide connected to the corresponding laser or white light source was immersed into the blood. The irradiation of 2.5 mW was applied for 30 min and samples were taken each 5 min for analysis. For SEM investigation erythrocytes were placed on metal plates covered with a thin layer of gelatin. After 30 s the plate was immersed into 2.5% glutaraldehyde solution for 1 h and was processed as described above.

SEM is an informative method of studying erythrocyte forms [5–8]. However this method needs special equipment and time associated with sample preparation and analysis. The "Thick Drop Express Method" - TDEM developed in our group, has been used for the evaluation of erythrocyte detoxification before and after haemoperfusion. Briefly, one or two drops of blood incubated in glutaraldehyde was immediately placed on a glass slide and covered with a cover glass. Erythrocytes number was counted using light microscopy (this procedure takes 10–15 min). The peripheral blood of 43 patients with myasthenia was analysed using this method. Eight patients underwent ELBI using the apparatus "Matrix –VLOK" (Russia) with special needles. Plasmapheresis was carried out in all 8 patients using a "Hemophonix" device. Complex effect of ELBI and plasmapheresis was studied in 6 patients. The control group comprised 21 patients. Erythrocytes with different forms were counted in a portion of blood with 1,000 red cells. Statistical analysis of the data was performed.

30.3 Results and Discussion

The luminal surface of aorta is folded, and the folds reflect the goffers of the inner elastic membrane. The aorta's intima is covered with an entire layer of endotheliocytes. The surface of these endotheliocytes is fine folded (Fig. 30.1a). The luminal surface of the femoral vein is covered by endotheliocytes, whose plasma membrane is also fine folded. The bounds which separate endotheliocytes appear as irregular lines (Figs. 30.1a–30.2a).

ELBI for 15 min causes alteration of endotheliocytes of the luminal surface of the aorta. The fine folds of their surface become smooth. The endotheliocytes swell and intercellular space is increased denuding the basal membrane. These changes have been noticeable within 1 h after irradiation and completely disappeared after 6 h.

Prominent changes in the cells have been revealed after 30 min of irradiation. Besides the oedema of the cytoplasm and nuclei swelling, crater-like erosions appeared on the luminal surface of the endotheliocytes (Fig. 30.1b). Intercellular spaces became wider, and fibrin thread and single erythrocytes were found in these spaces. In some zones the longitudinal folds of the intima were smoothed, but the endothelial layer remained intact. Such zones may correspond to the sub-endothelial oedema. These changes remained for 6 h after irradiation. One day later the microrelief of the aorta's intima returned to normal.

Irradiation for 60 min caused more damage. Partial detachment and desquamation of endotheliocytes from the basal membrane took place (Fig. 30.1c). Thrombocytes, fibrin threads and erythrocytes were found on the surfaces of denudated zones.

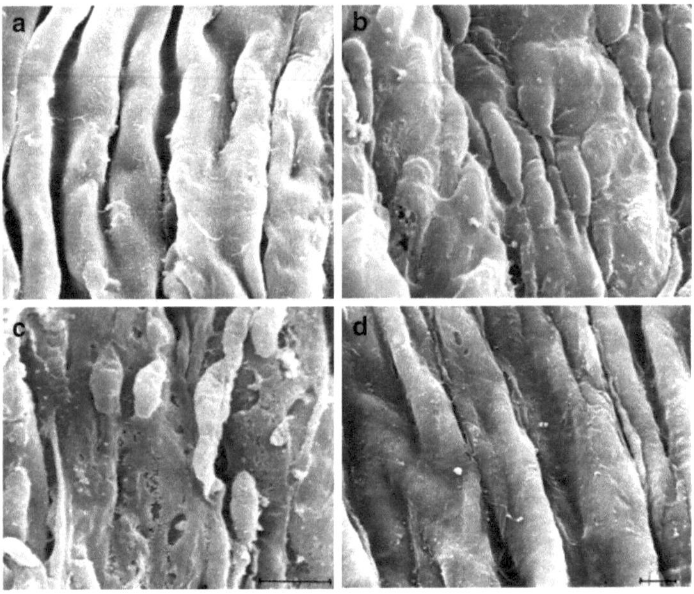

Fig. 30.1 Luminal surface of the rabbit's aorta intima after ELBI with HNL. (**a**). Microrelief of the luminal surface of intact aorta. (**b**). Microerosions and swellings of supranuclear parts of endotheliocytes after 30 min irradiation. (**c**). Desquamation of some endotheliocytes after 60 min irradiation. (**d**). Microrelief of the aorta intima two days after 60 min irradiation

These changes were considerably less noticeable 6 h after the irradiation and completely disappeared after two days (Fig. 30.1d). The formation of thrombi did not take place.

The irradiation of the vein for 15 min caused smoothing of the folds and wrinkles on the endotheliocyte surface. The cell swelling influenced the intercellular space which became wider (Fig. 30.2b).

Irradiation for 30 min resulted in an increase in the intercellular space and led to the formation of crater-like defects on the cell surface. The microrelief normalised 6 h later (Fig. 30.2c).

Irradiation for 60 min resulted in the desquamation of some cells from the basal membrane and the formation of denudated areas of the intima. The affected areas were covered with thrombocytes, erythrocytes and fibrin threads. But 1–2 days after irradiation the intima microrelief of the vein returned to normal. There were no thrombi formations either in the aorta or the vein.

Thus the effect of ELBI on the aorta and vein endotheliocytes depends on the duration of irradiation. Irradiation for 15 and 30 min caused reversible changes which were expressed in changes of the normal cell forms, appearance of crater-like depressions and surface defects, swelling of nuclei and oedema. Irradiation for 60 min had a more pronounced effect on the inner surface of blood vessels resulting in detachment of endotheliocytes from the basal membrane and their desquamation. Restoration of the endothelial structure after 15 and 30 min of laser irradiation

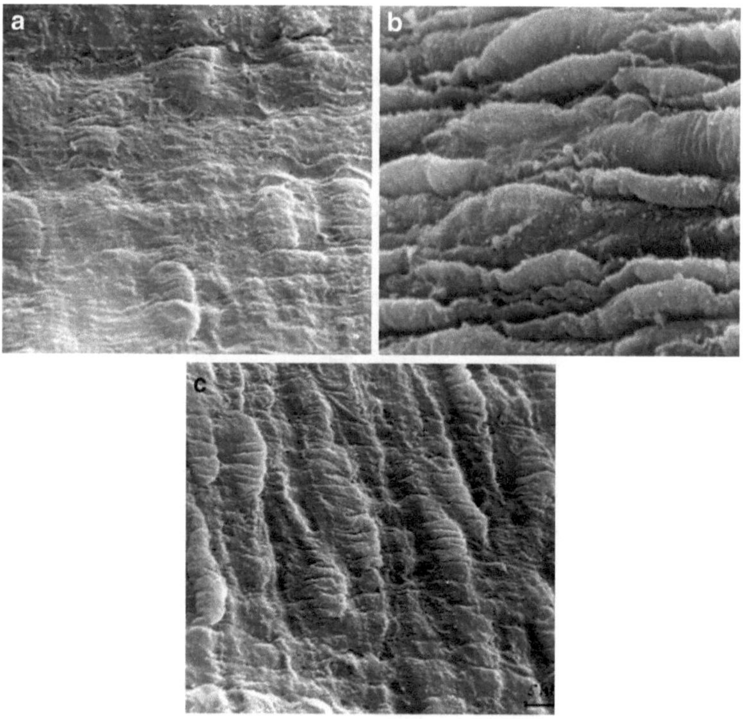

Fig. 30.2 Luminal surface of the rabbit's femoral vein after ELBI with HNL. (**a**). Microrelief of the luminal surface of intact vein. (**b**). Swelling of the supranuclear parts of endotheliocytes after 15 min irradiation. (**c**). Microrelief of the luminal surface of vein two days after 60 min irradiation

occurred within 6 h. After 60 min of irradiation the microrelief of the endothelial layer returned to normal one day later.

SEM is a more informative method of studying erythrocyte form. It allows examining changes in the erythrocyte shape and the surface microrelief [4–8].

Normal erythrocytes must retain their shape and elasticity, which is very important for the microcirculation. In normal conditions most erythrocytes have the form of discocytes (concave-concave disc) (Fig. 30.3a). The ability of discocytes to change their form depends on physical and chemical properties of their membranes. Discocytes transform into echinocytes when the volume of calcium ions in the cell increases and the volume of ATP decreases, or the level of bile acid in blood increases. The transformation of discocytes into stomathocytes is caused by increase of ATP concentration [4–8]. A study of erythrocytes after 60 min irradiation did not reveal any significant changes in the erythrocyte form. The dominant form of erythrocytes remained discocytes (Figs. 30.3b,c). Thus ELBI *in vivo* did not affect the erythrocyte form. Moreover, LILI prevented appearance of pathological forms of erythrocytes and may restore pathological forms into discocytes.

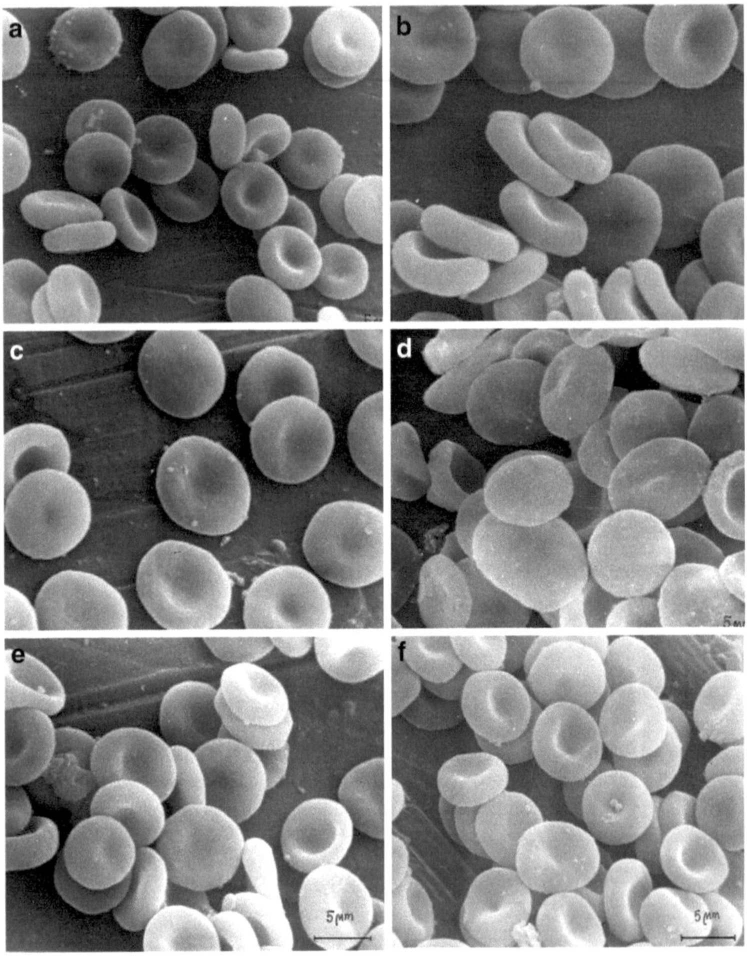

Fig. 30.3 Erythrocyte forms after irradiation with HNL and UVL. (**a**). Erythrocytes of control rabbit. (**b**). Erythrocytes after 60 min ELBI with HNL. (**c**). Erythrocytes after 60 min ELBI with UVL. (**d**). Erythrocytes after *in vitro* irradiation with white light. Transformation into stomatocytes. (**e**). Erythrocytes after *in vitro* irradiation with HNL. (**f**). Erythrocytes after *in vitro* irradiation with UVL

SEM investigations have shown that irradiation of blood with white light caused an increase in the number of stomatocytes transformed from erythrocytes. Before irradiation the volume of discocytes was $89.3 \pm 1.6\%$, echinocytes $8.2 \pm 0.5\%$ and stomathocytes $1.9 \pm 0.06\%$, and after 15 min irradiation the volume of discocytes decreased to $72 \pm 2.4\%$, but the volume of stomathocytes increased to $16.4 \pm 0.6\%$. The volume of echinocytes remained unchanged. Irradiation for 30 min caused an increase in the number of stomathocytes to $27.5 \pm 2.8\%$ (Fig. 30.3d).

HNL irradiation of blood did not cause any changes in volume of all above mentioned forms of erythrocytes. The same results have been obtained after the irradiation of blood with UVL (Figs. 30.3e,f). Thus LILI of blood resulted in better conservation of erythrocytes *in vitro*.

Myasthenia is accompanied by a significant increase in the number of pathological forms of erythrocytes such as echinocytes and stomatocytes, in peripheral blood, and so does plasmapheresis. Thus ELBI was conducted to decrease the number of pathological forms of erythrocytes and to increase the number of discocytes, which are normal erythrocytes. Treatment of patients with myasthenia by ELBI and plasmapheresis revealed significant differences in the ratio of discocytes, echinocytes and stomatocytes. ELBI decreased the level of pathological forms of erythrocytes and increased the level of discocytes (Figs. 30. 4 and 30. 5).

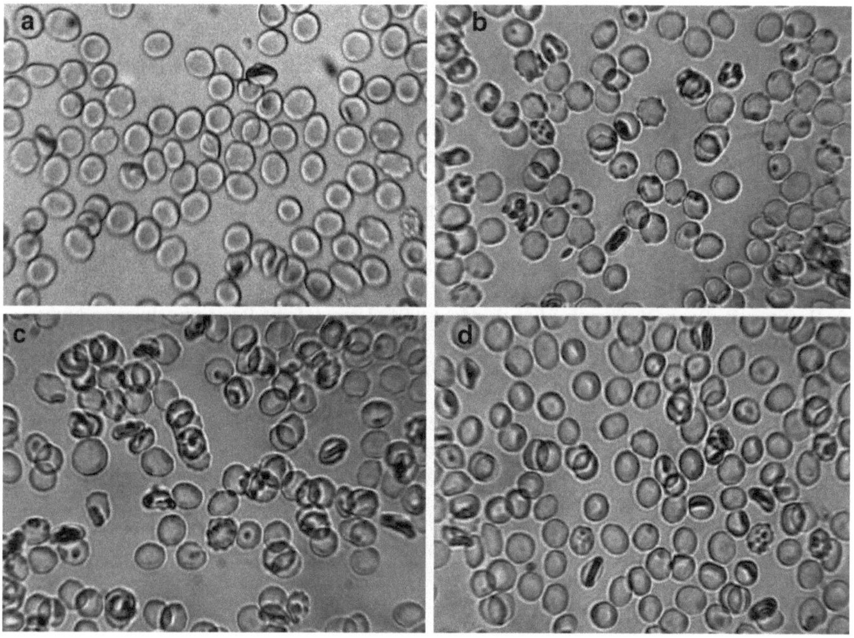

Fig. 30.4 Various forms of erythrocytes in "Thick Drop" at different conditions. (1). Control. Domination of discocytes in peripheral blood. 10×40. (2). Myasthenia. Numerous pathological forms of erythrocytes. 10×40. (3). Increase of the number of pathological forms of erythrocytes after plasmapheresis. 10×40. (4). Decrease of the number of pathological forms of erythrocytes after ELBI. 10×40

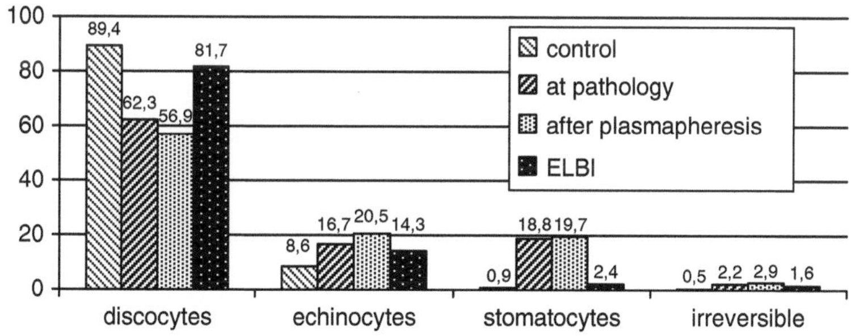

Fig. 30.5 The ratio of different forms of erythrocytes in the blood of patients with myasthenia after plasmapheresis and ELBI

30.4 Conclusion

Laser therapy in combination with efferent methods of detoxification effectively eliminates AChR antibodies from blood and restores an optimal ratio between discocytes and pathological forms of erythrocytes. On the basis of our data, plasmapheresis can be recommended for use together with the endovascular laser blood irradiation, ELBI in treatment of myasthenia. The duration of ELBI should not exceed 30 min.

References

1. Rosai J (ed) (2003) Ackerman's surgical pathology, vol 1 and 2, 9th edn. Mosby, New York
2. Cotran RS, Kumar V, Collins (2004) Pathologic basis of disease. W.B. Saunders Co, Philadelphia - London - New York, p 1426
3. Actual aspects of extracorporeal blood purification (2008) Materials of the 6th International Conference. Moscow, Russia, p 93
4. Baybekov IM, Mavlyan-Khodjaev RSh, Erstekis AG, Moskvin SV (2008) Erythrocytes in norm, pathology and under laser influence. Triada Publ, Moscow, Russia, p 255
5. Hoffman R, Benz EJ, Shattik SJ et al (eds) (2001) Hematology. Basic principles and practice. Churchill Livingstone, New York, p 1970
6. Kozisnets GI, Visotsky VV, Pogorelov VM (2008) Blood and infection. Triada Publ, Moscow, Russia, p 255
7. Novoderjkina JK, Shishkanova ZG, Kozisnets GI (2004) Configuration and surface of blood cells in norm and pathology. Triada Publ, Moscow, Russia, p 152
8. Novitsky VV, Ryazantseva NV, Stepovaya EA (2003) Atlas of clinical pathomorphism of erythrocytes. Tomsk, Russia, p 288

Chapter 31
Efficacy of Modified Hemosorbents Used for Treatment of Patients with Multi-Organ Insufficiency

B.A. Saidkhanov, A.R. Gutnikova, S.H.Z. Kasimov, M.T. Azimova, L.G. Bajenov, and N.A. Ziyamuddinov

Abstract The treatment of patients with multiple organ failure is one of the most complex problems of modern medicine. The possibility to directly control physicochemical characteristics of medical sorbents using different technologies and chemical modification, in particular surface oxidation, is one of the approaches used to improve efficacy of hemosorption. The developed technique of oxidative sorbent modification by treatment with a solution of neutral anolite was used to modify the polymer pyrolyzed active carbon SKN-2 K. The modified hemosorbent was used to treat 31 patients with postoperative complications which led to multi-organ deficiency. The positive clinical outcomes included decrease of signs of intoxication syndrome, health improvement, and improvement in biochemical parameters after just one session of hemosorption. The reduction in the level of endogenous intoxication markers was statistically significant after the second session. It was established that the developed hemosorption technique allows the increase in the efficacy of biotransformation and elimination of toxic metabolic products, and stimulates cellular and humoral immune response. The hemosorption performed through a modified sorbent showed a favourable effect on the main parameters of the homeostasis system. The neutral anolite possesses anticoagulant and anti-aggregation properties. This allows for a reduction in heparin dosage during the procedure with the modified sorbent, therefore minimizing homeostasis system complications during the course of detoxification therapy. The total duration of the treatment was reduced by 41% and the hospitalisation period was 4.8 times shorter in comparison with the control group.

Keywords Hemosorption • Multi-organ failure • Activated carbon

---

B.A. Saidkhanov (✉), A.R. Gutnikova, S.H.Z. Kasimov, M.T. Azimova,
L.G. Bajenov, and N.A. Ziyamuddinov
V.Vakhidov Republican Specialised Center of Surgery, Tashkent, Uzbekistan
e-mail: bois_485@mail.ru

S. Mikhalovsky and A. Khajibaev (eds.), *Biodefence*, NATO Science for Peace and Security Series A: Chemistry and Biology, DOI 10.1007/978-94-007-0217-2_31,

31.1 Introduction

The treatment of patients with multiple organ failure is one of the most complex problems of modern medicine. The basic trigger of multiple organ failure syndrome is an excessive accumulation of endogenous toxins in the body and inability to excrete them by normal physiological routes. Therefore, there is a real need for the application of methods of detoxification therapy, such as extracorporeal techniques of hemodialysis, hemofiltration and hemoperfusion, or hemosorption. Hemosorption (HS) is an effective method of metabolic correction. It is fast and efficient in reducing the toxic load, and provides a favorable background for restoration of normal physiological metabolic reactions.

At the same time some clinicians consider hemosorption to be an aggressive method of efferent therapy, viewing the main obstacle for its wider use in medical practice in the complications associated with the development of a generalized inflammatory process. The main role in its genesis belongs to induction of blood humoral and cellular systems, particularly systems of contact activation as a consequence of interaction with a hemosorbent [1]. A number of researchers also indicate a substantial degree of blood damage as it passes through the sorbent, which results in the reduction of platelets and red blood index.

One of the ways of improving efficiency and safety of hemosorption is to modify physical and chemical properties of sorbents to increase their biocompatibility. The surface chemical oxidation of medical carbon adsorbents has been assessed as one of the promising methods of sorbent modification. This method allows the increase in the quantity of functionally active groups on the carbon surface and brings new properties and sorption mechanisms of detoxification [2–5]. At present there is a lot of controversy surrounding possible effects of surface oxidation of carbons on their biocompatibility: it is thought that oxidation of carbon sorbents is accompanied by reduction of blood damage during the sorption procedure [6], but this view is contradicted by other researchers [7].

The discrepancy of literature data and the urgency of this problem have induced us to study the hemosorption effects of the modified sorbents on the condition of patients with multiple organ failure.

31.2 Experimental

Extracorporeal hemosorption on modified activated carbon hemosorbent was used in 31 patients (16 males and 15 females), 15–74 years of age (mean 36.2 ±3.1), who required intensive care in the postoperative period. All patients were treated in the City Hospital of Yangiyol, Uzbekistan, and were operated due to pathology of an abdominal cavity ($n=15$), purulent inflammatory diseases of soft tissues ($n=11$) and surgical pathology of genitals ($n=5$). The procedure of extracorporeal detoxification was required in 6 patients due to serious endogenous intoxication with progression of hepatic and renal insufficiency, and in 16 patients due to peritonitis.

Postoperative complications included incompetence of seams of an anastomosis, sepsis, and hepatitis in 5 patients; and accompanying diseases such as cardiovascular insufficiency, diabetes and cirrhosis were found in 4 patients. The control group ($n=25$) was generated by a random sampling of case histories from a set of patients with a similar pathology, who were treated in our clinic according to standard hemosorption procedure using a non-modified hemosorbent. Both groups were comparable by gender distribution and age of the patients.

The course of treatment consisted of two or three HS sessions with one day intervals. Hemosorption was carried out using a roller pump AKST-3 (Russia). Polymer pyrolyzed activated carbon hemosorbent SKN-2 K, modified by oxidation, was used. The hemoperfusion column was connected to a veno-venous contour. The flow rate of blood perfusion through the column was 80–100 mL/min, and duration of the first hemoperfusion session was 40–50 min. Oxidative modification of the hemosorbent SKN-2 K was carried out using the technique developed by the authors. Briefly, immediately before the HS session, two liters of neutral anolite solution ON were perfused through the hemoperfusion column for 30 min. The ON anolite was obtained by electrochemical activation of a sodium chloride solution using "STEL-MT-1C" electrochemical unit (Russia). The concentration of the active chlorine generated in the solution was 300 ± 50 mg/L, pH $=6.5\pm0.5$. The efficiency of treatment was judged by a decrease in the patients' subjective complaints, clinical symptoms of the disease and improved results of the laboratory tests. The laboratory tests were performed on patients' admission to the hospital, after the 1st hemosorption session and 24 h after the 2nd or 3rd session. Immunoglobulins were measured using radial immunodiffusion in agar gel, and other parameters of homeostasis, immune and humoral response were measured in blood smears using standard laboratory protocols.

31.3 Results and Discussion

The severity of the initial clinical condition of patients in both groups was established by the biochemical and hematological indices in laboratory tests. Prior to hemosorption sessions all patients had substantial accumulation of endogenous toxic metabolites in their blood plasma due to the functional damage of vital organs. The majority of patients suffered from azotemia and bilirubinemia with the prevalence of direct fraction of bilirubin. Laboratory test revealed that 54% of patients had cholemic intoxication with the clinical signs of hepatic insufficiency, and 27% of patients had a disorder of nitrogen, protein and carbohydrate metabolism with characteristic signs of general toxemia.

The assessment of basic hematological indicators and endotoxemia blood indices such as creatinine, urea and bilirubin in patients treated by standard hemosorption procedure revealed the insufficiency of its detoxification effect. Only after three hemosorption sessions (HS) were positive clinical dynamics and reduction of endotoxemia indices seen in patients of the control group. In the treatment group positive clinical dynamics, reduction of endotoxemia indices and reduction of intoxication syndrome were achieved faster and to a greater extent than in the control group.

It was suggested that the ON solution possesses hypocoagulation properties [8, 9], therefore an additional study was undertaken to assess the effect of hemoperfusion through the modified carbon sorbent on the blood coagulation system and key homeostasis parameters. Tendency for normalization of blood indices in patients of the treatment group was noticeable after the first HS session, and after the second session full normalization was evident (Table 31.1).

The immune system in the majority of patients was compromised by the initial condition (Table 31.2), as was evident by suppression of immunocompetent cells though it was not reflected in production of immunoglobulins IgA and IgM.

As all the links and functions of the immune system are interconnected and depend on each other, a correlation analysis of the parameters studied was carried out. A significant decrease in CD3/CD8 parity was noted. The indices of Th/Ts and CD3/CD4 were within a normal range. The depression of the general pool of CD3 cells in the studied group does not change the parity between a subpopulation of T-cell helpers and the general pool of CD3 lymphocytes. Thus it can be assumed that CD4 cells preserve their immune-stimulating functions. The assessment of humoral immunity confirms this hypothesis. However the IgG level was lower and IgM and IgA levels were higher in the studied group when compared with the results for the control group. This can be explained by an autoimmune aggression characteristic of hepatic pathology such as chronic liver lesion, as IgA and IgM are involved in formation of the immune complexes deposited in liver cell sinusoids and membranes thus provoking a cytopathic effect.

Studying nonspecific immunity we noted the suppression of corresponding parameters of the immune system. The phagocytic activity of neutrophils (FAN) was considerably decreased which could lead to the development of infection. After hemosorption the activation of the immune system was noted and a significant increase in CD3, CD4 and CD19 lymphocyte numbers were seen. The level of

Table 31.1 Effect of hemoperfusion through the modified activated carbon sorbent on the blood coagulation system

Stage of treatment	Fibrinogen, μg%	Fibrinolytic activity,%	Ht,%	Time of serum recalcification, seconds	Serum tolerance to heparin, min
Before hemo-sorption	1824.2±87.8	12.3±0.3	29.4±0.4	78.8±0.54	6′06″±10.2
After 1st session (SI)	1002±25.6	17.7±0.1	36.2±0.8	99.2±1.3	7′18″±11.3
After 2nd session (SII)	404.5±22	21.8±0.4	41.9±0.7	114.7±0.8	7′15″±10.5
SI-SII	$P<0.01$	$P<0.001$	$P<0.02$	$P<0.01$	$P<0.05$
SII-SIII	$P<0.001$	$P<0.01$	$P<0.05$	$P<0.01$	$P>0.05$
SI-SIII	$P<0.001$	$P<0.001$	$P<0.01$	$P<0.001$	$P<0.01$

Table 31.2 Indices of cellular and humoral immunity before and after hemosorption

Index	CD3,%	CD4,%	CD8,%	CD19,%	T_h/T_s	FAN,%	IgM, g/L	IgG, g/L	IgA, g/L
Before hemo-sorption	42.4±2.3	25.3±0.64	15.1±0.31	16.8±0.4	2.3±0.6	42.0±1.63	1.9±0.37	9.05±0.39	2.93±1.5
After 1st session	59.0±0.8	32.7±0.68	15.5±0.19	25.7±1.75	2.87±0.7	55.9±2.08	2.17±0.48	12.6±0.56	3.44±1.75
SI-SII	$P<0.001$	$P<0.001$	$P>0.05$	$P<0.02$	$P>0.05$	$P<0.02$	$P>0.05$	$P<0.01$	$P>0.05$
Healthy donors	65.4±2.1	34.6±1.12	16.3±0.8	29.4±1.31	2.12±0.2	61.9±2.1	1.1±0.1	12.0±0.6	1.5±0.2

T_h - helper T-cells (CD4), T_s - suppressor T-cells (CD8), FAN - phagocytic activity of neutrophils, CD3 - T-lymphocytes, CD19 - B-lymphocytes.

immunoglobulins of all three classes also tended to increase, however only IgM growth was significant. It is possible that due to hemosorption and decrease in the levels of toxins and immune complexes, unblocking of the lymphocyte receptors occurs. This increases the production of lymphokines and improves their effect on immune cells leading to activation of cellular and humoral immunity noted in our experiments. Nonspecific immunity, as judged by FAN index, was also raised significantly. This could benefit patients by protecting them from bacterial infection.

The immune system of patients with postoperative multiple organ failure is compromised, which is confirmed by the decrease of immunocompetent cells but not immunoglobulins IgA and IgM. Nonspecific immunity of these patients is also depressed. However, after extracorporeal blood purification had been performed, immune system stimulation was observed, which was higher than hemosorption specific indicators of cellular and humoral immunity.

A substantial number of clinicians consider the removal of products of abnormal blood metabolism by hemosorption as a major factor of its clinical outcome. However the effect of direct detoxification on pathological process could be compromised because not only toxic substances but some of the circulating immune complexes, immunocompetent cells and biologically active substances are also removed from the blood.

Hemosorption performed using the modified sorbent revealed a number of advantages over conventional hemoperfusion. These include positive dynamics of clinical characteristics expressed in reduction of complications, improvement of general health and main biochemical and immunological parameters. Normalization of blood indices and reduction of level of endogenous intoxication in patients of the treatment group was seen after the first hemoperfusion session and after the second session the full normalization was evident. The changes in the chemical structure of the modified sorbent underlie the positive clinical changes in patients who have undergone hemoperfusion through the modified sorbent. By treating the activated carbon with anolite ON, an inclusion of acid groups into the hemosorbent surface structure occurs, which provides additional oxidizing properties.

The described modified extracorporeal hemoperfusion promotes stimulation of cellular and humoral immunity and mobilization of protective systems of an organism. Therefore the HS through the modified sorbent is more effective and has an effect on the main parameters of the hemostasis system when compared with conventional techniques. This procedure of blood purification also acts as a replacement for the functions of a failed organ of the patient.

Modification of the activated carbon sorbent by neutral anolite solution in situ solves another important problem associated with the need to use anticoagulants for prevention of thrombosis within a hemosorbent. Oxidizing modification of carbon with ON solution considerably reduces the required doses of anticoagulants such as heparin or solutio glugicirum (a solution of 2% of sodium hydrocitrate and 3% glucose) and decreases the risk of postoperative complications associated with an imbalance of the coagulation system.

The described sorbent modification technique by using neutral anolite solution improves the efficiency of blood detoxification and improves treatment results in patients with the signs of an endogenous intoxication syndrome. The treatment duration was reduced by 41% using the modified hemosorbent in comparison with the control group. The hospitalization time was reduced 4.8-fold after hemosorption over the modified sorbent.

31.4 Conclusions

The described sorbent modification technique by using neutral anolite solution improves the efficiency of blood detoxification by hemosorption. It has a stimulating effect and improves treatment results in patients with multiple organ failure.

Hemosorption through the modified sorbent has a sparing effect on the homeostasis system and causes minimal adverse blood reactions when compared with conventional hemosorption.

References

1. Kuznetsov SY, Yankovsky OK, Burkov NV et al. (1997) Production of active forms of oxygen leucocytes as an integrated indicator of biocompatibility of haemosorbents. Efferent Therapy 2:46–50
2. Kardanov VZ, Petrosian EA, Pasechnikov VD et al. (2005) The estimation of efficiency of use of the haemosorbents modified with glutathion in treatment of an ischaemic syndrome - reperfusion extremities in experiment. Efferent Therapy 2:23–26
3. Kartel NT (1995) Possibilities of therapeutic action of medical sorbents on the basis of the activated coals. Efferent Therapy 4:11–18
4. Petrosian EA, Sergienko VI, Sukhinin AA (2001) Estimation of detoxification properties of the haemosorbents modified with sodium hypochlorite. Efferent Therapy 2:34–38
5. Petrosian EA, Zelenov VI, Sukhinin AA (2003) Comparative estimation of detoxication properties of haemosorbents after their modification with various agents. Efferent Therapy 4:27–30
6. Kartel NT (1998) Biocompatibility of carbon sorbents. Efferent Therapy 4:3–9
7. Batalov MI, Levin GY (2000) Oxidizing modification of fibrous carbon haemosorbents. Efferent Therapy 1:45–48
8. Kruchinskiy NG, Savelyev VA, Tepliakov AI et al (2002) Change of haemostasis equilibrium in a hemosorption session. Efferent Therapy 1:36–40
9. Kruchinskiy NG, Novikov DV, Akulich NV et al (2005) Application of a low-molecular heparin at carrying out of a hemosorption at patients of a therapeutic profile. Efferent Therapy 1:40–44

Index

S. Mikhalovsky and A. Khajibaev (eds.), *Biodefence*, NATO Science for Peace and Security Series A: Chemistry and Biology, DOI 10.1007/978-94-007-0217-2,

MIX
Papier aus verantwortungsvollen Quellen
Paper from responsible sources
FSC® C105338

If you have any concerns about our products,
you can contact us on
ProductSafety@springernature.com

In case Publisher is established outside the EU,
the EU authorized representative is:
Springer Nature Customer Service Center GmbH
Europaplatz 3, 69115 Heidelberg, Germany

Printed by Libri Plureos GmbH
in Hamburg, Germany